Wound Healing

George-Sorin Tiplica · Kirsi Isoherranen
Editors

Wound Healing

A Practical Approach

Springer

Editors
George-Sorin Tiplica
Department of Dermatology, Colentina
Clinical Hospital
Carol Davila University of Medicine
and Pharmacy
Bucharest, Romania

Kirsi Isoherranen
HUS Helsinki Wound Healing Centre
Helsinki, Finland

ISBN 978-3-031-84578-9   ISBN 978-3-031-84579-6 (eBook)
https://doi.org/10.1007/978-3-031-84579-6

This Springer imprint is published by the registered company Springer Nature Switzerland AG
The registered company address is: Gewerbestrasse 11, 6330 Cham, Switzerland

Contents

Introduction to "Wound Healing: A Practical Approach"

1

George-Sorin Tiplica and Kirsi Isoherranen

Abstract

Cutaneous wounds, resulting from skin integrity loss, pose a significant burden globally. Acute wounds, affecting all humans, are expected to heal. Chronic wounds—skin ulcers that fail to reduce by 50% in a timely manner—affect over 2.5% of the general population. In Europe, chronic wound care costs 2–4% of total healthcare expenditure. Wound care involves a multidisciplinary approach, connecting various specialists and healthcare professionals. Recognizing the absence of wound healing curricula in many European countries, the European Union of Medical Specialists (UEMS) collaborates with professional organizations such as the European Wound Management Association (EWMA) and the European Association of Fellows in Wound Healing (EAFWH) to address this gap. Aligned with the wound healing teaching curricula of MJC-WH UEMS, this book serves as a valuable resource for colleagues interested in chronic wound management. It covers various aspects of chronic wounds, offering solutions from wound healing experts. The chapters provide a succinct overview of general pathology, referencing the European Training Requirements (ETR). Clinical case presentations highlight practical aspects, emphasizing the multidisciplinary nature of wound care. As Europe's population ages, healthcare providers must consider chronic wounds within the broader context of patients' overall health. The collaborative effort of authors from different European countries underscores the importance of patient quality of life in wound care decisions.

G.-S. Tiplica (✉)
Dermatology 2, Colentina Clinical Hospital, Carol Davila University of Medicine and Pharmacy, Bucharest, Romania
e-mail: george.tiplica@umfcd.ro

K. Isoherranen
Wound Healing Centre, Helsinki University Hospital, Helsinki, Finland

G.-S.Tiplica and K. Isoherranen (eds.), *Wound Healing*,
https://doi.org/10.1007/978-3-031-84579-6_1

Keywords

Wound healing teaching • Wound healing ETR • Healthcare professionals • UEMS-MJC Wound Healing • EWMA • EAFWH

Cutaneous wounds defined by the loss of the skin integrity, represent a substantial burden for both patients and healthcare systems in all the countries around the globe. Acute wounds are affecting, in different forms, all humans sometime during their lifetime and are usually expected to heal. Chronic wounds, having an impaired healing process, often necessitate the intervention of medical care. More than 2.5% of the general population is suffering from chronic wounds [1] defined as skin ulcers that are not reducing their surface with 50% in a timely manner [2]. The estimated cost of chronic wound care in Europe is immense, being estimated at 2–4% of the total healthcare expenditure [3]. With those high and impacting epidemiological figures, wound care plays an essential part in medicine. The medical field responsible for wound diagnostics is multi-disciplinary, involving dermato-venereologists, plastic surgeons, vascular surgeons, infection disease specialists, general practitioners, endocrinologists, orthopaedists, oncologists and other specialists. The healing activities are performed in an inter-professional way, connecting doctors, nurses, podiatrists, nutritionists, dietitians, occupational therapists—to name just a few of the healthcare professions involved in wound care.

Acknowledging that in more than 80% of all European countries there is no specific wound healing curriculum implemented in the general curricula of the medical specialties that often deal with wounds, the European Union of Medical Specialists (UEMS) founded the Multidisciplinary Joint Committee—Wound Healing (MJC-WH) in 2018 with the major task of harmonization and synchronization of the medical field of wound healing in all EU countries [4]. In close collaboration with the European Wound Management Association (EWMA), the European Association of Fellows in Wound Healing (EAFWH) and other national and international medical societies, a series of scientific activities were started in order to promote the medical field of wound healing.

This book follows the wound healing teaching curricula of MJC-WH UEMS and aims to be a support for all colleagues interested in this medical field by presenting the many aspects of chronic wounds and the solutions provided by a group of wound healing experts. The chapters of the book are organized in a concise description of the general pathology with clear references to the wound healing European Training Requirements (ETR) followed by clinical case presentations selected by the authors to highlight important practical aspects demonstrating the multidisciplinarity of this medical field. Following their different pathogenic mechanisms the chronic wounds are presented in a practical approach with the discussion of clinical aspects, differential diagnosis and different treatment modalities. Special chapters are dedicated to the active wound-phase adapted dressings, negative pressure wound therapy, adjuvant therapies and to the innovative materials used to heal the wounds. Other books are addressing the chronic wounds too, including in Springer Nature collections; however, this book is unique in providing this close relation with the teaching activities comprehensively included in the training requirements. The updated ETRs are built on the learning goals and content of the Special Competence in Wound Management programme, which is a national specialist level educational initiative in wound care that is maintained by the Finnish Medical Association [5]. The learning goals of the programme were developed by a multidisciplinary oversight committee in 2022, and these goals incorporate several elements of the original ETRs for Wound Healing. In the next revision, Bloom's Taxonomy action verbs [6] and the CanMEDS Roles [7] will be introduced into the updated ETRs, which is a measure that can be seen as representing a further evolution of these goals. In the renewal process of the Wound Healing ETRs, the Editors acknowledge the kind support and hard work of Dr. Jaakko Viljamaa from Turku, Finland.

In a holistic approach, the Editors thought to present to the reader not only the difficulties encountered in chronic wounds management but also the existing possibilities that alleviates the sufferance of the patient and of their caregivers.

As the prevalence of chronic wounds increases with age, and in Europe the average age of the population is increasing, it is expected to encounter more frequently in clinical practice patients suffering with chronic wounds. The healthcare providers must be prepared to address the skin lesions in the context of the general health of the patient who might harbour other health conditions. Diabetes mellitus has a special connexion with wound healing, and those particular aspects are presented in a separate chapter of this book. The attitude towards infection of the wounds should demonstrate a justified approach, based on the patient health status and on the amount and virulence of the microorganisms. The therapy of those cases should rely on antiseptics, topical therapy and, when needed, on systemic antibiotics. Pressure ulcers pose a significant challenge for all practitioners; therefore, it is critical to evaluate the condition and to consider the proper prevention measures. Atypical wounds should be recognized and referred to dermato-veneorologists by other specialists involved in wound care. Also considered of relevance, the spectrum of blistering skin diseases requests the attention of the reader due to the severity of the health problems induced in skin failure.

The Editors searched to blend the different aspects of chronic wounds that are frequently encountered in clinical settings. Based on the UEMS ETRs for Wound Healing we invited authors from different European countries who brought not only their expertise but also their cultural experience. As a connecting string, all contributions are insisting on the patients' quality of life, a consideration that is essential when difficult decisions are made. Unfortunately, specialists in wound care are rarely involved in such difficult decisions induced by diabetes, pressure ulcers, blistering diseases or atypical wounds to name only few situations. We express our sincere gratitude for all the Chapter Editors and authors across Europe for their excellent contributions for this book. Again, the power of teamwork was demonstrated and surely will lead for future joint achievements as well.

We hope that this volume will enable an improved approach of the patients with chronic wounds and will inspire new generations of healthcare professionals dedicated to this field.

The Editors.

George-Sorin Tiplica
Bucharest, Romania

and

Kirsi Isoherranen
Helsinki, Finland

References

1. CK Sen 2023 Human wound and its Burden: updated 2022 Compendium of estimates Adv Wound Care 12 12 657 670 https://doi.org/10.1089/wound.2023.0150 PMID: 37756368
2. P Sheehan P Jones JM Giurini A Caselli A Veves 2006 Percent change in wound area of diabetic foot ulcers over a 4-week period is a robust predictor of complete healing in a 12-week prospective trial Plast Reconstr Surg 117 7 Suppl 239S
3. N Graves CJ Phillips K Harding 2022 A narrative review of the epidemiology and economics of chronic wounds Br J Dermatol 187 2 141 148 https://doi.org/10.1111/bjd.20692
4. The UEMS Multidisciplinary Joint Committee—Wound Healing. Available at: https://mjcwoundhealing.org/. Last accessed 01 May 2024.
5. Viljamaa J, Koljonen V, Isoherranen K. Wound care education from a medicine perspective. In: Kielo-Viljamaa E, Stolt M, Suhonen R, editors. Wound care education in nursing: a European Perspective. Springer; 2024. p. 109–17. https://doi.org/10.1007/978-3-031-53230-6_12
6. Armstrong P. Bloom's Taxonomy. Vanderbilt University Center for Teaching. 2010 [cited 6 May 2024]. Available: https://cft.vanderbilt.edu/guides-sub-pages/blooms-taxonomy/
7. CanMEDS: Better standards, better physicians, better care. [cited 6 May 2024]. Available: https://www.royalcollege.ca/ca/en/canmeds/canmeds-framework.html

Ischaemic Leg Ulcer

2

Annette Høgh, Daniel Mosgaard Sørensen, Anne Cathrine Nielsen, Ana Lamza, Tanja Planinšek Ručigaj, Mitra Sepehri, Hanne Birke Sørensen, Katariina Noronen, Arindam Bharadwaz, and Jaakko Viljamaa

All patients with a foot ulcer should have an objective assessment of their vascular status

Annette Høgh.

Abstract

In this chapter, nine cases are presented to describe the typical development of ischaemic leg ulcers focusing on the key point in diagnostics and treatment. The cases are selected to illustrate the importance of a holistic approach combined

A. Høgh (✉) · D. M. Sørensen · A. C. Nielsen
Department of Vascular Surgery, Regional Hospital of Viborg, Central Denmark Region, Viborg, Denmark
e-mail: Annette.hoegh@viborg.rm.dk

A. Lamza
Department of Vascular Surgery, Clinical Hospital, veti Duh", Zagreb, Croatia

T. P. Ručigaj
Head of the Dermatovenerology Clinic, University Medical Centre Ljubljana, Ljubljana, Slovenia

M. Sepehri
Videnscenter for Sårheling, Bispebjerg Hospital, Copenhagen, Denmark

H. B. Sørensen
Department of Vascular Surgery Kolding, South Denmark Region, Kolding, Denmark

K. Noronen
Department of Vascular Surgery, Helsinki University Central Hospital, Helsinki, Finland

A. Bharadwaz
Department of Radiology, Aarhus University Hospital, Aarhus, Denmark

J. Viljamaa
Department of Vascular Surgery, Turku University Hospital, Turku, Finland

G.-S.Tiplica and K. Isoherranen (eds.), *Wound Healing*,
https://doi.org/10.1007/978-3-031-84579-6_2

with a multidisciplinary set-up. Quick identification of a potential ischaemic component to a chronic wound is essential. The diagnosis of ischaemic leg ulcers is based on clinical characteristics combined with an objective and physical examination of the patient. Peripheral pulse palpation and measurement of the ankle brachial index (ABI) are first-line non-invasive hemodynamic screening for assessing the severity of the peripheral arterial disease (universal atherosclerosis, obstructing the circulation to the lower limbs leading to decreased oxygen inflow by which cell division and tissue survival are compromised and rest pain, necrosis and/or gangrene arise). Furthermore, aggressive local wound treatment both before and after revascularization is essential.

Keywords

Vascular assessment • Pain control • Amputation • Vascular reconstruction

Abbreviations

ABI	Ancle-brachial-index
ADP	Arteria dorsalis pedis
ATA	Arteria tibialis anterior
ATP	ArteriA tibialis posterior
CLTI	Chronic limb-threatening ischemia
CT	Computed tomographic
DM	Diabetes mellitus
ER	Emergency room
IPC	Intermittent Pneumatic Compression
IV	Intravenous
LDL-C	Low-density lipoprotein-cholesterol
MDT-DFU	Multidisciplinary team regarding-diabetic foot ulcers
MR	Magnetic Resonance
NPWT	Negative pressure wound therapy
PAD	Peripheral arterial disease
POBA	Plain old balloon angioplasty
PTA	Percutaneous transluminal angioplasty
PTFE	Polytetrafluoroethylene
SFA	Superficial femoral artery
$TCPO_2$	Transcutaneous oxygen pressure

Ischaemic Wound Cases, Introduction [1]

Chronic limb-threatening ischaemia (CLTI) is the end stage of peripheral arterial disease (PAD). Atherosclerosis obstructs the circulation of the lower limbs leading to decreased oxygen inflow by which cell division and tissue survival are compromised and rest pain, necrosis and/or gangrene arise. CLTI is associated with high frequency of mortality, cardiovascular events (ex: Myocardial infarction and stroke), minor and major amputation, persistent disability, and impaired health-related quality of life because of the presence of universal atherosclerosis. Although CLTI is widely believed to be a growing global health care problem, reliable epidemiological data is extremely limited.

Ischemic wounds are typically placed on the tiptoe or on bony protrusions on the foot, and representing as devitalized tissue or dry gangrene. The affected skin becomes chilly, dry and changes colour to dark purple and eventually turning into a black dry mummified area. Debridement of devitalized areas should be avoided as the body is unable to support the revision with autolysis and necrosis quickly regenerates. The process causes disabling pain combined with decreased mobility and disturbed sleep; if pain is absent or pain sensitivity is reduced, peripheral neuropathy should be considered. However, patients may have severe CLTI without symptoms, which can be related to their incapacity to walk far enough to reveal symptoms (e.g. heart failure) and/or reduced pain sensitivity (e.g. diabetic neuropathy).

Quick identification of a potential ischaemic component to a chronic wound is essential. The diagnosis is based on clinical characteristics combined with an objective and physical examination of the patient. Peripheral pulse palpation and measurement of the ankle brachial index (ABI) are first-line non-invasive hemodynamic screening for assessing the severity of PAD. All patients without pulse on the foot and/or $ABI \leq 0.7$ should be suspected for CLTI and urgently referred to a vascular specialist. With decreasing ABI the risk of iatrogenic skin damage due to compression therapy increases. However, compression therapy is still one of the keystones in treatment of chronic ulcers, independently of the underlying aetiology. With $ABI < 0.7$ modified compression under close clinical supervision is mandatory. Exceptional attention is needed among patients suffering from peripheral neuropathy to avoid skin damage triggered by compression therapy.

Imaging is a cornerstone in the planning of the revascularization and is used to map the extent of the atherosclerosis and afterwards used in the planning of the vascular surgery reconstruction of the blood flow to the affected area. Following revascularization the treatment-focus can return to standard wound care. Re-established tissue oxygenation predisposes to infection and oedema, why debridement and compression therapy now is vitally important to facilitate wound healing.

Assessment of vascular status is mandatory to optimize wound care. Referral to a vascular specialist or a multidisciplinary approach may be needed. Furthermore, aggressive local wound treatment both before and after revascularization is essential.

Endovascular therapy has emerged as a standard therapy in the treatment of CLI, offering minimally invasive approaches to restore blood flow to ischaemic limbs. While the primary goal of endovascular intervention is revascularization, its impact on wound healing in CLI patients cannot be underestimated, as wound healing after endovascular therapy is crucial for optimizing patient care and enhancing clinical outcomes in this challenging patient population.

In this chapter, nine cases are presented to describe the typical development of ischaemic leg ulcers focusing on the key point in diagnostics and treatment. The cases are selected to illustrate the importance of a holistic approach combined with a multidisciplinary set-up. Furthermore, the cases are in line with the learning objectives of the Wound Healing MJC UEMS standards concerning training requirements for all medical specialties, which include wound healing in their curricula.

Case 2.1. Minor (Spontaneous) Amputation

Introduction

A 69-year-old male with a background of curative colon cancer resection, diabetes mellitus (DM), hypertension and hypercholesterolemia was presented at the department of vascular surgery. His main symptom was prompt onset of severe pain in the first and fifth toe on the left lower limb through five weeks. The fifth toe turned black after two weeks from pain debut (Fig. 2.1). Furthermore, the patient developed claudication (walking distance < 200 m) and rest pain eased by positioning the leg downwards during bed rest. Ankle-brachial pressure prior to consultation showed left sided ABI of 0.44 (ankle pressure 60 mmHg and toe pressure 33 mmHg). There was a detectable pulse in the femoral and popliteal artery, but no pulses on the foot.

From the patient history and physical examination (dry gangrene, cyanotic toe, claudication), other causes of dry gangrene (ex. frostbite, trauma) could be excluded, and the arterial occlusive disease was suspected as the aetiological factor in this patient.

Treatment

CT angiography showed occlusion and severe atherosclerosis of the superficial femoral artery (SFA) at level of Hunter's channel which reopened at the popliteal artery (Fig. 2.2). Patient was offered revascularization by a short venous bypass around the occlusion.

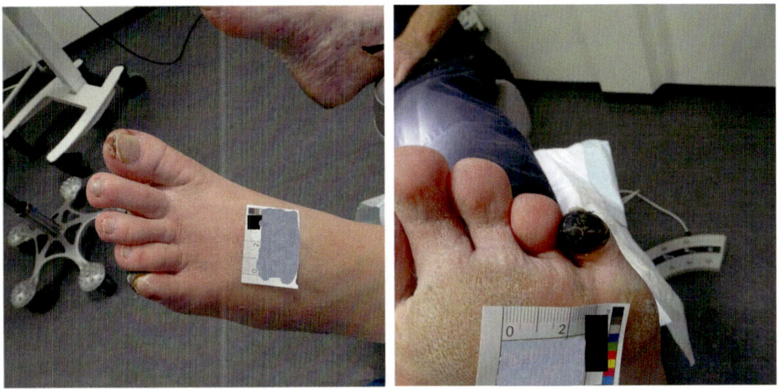

(a) (b)

Fig. 2.1 Dry gangrene on the 1th and 5th right toe, at the day the patient was offered vascular reconstruction. (a) anterior view; (b) posterior view

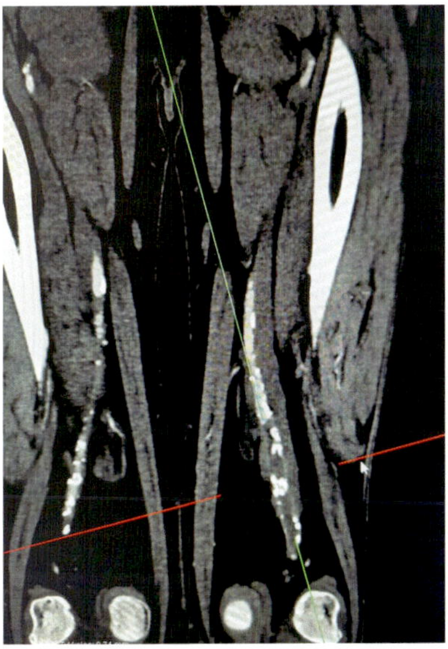

Fig. 2.2 CT angiography (coronal plane) showed occlusion and severe atherosclerosis of the superficial femoral artery (SFA) at level of Hunter's channel which reopened at the popliteal artery

In the timespan between diagnosis and revascularization, the patient was offered optimized wound treatment including customized offloading footwear, along with infection and pain control. Furthermore, a homecare nurse managed the continuity of wound treatment.

The revascularization was successful with restoration of the pulse in the dorsal pedal artery (ADP). Following four days, the distal necrotic part of the fifth toe was partly rejected from the vital part of the toe. The patient was offered minor amputation, which left the proximal fifth toe with healthy vital tissue and point

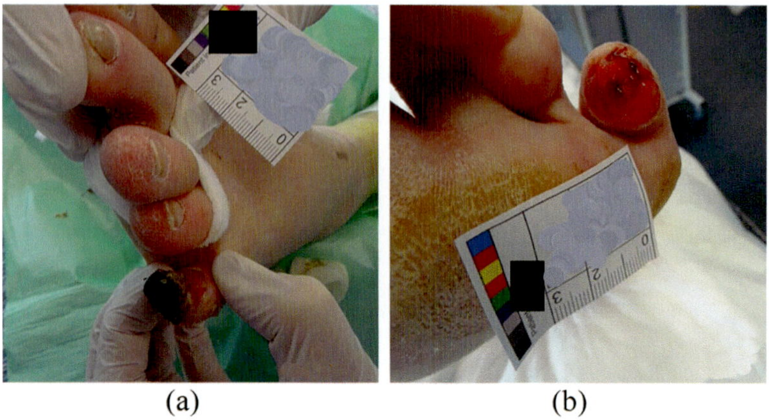

Fig. 2.3 The process of spontaneous amputation, (a) 7 days and (b) 11 days after vascular reconstruction. 100% epithelialization was obtained on the 41th postoperative day

bleeding from edges. Patient was discharged from hospital two days after minor amputation with close follow up, as initiated before surgery (Fig. 2.3). Nine days after discharge the patient was seen in the wound care center with progress in wound healing (hypergranulated tissue), and treatment with group III steroid cream was added to the standard care a few times. 1 month after follow-up the wounds (including the first toe) were completely healed.

Discussion

Revascularization in patients with CLTI is the direct method for achieving functional limb salvage and improved quality of life [2]. Most patients require a minor amputation to remove distal necrotic tissue (dry or wet gangrene often combined with infection) to restore a functional limb [2].

Loss of blood supply to body tissue leads to necrosis. Demarking of dry gangrenous tissue occurs in the following process of spontaneous amputation [3, 4]. Dry gangrene can progress into wet gangrene and possibly infection which can progress into fatal consequences, unless minor amputation is carried out and infection is treated [3]. Treatment with minor amputation requires sufficient arterial perfusion and appropriate offloading which are the major principles of preserving foot function. DM patients with concomitant CLTI have significantly higher risk of re-amputation at higher level [2]. One-year and 5-year mortality rates after minor amputation are relatively high by 16% and 25% respectively for patients with ischemia and even higher in DM patients with a 5-year mortality > 50% [2].

Overall, minor amputation is essential in wound management/debridement in patients with CLTI with gangrene and require sufficient distal arterial perfusion (revascularization), offloading, pain treatment and infection treatment for adequate healing.

Case 2.2. Minor Amputation May Reduce the Risk for Major Amputation

Introduction

A 74-year old man presented in an outpatient clinic with dry gangrene of the second and fourth toe of his left foot. The changes started after minor injury, while gardening. He had a history of hypertension and was on intermittent haemodialysis for kidney failure. Otherwise, he was in good physical condition. His pain level was 7/10 on NRS score. He did not complain of typical claudication pain while walking yet admitted that he wasn't walking longer distances anymore.

Clinical Findings

Immediately we assessed the distal blood pressure in the affected leg. The ABI was 0.4 for the left leg and 0.7 for the right leg. MSCT angiography was done next and showed calcification of calf arteries, often seen in patients on chronic haemodialysis [5]. As no runoff in the arterial system was present and thereby no opportunity to reconstruct the circulation to the foot, our vascular team decided that the patient was not suitable for revascularization procedures; neither open surgery nor endovascular treatment. As expected, laboratory results showed elevated kidney function markers and lipid levels combined with low levels of albumins and proteins. On inspection his foot was euthermic, gangrene on his toes was dry, with no signs of spreading or infection that could progress to the rest of the foot. The oedema of the foot and calf was noticeable (Fig. 2.4).

Treatment

Conservative approach was applied with regular washing of the foot and the use of dry dressings. Mild compression therapy with short stretch bandages was applied with sub-bandage pressure of 20 mmHg. Oral nutritional supplementation using high protein readily available drinks with the addition of glutamine and arginine was provided [6]. 40 mg of atorvastatin was prescribed to accomplish targeted C-LDL levels of 1.8 mmol/L [7]. Strict hypertension control, as per guidelines, was not achieved, which is often the case in patients on chronic haemodialysis. The patient came to have a regular check-up in our outpatient clinic and when almost

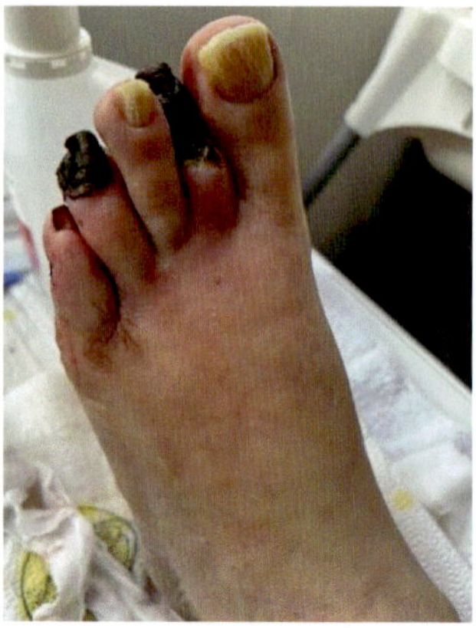

Fig. 2.5 Four weeks later. Minor amputation of the left 2nd toe is healed on a conservative wound treatment strategi despite low ABI

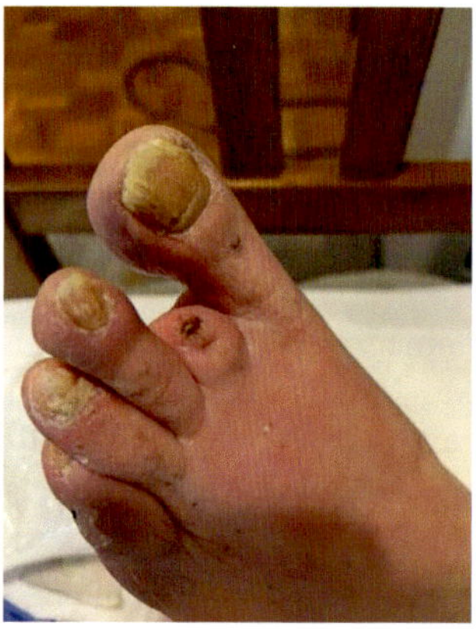

Fig. 2.4 First visit in outpatient clinic. Vascular reconstruction is not possible

autoamputation of the toe was achieved, we performed a precise surgical amputation. Afterwards a small clean wound remained and was treated with alginate dressing until final closure two weeks after the minor amputation (Fig. 2.5). During the whole treatment, as well as after the wound closure, the patient was encouraged to wear appropriate shoes with orthopedic insoles to off-load the wound area. Supervised physical therapy was performed daily.

Discussion

Ischaemic changes and ulcerations on the feet/lower extremities, without the possibility to optimize the blood circulation by surgical revascularization, do not always lead to major amputation. Meticulous conservative wound treatment strategy with appropriate foot and wound care including offloading shoes or devices can lead to wound healing [8]. In the case of dry gangrene of the toe or a wound covered with dry eschar, due to absence of adequate arterial inflow, it is recommended to omit wound debridement and treat the wounds with dry dressings until they loosen on its own. Debridement of a dry ischaemic wound, will only enlarge the wound area and may worsen the ischaemia in the area by increasing the metabolic demand. Furthermore, dry eschar protects the wound from infection and has a "scab" effect that promotes epithelization beneath the necrotic tissue [9].

Control of risk factors is of utmost importance (ex. optimization of medical treatment of hypertension, glycaemia, and/or lipidemia). Adequate nutritional support can be a decisive factor in the wound healing process. Conservative wound care strategy to patients suffering from lower extremity ischaemic wounds is successful in more than two-thirds of the patients. The failure of conservative management does not increase mortality or amputation rates [10].

Case 2.3. Multifactorial Causes to Prolonged Healing; Never Give up

Introduction

An 82-year-old woman (heavy smoker) with known hypertension, ischemic heart disease and claudication (former endovascular treatment and bilateral stenting bilateral in a. iliaca communis) was referred to the Department of Vascular Surgery due to CLTI. The patient had a wound-history of two months progression of a large infected, painful ulcer developed after a trauma. Treatment with IV and oral antibiotics (but no compression) was initiated early in the treatment course.

Clinically the wound size was estimated to 10 × 7 cm with dry necrosis and clinical signs of infection (Fig. 2.6a). No palpable pulses were present in the foot, left ankle/toe pressure showed 41.9/17.3 mmHg, respectfully (ABI of 0.42). The patient had no diabetes and only a small degree of peripheral oedema. Other types of leg ulcers; e.g. vasculitis, neoplasma, venous ulcers were excluded [2].

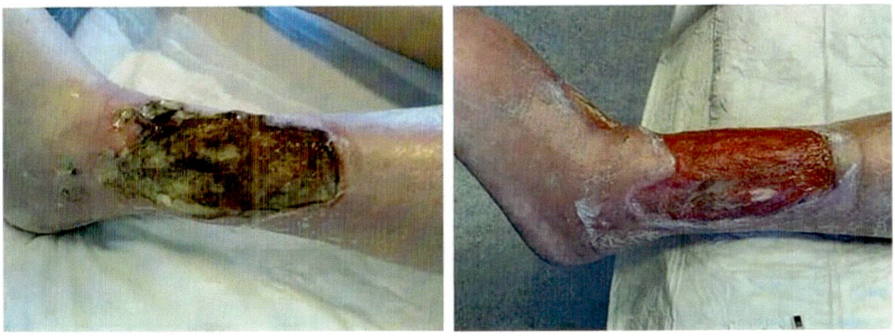

(a) (b)

Fig. 2.6 **a** Wound with multi factorial causes containing a significant arterial component. **b** After revascularization and control of infection and removal of necrosis NPWT was initiated

Treatment

Revascularization was planned after CT angiography with in situ bypass surgery (v. saphena magna to ATP). A very close cooperation between vascular, orthopedic and plastic surgeons enabled a good outcome for this patient despite complications [11, 12]. Compression bandaging was used to reduce postoperative oedema and to reduce secretion from the surgical site.

After successful revascularization, the patient was referred to the Wound Healing Center for surgical wound revision, including excision of necrotic tendons in the wound bed (tendon of hallucis longus, proximal part of the tibialis anterior tendon and the peroneus longus tendon). NPWT was implemented one day after surgery, followed by positive signs of healing (ex. granulation tissue, reduction of oedema, and secretion and wound pain) (Fig. 2.6b).

Nine days later the patient suddenly got high fever and hypotension. Septic shock was suspected and she was transferred to the semi-intensive care (pressor drugs, IV antibiotics and resuscitation). Blood samples showed bacteremia and the main focus was the old trauma wound bed and the scar after revascularization on the medial side of the leg. An ultrasound examination of the surgical scar confirmed abscess leading to reoperation (removal of purulent secretion and old hematoma) in the Department of Vascular Surgery.

Postoperatively the patient's wounds and infection were treated at the Wound Healing Center. Three months after revascularization a duplex ultrasound identified stenosis in the distal in-situ anastomosis leading to reoperation to prevent reconstruction failure.

A significant increase in perfusion to the leg and foot was achieved (left ankle/toe pressure showed 136/54 mmHg, ABI of 1.02). The patient was now offered additional surgical revision of the wound(s) and split skin transplantation combined with Matriderm® (an acellular dermal matrix) on the vital part of the tendon with split skin on top [13], resulting in a 95% healing of the area (Fig. 2.7a, b).

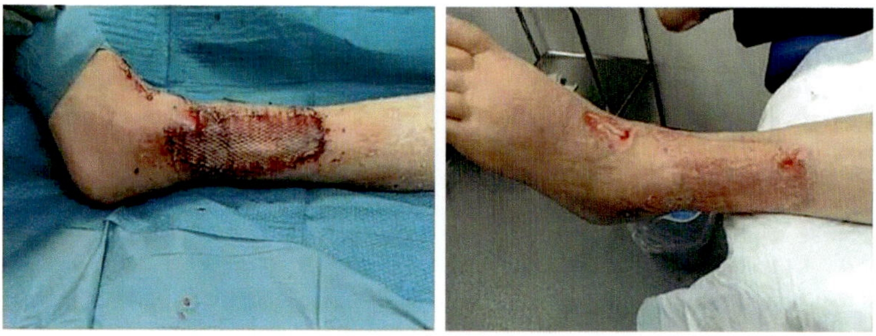

(a) (b)

Fig. 2.7 **a** 3 months after revascularization the patient needed reoperation to prevent vascular reconstruction failure. An additional surgical revision of the wound(s) and split skin transplantation was preformed. Matriderm® (an acellular dermal matrix) was applied on the vital part of the tendon with split skin on top. **b** 4 weeks after split skin transplantation

At the time of surgery, the patient had reduced smoking dramatically and had a high adherence to the postoperative wound treatment including bandages, compression and an aircast to immobilize the ankle joint. Reduced function, especially dorsi flexion of the foot, was a consequence of the removed tendons. But importantly, the patient kept her leg and is now well mobilized without any assistive devices.

Discussions

Successful wound management revolves around a multidisciplinary approach combined with determination of the wound etiology [11, 12]. A very close cooperation between vascular, orthopedic and plastic surgeons enabled a good outcome for the patient. In this case, despite complications with infection, near-occlusion of the in situ graft and septic shock, the outcome was successful.

Focus on the aetiology is essential in all parts of the patient care along with the fact that focus may change. Additionally, modifiable risk factors may be addressed to achieve wound healing and pain relief. In this case, smoking was a big issue as smoking dramatically reduces the arterial blood supply to the wound. As healthcare professionals, we need to support the patient in accepting smoking cessation as a part of the treatment in total.

Case 2.4. Both Macro- and Micro-circulation Are Crucial

Introduction

A 74-year-old male with hypertension, atrial fibrillation and DM. After 35 years of smoking, he stopped smoking 15 years ago. He lives with his wife and uses a walking aid outside the home. No claudication or signs of rest pain in the anamnesis. The patient arrives at the hospital due to chronic oedema of both lower limbs and now acutely presents a necrotic second toe on the right foot (Fig. 2.8a).

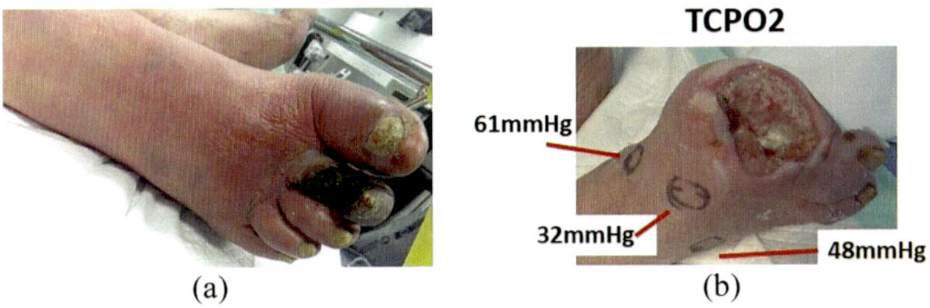

Fig. 2.8 (**a**) At arrival to the hospital, a necrotic toe was observed; (**b**) measurement of the microcirculation as a tool to predict the need for further surgery

Femoral pulse was palpable, but neither the ADP nor the ATP were found. Infection parameters were elevated (CRP 102, temperature of 37.5 °C). MRA imaging showed a stenosis in the SFA, and more important a severe crural arterial disease with occlusions in the ATA and ATP and a stenotic fibular/peroneal artery.

Treatment

Immediate toe amputation was performed due to infection. During the surgery, it also became clear that the first toe was affected and consequently amputated with the surgical wound left open.

The next day endovascular intervention with angioplasty to SFA and peroneal artery was performed resulting in good collateral supply to the foot, where plantar artery was patent.

At day 3, due to insufficient healing; NPWT was initiated. After two rounds of NPWT the wound intensified. Debris was building up, bone was exposed. TCPO2 measurements (Fig. 2.8b) were performed to verify the healing potential followed by a transmetatarsal amputation and surgical wound closure.

During a couple of days, the plantar side of the wound went cold and ischaemia was obvious (Fig. 2.9a). On bedside ultrasound examination, a patent distal ATP was still seen. A good quality unilateral great saphenous vein was found and a bypass from distal popliteal artery to distal ATP was performed. Postoperatively, the patient suffered from congestive heart failure leading to oedema in both lower legs, complicated wound healing. With a patent graft and diligent local wound treatment including intensive oedema control, the wound was nearly healed after 5 months. (Fig. 2.9b) Patient was ambulatory and referred to foot therapist for customized footwear.

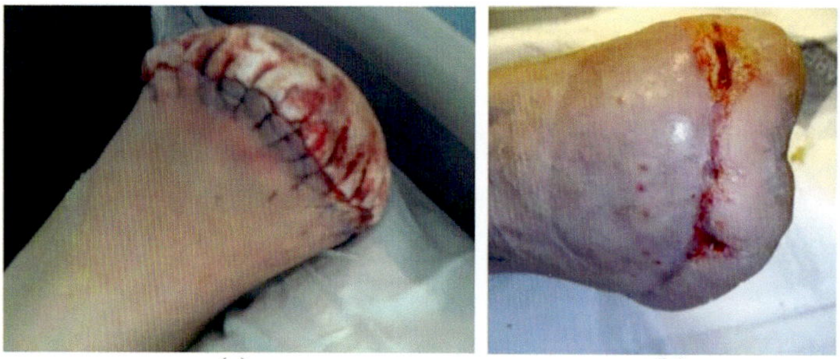

(a) (b)

Fig. 2.9 (**a**) New development of ischemia and a new revascularization procedure was planned; (**b**) 5 months after the vascular reconstruction

Discussion

Ischemia in diabetic patients is often diagnosed for the first time in a situation where foot infection is present. Most often, the crural arteries are affected [14] as in this case. Whenever there is an infection involved in suspected ischemic diabetic foot ulcer, urgent evaluation is recommended to determine the timing of revision and revascularization [15]. Typically, revision surgery is performed immediately to stop the infection from progressing and revascularization is done afterwards, whereas in a chronic wound situation revascularization is usually performed first and preferably within 2 weeks after ischemia is detected [16].

Endovascular treatment is in many cases the first option for revascularization aiming to achieve adequate perfusion to the wound area. After revascularization, the perfusion should be evaluated repeatedly when signs of poor healing arise, as restenosis and occlusion sometimes occur. TCPO2 (measurement of micro circulation in the skin) has been shown to be fairly reliable in predicting wound healing among diabetics [17], but the method does have some pitfalls. Measurement sites should be on "healthy" skin without infection or swelling. Tendons and bony structures may also affect the results.

There has been a massive debate of whether endovascular treatment or open surgery should be chosen as the first-line treatment for patients with CLTI. According to a recent large randomized trial [18, 19] open surgery is superior when the patient has a suitable vein graft material. However, the two different treatment methods are not necessarily competing methods, but rather complementing each other, as was the case with our patient, where PTA to SFA made the needed bypass shorter.

Diabetic foot with ischemic tissue loss always presents a challenge to the treating physicians from the diagnosis to the need for rapid vascular evaluation, revascularization, on to follow up and wound management in order to gain limb salvage; thereafter further focus is needed on appropriate footwear and foot care to prevent tissue defects from reoccurring.

Case 2.5. Osteomyelitis Treatment Needs a MDT Approach

Introduction

A 65-year-old gentleman with DM, hypertension, hypercholesterolemia and sarcoidosis was referred to our MDT-DFU. The patient had not experienced walking related pain neither rest pain from his legs prior to the referral. His ulcer was located over the base of the right fifth metatarsal bone. The ulcer had been present for about 4 weeks with progression of wound size and tissue loss.

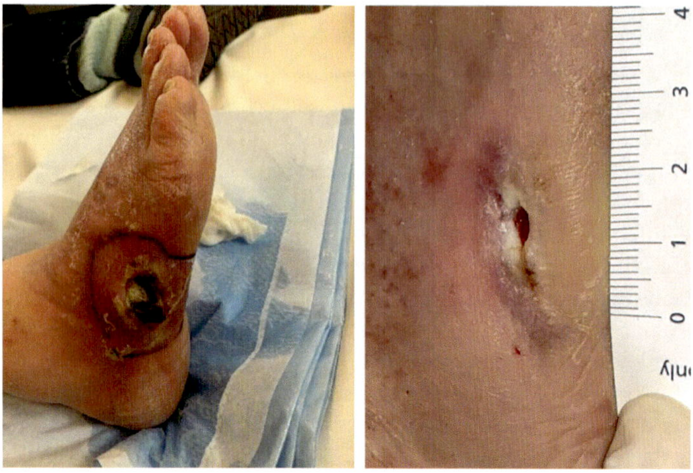

(a) (b)

Fig. 2.10 (**a**) Diabetic foot ulcer with osteomyelitis corresponding basis of the right 5th metatarsal bone at a man, 65 years of age, with DM, hyposensitivity and peripheral ischemia; (**b**) Healing 6 months after intensive wound treatment and revascularization (two procedures)

Clinical Findings

At the physical examination good quality pulse was found in the femoral arteries but no palpable pulses at the right foot. Usually, we only measure toe pressure in patients with known diabetes as we expect an ankle measurement to be false high due to medial calcific sclerosis in the peripheral arteries on the ankle level. In this case, the blood pressure at the right first toe was 52 mmHg. Furthermore, a significantly reduced sensitivity was found on both feet. The ulcer measured 4.2 cm × 2.8 cm with a depth of 2 cm in a plantar cavity containing necrotic tissue with a central area with positive "probe to bone" test, indicating osteomyelitis [20] (Fig. 2.10a).

Altogether, the wound was classified as a neuropathic wound on a hyposensitive diabetic foot with lack of healing due to ischaemia. An MRI-angiography confirmed a stenosis at the proximal part of the deep femoral artery and a 14 cm long stenotic area in the SFA. The ATA was occluded, the PTA and the peroneal artery had multiple stenosis. Additionally, another MR scan confirmed osteomyelitis of the base of the 5th metatarsal bone and the cuboid bone.

Treatment

The glycaemic control and antibiotic treatment was optimized. Antibiotic treatment was primarily given intravenously in high doses in accordance with the microbial findings attending sensitivity and resistance patterns.

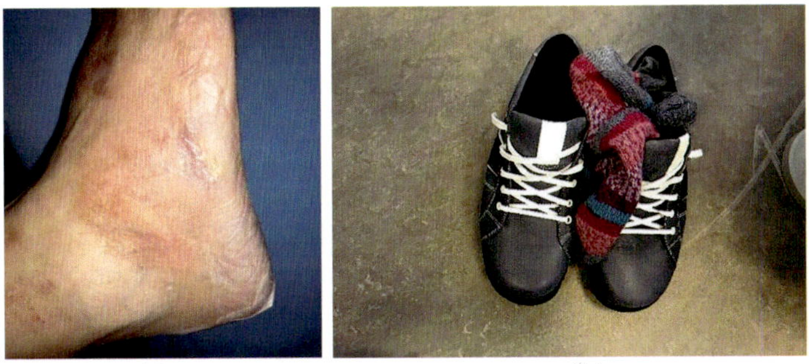

(a) (b)

Fig. 2.11 (**a**) Complete healing of neuropathic wound on a hyposensitive diabetic foot with ischemia and osteomyelitis 12 months after primary referral; (**b**) custom made shoes with the possibility of offloading, a very important part of the treatment but also a way to reduce the risk of recurrence

Revascularization was performed by open endarterectomy in the left groin in combination with endovascular treatment with a stent proximally in SFA, and balloon dilatation in the rest of SFA, the peroneal artery and PTA. Intensive wound treatment was initiated including: Surgical and maggots wound debridement, NPWT, offloading with felt. After healing was achieved, costume made shoes were manufactured (Fig. 2.11b).

Most controls in the follow-up period were performed by use of telemedicine between the primary wound nurse and the wound specialists in the MDT-DFU at the hospital. At follow-up in the MDT-DFU the toe pressure was found reduced, leading to repetition of the endovascular part of the revascularization procedure, approximately 41/2 month after the primary procedure.

7 months after the first visit in the MDT-DFU, the wound was reduced to 4 mm by 2 mm (Fig. 2.10b) but 8 days later, a massive deterioration was seen. The offloading was intensified, and the peripheral endovascular treatment was performed for the third time. Three months later a complete healing of the wound was obtained (Fig. 2.11a). No recurrence has been seen in the following 18 months during which the patient has been living a very active life. He and his wife are performing daily inspections of his feet.

Discussions

When dealing with a combined ischaemic and diabetic foot ulcer it is of utmost importance to understand all the different aspects of the aetiology and the demands for healing, calling for a MDT-DFU set-up [15, 21]. Medical treatment of osteomyelitis cannot stand alone, if we wish to avoid major amputation. Without the three times of revascularization together with intensive wound treatment, glycaemic control, and antimicrobial treatment combined with parallel optimal offloading, healing could not have been obtained.

The most important aspect, nevertheless, is the patient himself: The treatment must be planned in full common agreement with the patient. He must recognize all he needs to invest, and he has to accept that there is no guarantee of success [22].

Case 2.6. Keep Fighting Oedema

A 74-year-old male was referred from his general practitioner to a wound center, embedded in a department of vascular surgery, due to CLTI resulting in severe pain from a heel ulcer during low activities, at rest, and through the night. The patient had a background of DM, hypertension, hypercholesterolemia and experienced a two-month progression of a left heel fissure that progressed into an ulcer. Furthermore, the patient had leg oedema and hyperemic toes with edematous bullae on the first, second and third toe. Heel ulcer size was 1 × 1 cm, superficial, with no signs of infection and with well-defined edges and moderate moisture (Fig. 2.12). There was no detectable pulse from the level of the popliteal artery and periphery. The left ankle/toe pressure showed 48/12 mmHg (ABI 0.32).

The patient's anamnesis and the findings from the physical examination (severe pain, ulcer, pale foot, low ABI, no distal pulse) indicated CLTI. Furthermore, the patient had peripheral oedema combined with a component of diabetic neuropathy. All these etiological factors led to the ulcer in the heel and bullae formation on toes.

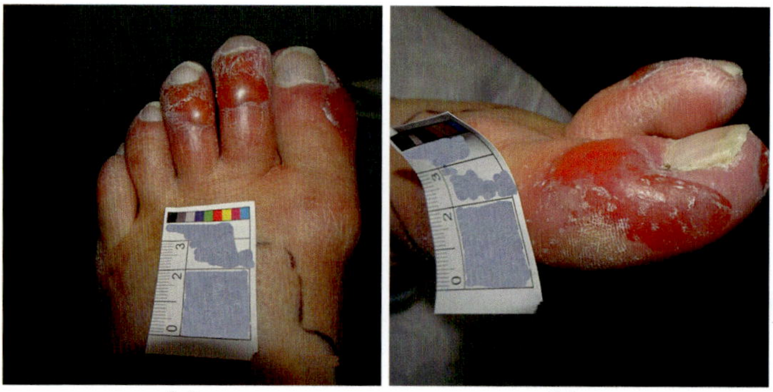

(a) (b)

Fig. 2.12 In addition, to severe rest pain the patient had leg oedema and hyperaemic toes with edematous bullae on the 1st to 3rd toe **(a)** dorsal aspect; **(b)** lateral aspect

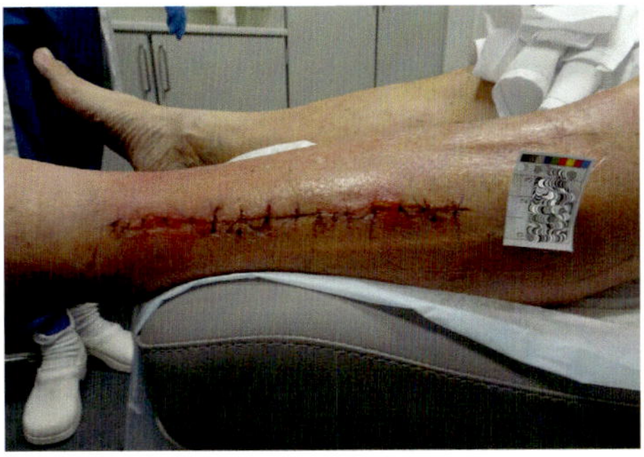

Fig. 2.13 Oedema in the scar region after revascularization

Treatment

Revascularization was planned after CT angiography showing occlusion from the beginning of the popliteal artery and several stenoses on the leg arteries. Only the distal ATA was graftable and the patient was offered revascularization by in situ bypass.

Until vascular surgery was performed, the patient was offered wound treatment, including compression therapy with inelastic bandages, customized offloading footwear and pain medication.

The revascularization was successful followed by restoration of pulse in the dorsal pedal artery. The following postoperative days, the compression therapy was intensified by combining inelastic bandages with intermittent pneumatic compression (IPC) due to massive postoperative oedema. Furthermore, NPWT was used in the lower leg because of lymphatic drainage from the surgical sites (Fig. 2.13).

The patient was discharged after eight days with planned follow-up in the wound care center after 12 days. Until follow-up, a homecare nurse provided wound care, including daily application of short-stretch compression bandages, prophylactic antibiotics, offloading, pain medication and moist wound care three times a week. The toe ulcers were healed completely and the ulcer in the heel was almost healed. The patient was still suffering from post-operative oedema and needed continued daily application of inelastic bandages.

Discussion

Wound care management depends on the aetiology and involvement of a multidisciplinary team to improve wound healing and decrease amputations [23]. CLTI consisting of intractable rest pain, tissue loss and hence wounds or/and gangrene is associated with limb amputation, high mortality and a significant economic burden to society [2, 23]. Revascularization with bypass surgery around the blockage in leg arteries is a cornerstone to prevent amputation and increase healing of wounds alongside conservative wound care management (off-loading, oedema and infection treatment, revascularization etc.) [24].

Compression therapy is important both in the pre- and post- revascularization period to prevent oedema and to optimize wound healing [24]. Peripheral oedema is a common component to CLTI as well as other concomitant competitive diseases, e.g. chronic kidney disease or heart failure.

Among CLTI patients, the patients often choose sitting position rather than supine during the night, thus increasing leg blood pressure and oxygen supply in tissue, which reduces pain. However, sitting position also increases venous pressure inducing oedema which compromises wound healing. Oedema causes increased distance between the cells due to distention of the interstitial space, which further compromise oxygen delivery and may aggravate hypoxia in already critically ischemic peripheral tissue [25, 26]. Compression therapy to CLTI is often avoided, in fear of compromising the circulation and acceleration of pain and ischemic wound formation. It is important to acknowledge that there is no harm from mild/moderate compression (18–21 mmHg ankle pressure) to patients with PAD (ABI > 50 mmHg) [27].

In the postoperative period after revascularization of the lower limbs, patients often suffer from reperfusion oedema, which may delay wound and scar healing if not treated. Daily application of compression therapy with inelastic bandages is effective. Further addition of IPC optimizes the oedema treatment [2, 28] as IPC increases arterial blood flow in the distal limb by an arteriovenous pressure gradient stimulating endothelial vasodilators [2, 28].

Conclusion

Fighting oedema is essential according to wound healing time, cicatricial healing, accelerating mobilization and reducing pain. In addition, moderated compression as inelastic bandages optionally combined with IPC, is important in wound care management in the pre- and postoperative period in patients with CLTI / ischaemic wounds and concomitant competitive diseases.

Case 2.7. The Assessment of Peripheral Arterial Circulation is Necessary

Introduction

A 76-year old female was referred to our outpatient clinic for vascular surgery by her general practitioner. During the past two months, ulcers had developed on the dorsum of the 1st, 2nd, and 5th right toe. Furthermore, the patient experienced rest pain in the right leg occurring several times every night, eased only by standing up or leaving the leg hanging from the bedside. Comorbidities were hypertension, hypercholesterolemia and osteoporosis. The patient had been a smoker for many years and was recently widowed, but managed daily routines without any help.

Clinical Findings

At the clinical examination, we found the entire distal foot to be hyperaemic and cold. The pulse was palpable only over the common femoral artery (in the groin), more week on the symptomatic leg, and no pulses were found more distally. Ultrasonically, blood flow was only detectable until 15 cm proximally from the knee joint. Distal blood pressure on the relevant extremity was 46 mmHg on ankle and 17 mmHg on toe levels (ankle-brachial-index 0.35).

There were no oedema or ulcers proximal on the leg and the patient was not prescribed any medication that could enhance wound formation, such as steroids. The position of the ulcers, the low distal blood pressure, no signs of infection and typical anamnestic risk factors for developing atherosclerosis made the diagnosis of CLTI plausible.

Treatment

A CT-angiography revealed multiple stenosis in the right external iliac artery. Additionally, the SFA was totally occluded and had been so for a long time, as contrast was seen to fill the popliteal artery via collateral arteries. First treatment was endovascular revascularization with stents of the external iliac artery, after which a direct angiography showed open lumen until the proximal part of the SFA and contrast filled the popliteal artery via collateral arteries. The patient was discharged to the care of nurses, representing the primary healthcare system. A plan for wound treatment and pain relief was made. However, worsening of the wounds and pain precipitated consultation 15 days postoperatively (Fig. 2.14).

The patient was rehospitalized and only anesthesia administered epidurally provided sufficient pain relief. Additional revascularization was needed and an

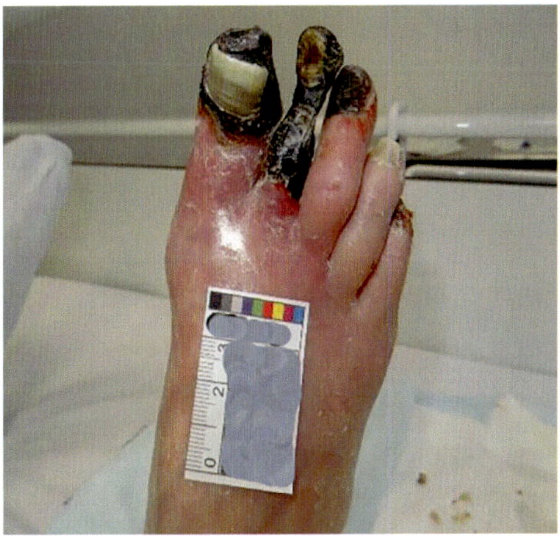

Fig. 2.14 Days postsurgery, gangrene had worsened and amputation is inevitable

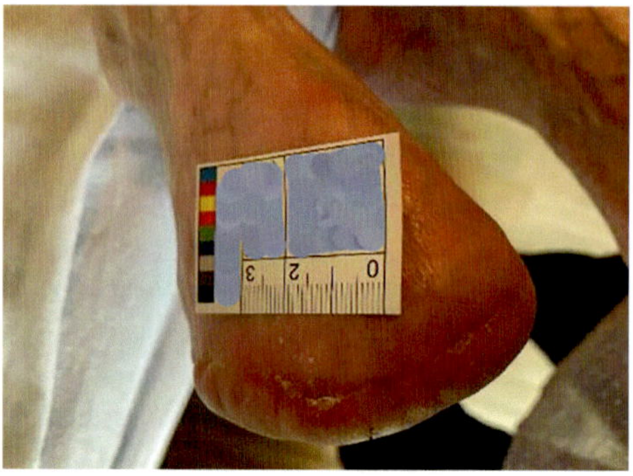

Fig. 2.15 Functional result after forefoot amputation, final control 5 months after vascular reconstruction

intercomposite bypass was grafted from the common femoral artery to the proximal ATA followed by an amputation of the forefoot.

Six days later the patient was discharged with tolerable pain and good signs of wound healing followed by a period of physiotherapy at a rehabilitation unit and continuing wound treatment. The patient was able to walk short distances. After three weeks, sutures were removed and antibiotic treatment was discontinued. Offloading of the foot was ensured with customized insoles and shoes specially designed to fit the amputated foot (Fig. 2.15).

Discussion

CLTI presents the end stage of PAD [29] and is associated with very high rates of co-morbidity and mortality due to universal arteriosclerosis [30, 31]. Mortality rates increase if minor or major amputations are added – increasing the more proximal the amputation level is located [32].

This present case points out that multidisciplinary cooperation and close monitoring of the patient with well-timed surgical treatment, can lower the amputation level on an extremity leading to great benefit for the patient [31, 32]. Optimal medical management of arteriosclerosis (statines, antiplatelet medicine, smoking cessation and walk training) may postpone the consequence of CLTI that further emphasizes the need of multidisciplinary collaboration in the care of CLTI patients.

Case 2.8. Ischemia and Neuropathy; a Bad Cocktail

Introduction

A 57-year-old male was transferred to our Department of Vascular Surgery after admission to the ER due to gangrene of his left foot. Moreover, the patient had a history of DM, hypertension, dyslipidemia and underwent cardiac intervention after myocardial infarction (Coronary angioplasty inclusive stent placement). His

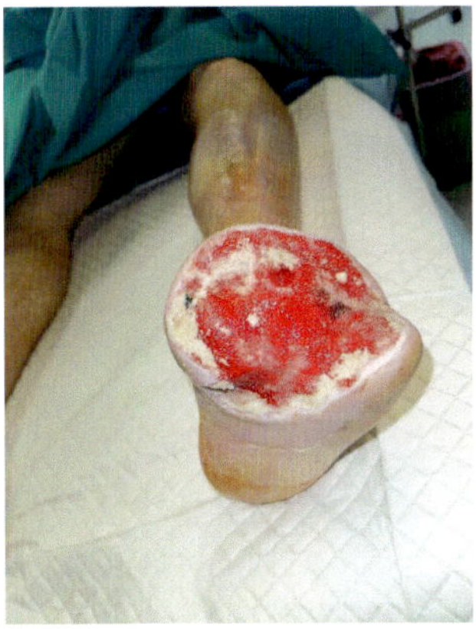

Fig. 2.16 Emergency transmetatarsal amputation followed by vascular assessment

everyday medical treatment included metformin, acetylsalicylic acid, statins and antihypertensive drugs. Laboratory tests showed high levels of leukocytes, blood glucose, creatinine and CRP. Emergency transmetatarsal amputation of the forefoot was performed at admission and broad-spectrum antibiotic and other symptomatic therapy was initiated immediately (Fig. 2.16).

Clinical Findings

On the first day after admission, CT angiography of abdominal aorta, pelvic and lower extremity arteries was performed. It detected occlusion of the left SFA. The ABI was 0.4 for the left leg and 0.8 for the right leg. After forefoot amputation, on the first dressing change, the remnants of the left foot looked ischaemic, with no significant bleeding, but with no signs of gangrene progression. Decision was made to perform a vascular reconstruction to increase the oxygen supply to the wound area of the amputation.

Treatment

The patient's great saphenous vein was not suitable as a graft; why a polytetrafluoroethylene (PTFE) vascular graft was used to by-pass the occlusion of the SFA. Surgery was performed in general anesthesia. At the end of the procedure, additional surgical excision of the left foot was done, and NPWT was applied. The NPWT system was changed three times, with one additional debridement on the first change, before healthy granulation tissue appeared. Then a decision was made to cover the remaining wound with a dermal substitute (Matriderm®) combined with a split-skin graft.

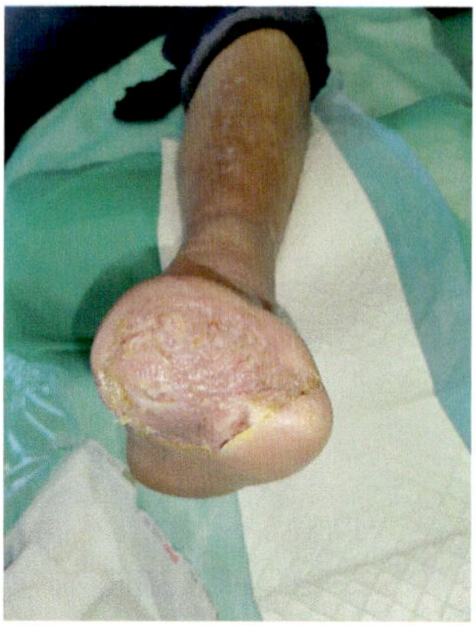

Fig. 2.17 Wound healing after vascular reconstruction, NPWT treatment and split-skin graft

Cardiologists and endocrinologists were consulted to optimize the medical treatment of the patient, because of the history of prior myocardial infarction and poorly regulated diabetes.

Conclusion

Complete healing of the left foots' remnant was achieved after three weeks of hospital stay and two weeks rehabilitation at home. The patient was provided with orthopedic shoes and was able to go back to work (Fig. 2.17).

In this case we have a patient with foot gangrene due to a combination of diabetic neuropathy and peripheral arterial disease. Unfortunately, there are still a lot of patients coming to the ER presenting like this [33, 34]. Patients with DM lack education about the importance of regular self-examination of their feet. Physicians also do not pay enough attention to their patients' feet and the necessary education of the patient on the topic. Likewise, peripheral arterial disease is also underdiagnosed and untimely treated [34, 35].

Since this was a patient still employed and otherwise in good physical condition, our goal was to enable him to get back to work and his normal life as soon as possible. Usually, after transmetatarsal amputation on infected foot, the remnant wound is left to heal with formation of granulation tissue and epithelialization following the principles of moist wound healing, reflected in the choice of wound dressings [36, 37]. The downside of this approach is the time consumed in addition to complications with secondary infection and subsequent the need for re-amputation at a higher level. Infection, in this case, could be potentially hazardous, because infection in a synthetic vascular graft is close to incurable and may lead to above knee amputation with an increased risk of sepsis and death. To achieve a faster healing we decided to use NPWT on foot remnant followed by reconstruction with dermal substitute and split-skin graft [38]. Technique with dermal substitute provides healing with minimal scarring and tissue that better endures pressure from walking and consequently prevents new ulcer formation [39].

Case 2.9. Below-the-Knee Plain Old Balloon Angioplasty (POBA) Contributing to the Healing of Dry Gangrene of the Toe

Introduction

A 75-year-old man with type-II diabetes and arteriosclerotic changes of the lower extremities presented with signs and symptoms of critical limb ischemia of left lower limb. He had a non-healing ulcer of the second toe and rest-pain (9–10 on Visual Analogue Scale/ Numeric Rating Score where 0 = no pain, 10 = worst possible pain).

Diagnostic

The patient had adequate inguinal and popliteal pulses, but no perceptible pulse at ankle, including the dorsal pedis artery. Left toe pressure was 30 mm Hg. CT angiography revealed occlusion of the tibialis anterior, dorsalis pedis and plantaris arteries, and severe stenosis in tibialis posterior artery. Digital Subtraction Angiography performed during the endovascular treatment confirmed the findings of the CT scanning. Perfusion to the foot was significantly reduced, and the foot arcades and digital arteries were not well-visualized (Fig. 2.18).

Treatment

PTA was performed using antegrade approach. The occlusion in the anterior tibial and dorsalis pedis arteries were opened using 2.5 mm and 2.0 mm plain old balloon angioplasty (POBA) respectively. The stenosis and occlusion in the posterior tibial and plantar arteries respectively were similarly treated by 2.5 mm and 2.0 mm POBA. Final angiography revealed well-perfused left foot and all three open leg arteries and foot arcades. During the postoperative period, the patient had significant reduction of pain (2–3 on Visual Analogue Scale/Numeric Rating Score) with concomitant reduction of the use of analgesia. The ulcer at the tip of the toe started showing signs of healing. At two months, there was complete healing of the toe ulcer, and the patient was ambulant.

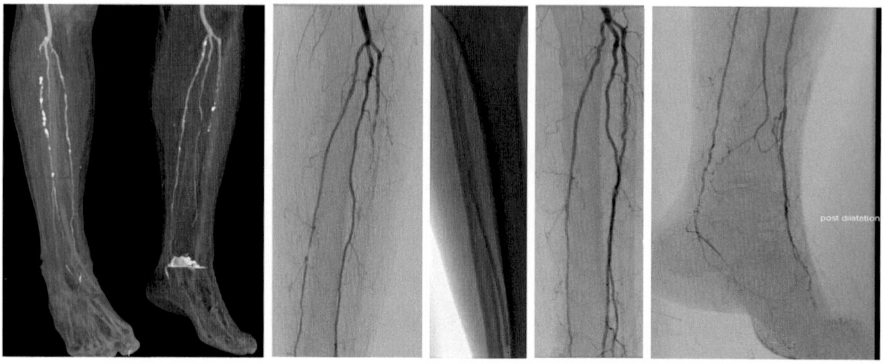

Fig. 2.18 Chronic limb threatening ischemia. CT angiography and Digital Subtraction Angiography reveal occlusion of tibialis anterior and dorsalis pedis arteries, and severe short stenosis of tibialis posterior artery and occluded plantaris artery (a, b). Plain balloon angioplasty (POBA) (c), post POBA angiographies show complete revascularization of all three leg arteries (d) and arcades of the foot (e)

Discussion

The anterior and posterior tibial arteries supply the angiosomes perfusing the toe areas. While the anterior tibial artery and its continuation, the dorsalis pedis artery supply the dorsal aspect of the toes, the plantar artery, which is the continuation of posterior tibial artery, supply the plantar aspect of the toes. After POBA of the leg and foot arteries there was adequate flow in the foot-angiosomes, including the toe areas, leading to healing of the toe ulcer (Fig. 2.19). PTA is widely used as a first-line treatment for revascularization of CLTI, which is the most advanced stage of PAD and is defined as rest pain and/or ulceration of lower limb of more than two weeks duration [40]. These patients are at a higher risk of major lower extremity amputation and premature death. The one-year risk of major lower extremity amputation in patients with CLTI exceeds 15–20% and the five-year all-cause mortality rate is approximately 50% [41]. It is therefore extremely important to treat these patients urgently, where both by-pass graft and PTA are deemed to be suitable options. A recent randomized control trial (RCT, BEST-CLI trial) concluded that a major adverse limb event (MALE) such as major lower extremity amputation or death is significantly lower after open surgical by-pass compared to endovascular treatment (PTA), where adequate long saphenous vein segment is available. However, with inadequate long saphenous vein, results of both open surgical by-pass and PTA are comparable [42]. Another retrospective study comparing open surgical by-pass with PTA showed improved wound healing, higher freedom from restenosis, improved patency rates, significantly fewer re-interventions, and higher survival at six-month for open by-pass compared to PTA [43]. The saphenous vein may not always be available for in-situ by-pass for various reasons, in these

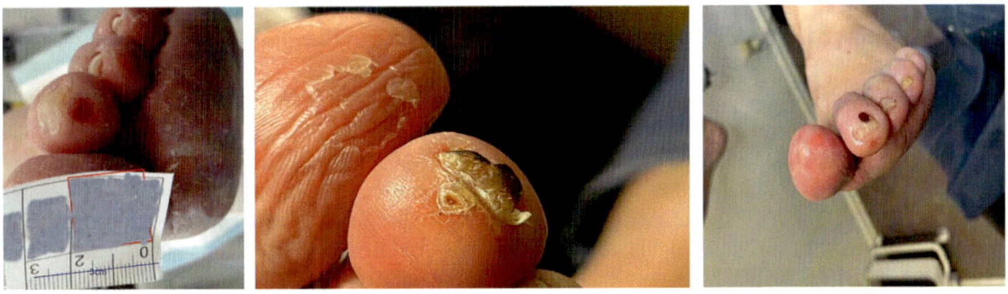

(a) (b) (c)

Fig. 2.19 (**a**) Pre-revascularisationt, (**b**) 2-weeks post-revascularisation and (**c**) 1-month post-revascularisationt clinical photos of the foot, showing complete healing of toe ulcer after PTA of leg and foot arteries.

cases PTA remains as a available strategy. PTA can be employed as POBA or with drug-eluting balloon impregnated with Paclitaxel/Sirolimus. The ACHILLES RCT trail showed accelerated wound healing and improved quality of life with drug eluting stent for below the knee lesions [44]. Other studies have shown improved results with PTA, where endovascular revascularization is directed according to the involved angiosome [45–47].

References

1. Isoherranen K, Montero EC, Atkin L, Collier M, Høgh A, Ivory JD, Kirketerp Møller K, Meaume S, Ryan H, Stuermer EK, Tiplica GS, Probst S. Lower leg ulcer diagnosis & principles of treatment. Including recommendations for comprehensive assessment and referral pathways. J Wound Manage. 2023;24(2 Supl):s1–76. https://doi.org/10.35279/jowm2023.24.02.sup01
2. Conte MS, Bradbury AW, Kolh P, White JV, Dick F, Fitridge R, et al. Global vascular guidelines on the management of chronic limb-threatening ischemia. Eur J Vasc Endovasc Surg. 2019;58(1s):S1–S109.e33.
3. Al WA. Autoamputation of diabetic toe with dry gangrene: a myth or a fact? Diabetes Metab Syndr Obes. 2018;11:255–64.
4. Kinlay S. Management of critical limb ischemia. Circ Cardiovasc Interv. 2016;9(2):e001946.
5. Düsing P, Zietzer A, Goody PR, Hosen MR, Kurts C, Nickenig G, Jansen F. Vascular pathologies in chronic kidney disease: pathophysiological mechanisms and novel therapeutic approaches. J Mol Med (Berl). 2021;99(3):335–48.
6. Saeg F, Orazi R, Bowers GM, Janis JE. Evidence-based nutritional interventions in wound care. Plast Reconstr Surg. 2021;148(1):226–38.
7. Rymer JA, Swaminathan RV, Aday AW, Patel MR, Gutierrez JA. The current evidence for lipid management in patients with lower extremity peripheral artery disease: what is the therapeutic target? Curr Cardiol Rep. 2021;23:1–7.
8. Chiriano J, Bianchi C, Teruya TH, Mills B, Bishop V, Abou-Zamzam AM Jr. Management of lower extremity wounds in patients with peripheral arterial disease: a stratified conservative approach. Ann Vasc Surg. 2010;24(8):1110–6.
9. Anghel EL, DeFazio MV, Barker JC, Janis JE, Attinger CE. Current concepts in debridement: science and strategies. Plast Reconstr Surg. 2016;138(3 Suppl):82S-93S.

10. van Reijen NS, Hensing T, Santema TKB, Ubbink DT, Koelemay MJW. Outcomes of conservative treatment in patients with chronic limb threatening ischaemia: a systematic review and meta-analysis. Eur J Vasc Endovasc Surg. 2021;62(2):214–24.
11. Moore Z, Butcher G, Corbett LQ, et al. AAWC, AWMA, EWMA position paper: managing wounds as a team. J Wound Care. 2014;23(5 Suppl.):S1–38.
12. Flores AM, Mell MW, Dalman RL, Chandra V. Benefit of multidisciplinary wound care center on the volume and outcomes of a vascular surgery practice. J Vasc Surg. 2019;(70):1612–19.
13. Kanapathy M, Smith OJ, Hachach-Haram N, Bystrzonowski N, Mosahebi A, Richards T. Systematic review and meta-analysis of the efficacy of epidermal grafting for wound healing. Int Wound J. 2017;14(6):912–28.
14. Graziani L, Silvestro A, Bertone V, Manara E, Andreini R, Sigala A, et al. Vascular involvement in diabetic subjects with ischemic foot ulcer: a new morphologic categorization of disease severity. Eur J Vasc Endovasc Surg. 2007;33(4):453–60.
15. Fitridge R, Chuter V, Mills J, Hinchliffe R, Azuma N, Behrendt C-A, et al. The intersocietal IWGDF, ESVS, SVS guidelines on peripheral artery disease in people with diabetes mellitus and a foot ulcer. J Vasc Surg. 2023;78(5):1101–31.
16. Noronen K, Saarinen E, Albäck A, Venermo M. Analysis of the elective treatment process for critical limb ischaemia with tissue loss: diabetic patients require rapid revascularisation. Eur J Vasc Endovasc Surg. 2017;53(2):206–13.
17. Catella J, Long A, Mazzolai L. What is currently the role of $TcPO_2$ in the choice of the amputation level of lower limbs? A Compr Rev J Clin Med. 2021;10:1413.
18. Špillerová K, Settembre N, Biancari F, Albäck A, Venermo M. Angiosome targeted PTA is more important in endovascular revascularisation than in surgical revascularisation: analysis of 545 patients with ischaemic tissue lesions. Eur J Vasc Endovasc Surg. 2017;53(4):567–75.
19. Faber A, Menard MT, Conte MS, Kaufman JA, Powell RJ, Choudhry NK et al. BEST-CLI Investigators. Surgery or endovascular therapy for chronic limb-threatening ischemia. N Engl J Med. 2022;387(25):2305–2316.
20. Calvo-Wright MDM, Álvaro-Afonso FJ, López-Moral M, García-Álvarez Y, García-Morales E, Lázaro-Martínez JL. Is the combination of plain X-ray and probe-to-bone test useful for diagnosing diabetic foot osteomyelitis? A systematic review and meta-analysis. J Clin Med. 2023;12(16):5369.
21. Berchiolli R, Bertagna G, Adami D, Canovaro F, Torri L, Troisi N. Chronic limb-threatening ischemia and the need for revascularization. J Clin Med. 2023;12(7):2682. https://doi.org/10.3390/jcm12072682. PMID: 37048765; PMCID: PMC10095037
22. Gethin G, Touriany E, van Netten JJ, Sobotka L, Probst S. The impact of patient health and lifestyle factors on wound healing, part 1: stress, sleep, smoking, alcohol, com mon medications and illicit drug use; J Wound Management, 2022;23(1 Suppl 1, pt 1):S1–41; https://doi.org/10.35279/jowm2022.23.01.sup01.01.
23. Chung J, Modrall JG, Ahn C, Lavery LA, Valentine RJ. Multidisciplinary care improves amputation-free survival in patients with chronic critical limb ischemia. J Vasc Surg. 2015;61(1):162–9.
24. Powers JG, Higham C, Broussard K, Phillips TJ. Wound healing and treating wounds: Chronic wound care and management. J Am Acad Dermatol. 2016;74(4):607–25; quiz 25-6.
25. Mponponsuo K, Sibbald RG, Somayaji R. A comprehensive review of the pathogenesis, diagnosis, and management of diabetic foot infections. Adv Skin Wound Care. 2021;34(11):574–81.
26. Khiabani HZ, Anvar MD, Stranden E, Slagsvold CE, Kroese AJ. Oedema in the lower limb of patients with chronic critical limb ischaemia (CLI). Eur J Vasc Endovasc Surg. 1999;17(5):419–23.
27. Stücker M, Danneil O, Dörler M, Hoffmann M, Kröger E, Reich-Schupke S. Safety of a compression stocking for patients with chronic venous insufficiency (CVI) and peripheral artery disease (PAD). J Dtsch Dermatol Ges. 2020;18(3):207–13.
28. Pawlaczyk K, Gabriel M, Urbanek T, Dzieciuchowicz Ł, Krasiński Z, Gabriel Z, et al. Effects of intermittent pneumatic compression on reduction of postoperative lower extremity Edema

and normalization of foot microcirculation flow in patients undergoing arterial revascularization. Med Sci Monit. 2015;21:3986–92.
29. Conte MS, Bradbury AW, Kolh P, White JV, Dick F, Fitridge R, Mills JL, Ricco JB, Suresh KR, Murad MH; GVG Writing Group. Global vascular guidelines on the management of chronic limb-threatening ischemia. J Vasc Surg. 2019;69(6S):3S-125S.e40. https://doi.org/10.1016/j.jvs.2019.02.016. Epub 2019 May 28. Erratum in: J Vasc Surg. 2019;70(2):662. PMID: 31159978; PMCID: PMC8365864.
30. Ventoruzzo G, Mazzitelli G, Ruzzi U, Liistro F, Scatena A, Martelli E. Limb salvage and survival in chronic limb-threatening ischemia: the need for a fast-track team-based approach. J Clin Med. 2023;12(18):6081. https://doi.org/10.3390/jcm12186081.
31. Sorber R, Dun C, Kawaji Q, Abularrage CJ, Black JH 3rd, Makary MA, Hicks CW. Early peripheral vascular interventions for claudication are associated with higher rates of late interventions and progression to chronic limb threatening ischemia. J Vasc Surg. 2023;77(3):836-847.e3. https://doi.org/10.1016/j.jvs.2022.10.025.
32. Berchiolli R, Bertagna G, Adami D, Canovaro F, Torri L, Troisi N. Chronic limb-threatening Ischemia and the need for revascularization. J Clin Med. 2023;12(7):2682. https://doi.org/10.3390/jcm12072682.
33. Edmonds M, Manu C, Vas P. The current burden of diabetic foot disease. J Clin Orthop Trauma. 2021;8(17):88–93.
34. Azhar A, Basheer M, Abdelgawad MS, Roshdi H, Kamel MF. Prevalence of peripheral arterial disease in diabetic foot ulcer patients and its impact in limb salvage. Int J Low Extrem Wounds. 2021;18:15347346211027064.
35. Lavery LA, Oz OK, Bhavan K, Wukich DK. Diabetic foot syndrome in the twenty-first century. Clin Podiatr Med Surg. 2019;36(3):355–9. https://doi.org/10.1016/j.cpm.2019.02.002. Epub 2019 Apr 8.
36. Rümenapf G, Morbach S, Rother U, Uhl C, Görtz H, Böckler D, Behrendt CA, Hochlenert D, Engels G, Hohneck A, Sigl M; Kommission PAVK und Diabetisches Fußsyndrom der DGG e. V.. Diabetisches Fußsyndrom—Teil 2 : Revaskularisation, Behandlungsalternativen, Versorgungsstrukturen, Rezidivprophylaxe [Diabetic foot syndrome-Part 2 : Revascularization, treatment alternatives, care structures, recurrency prophylaxis]. Chirurg. 2021;92(2):173–186. German.
37. Fejfarová V, Koliba M, Jirkovská J, Kůsová H, Piťhová P, Jirkovská A, Jep BSPSČČ, Szabo M. Podiatric care from diabetologists point of view. Vnitr Lek. 2022;68(E-7):3–10. English.
38. Weck M, Slesaczeck T, Rietzsch H, Münch D, Nanning T, Paetzold H, Florek HJ, Barthel A, Weiss N, Bornstein S. Noninvasive management of the diabetic foot with critical limb ischemia: current options and future perspectives. Ther Adv Endocrinol Metab. 2011;2(6):247–55.
39. Chiesa R, Astore D, Frigerio S, Garriboli L, Piccolo G, Castellano R, Scalamogna M, Odero A, Pirrelli S, Biasi G, Mingazzini P, Biglioli P, Polvani G, Guarino A, Agrifoglio G, Tori A, Spina G. Vascular prosthetic graft infection: epidemiology, bacteriology, pathogenesis and treatment. Acta Chir Belg. 2002;102(4):238–47.
40. Lee RE, Patel A, Soon SXY, Chan SL, Yap CJQ, Chandramohan S, Tay LHT, Chong TT, Tang TY. One year clinical outcomes of Rutherford 6 chronic limb threatening ischemia patients undergoing lower limb endovascular revascularisation from Singapore. CVIR Endovasc. 2022;5(1):32. https://doi.org/10.1186/s42155-022-00306-1.PMID:35792985;PMCID:PMC9259774.
41. Duff S, Mafilios MS, Bhounsule P, Hasegawa JT. The burden of critical limb ischemia: a review of recent literature. Vasc Health Risk Manag. 2019;15:187–208. https://doi.org/10.2147/VHRM.S209241.
42. Farber A, Menard MT, Conte MS, Kaufman JA, Powell RJ, Choudhry NK, Hamza TH, Assmann SF, Creager MA, Cziraky MJ, Dake MD, Jaff MR, Reid D, Siami FS, Sopko G, White CJ, van Over M, Strong MB, Villarreal MF, McKean M, Azene E, Azarbal A, Barleben A, Chew DK, Clavijo LC, Douville Y, Findeiss L, Garg N, Gasper W, Giles KA, Goodney PP, Hawkins BM, Herman CR, Kalish JA, Koopmann MC, Laskowski IA, Mena-Hurtado C,

Motaganahalli R, Rowe VL, Schanzer A, Schneider PA, Siracuse JJ, Venermo M, Rosenfield K. BEST-CLI investigators. Surgery or endovascular therapy for chronic limb-threatening Ischemia. N Engl J Med. 2022. https://doi.org/10.1056/NEJMoa2207899. Epub ahead of print. PMID: 36342173.
43. Darling JD, McCallum JC, Soden PA, Korepta L, Guzman RJ, Wyers MC, Hamdan AD, Schermerhorn ML. Results for primary bypass versus primary angioplasty/stent for lower extremity chronic limb-threatening ischemia. J Vasc Surg. 2017;66(2):466–75. https://doi.org/10.1016/j.jvs.2017.01.024. Epub 2017 Mar 6. PMID: 28274753; PMCID: PMC5524588.
44. Katsanos K, Spiliopoulos S, Diamantopoulos A, Siablis D, Karnabatidis D, Scheinert D. Wound healing outcomes and health-related quality-of-life changes in the ACHILLES trial: 1-year results from a prospective randomized controlled trial of infrapopliteal balloon angioplasty versus sirolimus-eluting stenting in patients with ischemic peripheral arterial disease. JACC Cardiovasc Interv. 2016;9(3):259–67. https://doi.org/10.1016/j.jcin.2015.10.038. Epub 2016 Jan 6 PMID: 26777329.
45. Kabra A, Suresh KR, Vivekanand V, Vishnu M, Sumanth R, Nekkanti M. Outcomes of angiosome and non-angiosome targeted revascularization in critical lower limb ischemia. J Vasc Surg. 2013;57(1):44–9. https://doi.org/10.1016/j.jvs.2012.07.042. Epub 2012 Oct 9 PMID: 23058724.
46. Söderström M, Albäck A, Biancari F, Lappalainen K, Lepäntalo M, Venermo M. Angiosome-targeted infrapopliteal endovascular revascularization for treatment of diabetic foot ulcers. J Vasc Surg. 2013;57(2):427–35. https://doi.org/10.1016/j.jvs.2012.07.057. Epub 2012 Dec 7 PMID: 23219512.
47. Shehata MMS, Abdelmalek WF, Kamel AN, Mohamed NM, Ahmed AM. Evaluation of wound healing after angiosome-directed infrapopliteal endovascular angioplasty in critical limb ischemia. Egypt J Surg. 2020; 39(4):1170–82. https://doi.org/10.4103/ejs.ejs_215_20.

Venous Leg Ulcers

3

Elena Conde Montero, Kevin Díez Madueño,
Ana Simón Gozalbo, Celia Horcajada Reales, Iulia Elena Negulet,
José Navarro Pascual, Elisa María Gómez González,
Viktorija Rogova, Ionela Manole,
and Jesús Manuel Borbujo Martínez

Abstract

Venous ulcers can be a therapeutic challenge and the practical keys to their proper management are not always included in clinical guidelines. In this chapter you will understand how to diagnose a venous ulcer, the importance of adequate diagnosis and etiological treatment, always consulting a vascular surgeon and with appropriate compression therapy tailored to the individual, anti-inflammatory treatments such as corticosteroids or zinc oxide, the value of spacing out dressing changes, and the benefits of advanced therapies such as punch grafting and negative pressure therapy to promote closure of hard-to-heal wounds.

E. Conde Montero (✉) · K. Díez Madueño · A. Simón Gozalbo
Dermatology Department, Hospital Universitario Infanta Leonor y Virgen de la Torre, Madrid, Spain
e-mail: elenacondemontero@gmail.com

C. Horcajada Reales · J. M. Borbujo Martínez
Dermatology Department, Hospital Universitario de Fuenlabrada, Madrid, Spain

I. E. Negulet · I. Manole
Department of Dermatology 2, Carol Davila University, Colentina Clinical Hospital, Bucharest, Romania

J. Navarro Pascual
Dermatology Department, Hospital General Universitario Reina Sofía, Murcia, Spain

E. M. Gómez González
Dermatology Department, Clínica de Navarra, Pamplona, Spain

V. Rogova
Dermatology Department Veselibas Centrs 4, Riga, Latvia

G.-S.Tiplica and K. Isoherranen (eds.), *Wound Healing*,
https://doi.org/10.1007/978-3-031-84579-6_3

Keywords

Venous leg ulcer • Chronic venous insufficiency • Phlebo-lymphedema • Punch grafting • Compression therapy • Obesity • Necrotic tissue • Doppler ultrasound • Nutrition • Treatment of venous reflux • Endovenous treatments

Introduction

All signs and symptoms of venous disease are related to venous hypertension, i.e., an increase in ambulatory venous pressure (absence of proper venous return during walking) [1].

The term chronic venous insufficiency should be reserved for the description of more advanced disease, beginning with venous edema (C_3), but more commonly in conditions where skin changes (C_4) or ulceration ($C_{5\text{-}6}$) have taken place, as defined in the Clinical, Etiological, Anatomical, and Pathophysiological (CEAP) classification system [2].

In many cases, especially in cases with poor mobility, obesity and deterioration of calf muscle pump, chronic venous insufficiency is often accompanied by secondary lymphatic malfunction (if venous return fails, the lymphatic system eventually deteriorates) [3].

Doppler ultrasound is essential in the diagnosis of chronic venous insufficiency.

Chronic wounds in the lower limbs constitute an important public health problem both due to their prevalence and the associated economic costs [4].

Compression therapy can be considered the mainstay of aetiological treatment of venous ulcers. However, in all cases it will be essential to find out whether there is a clinically significant venous reflux in the extremity which should be early ablated with endovenous techniques, such as thermoablation and sclerotherapy, to eliminate incompetent veins causing venous hypertension, and consequently, promote wound healing [5]. Nevertheless, in real life this referral may take time and should never prevent the clinician from starting early compression therapy.

In addition, physical exercise (including heel raises and walking) and anti-oedema measures (during rest, keeping the legs as elevated as possible) are essential [6].

In patients with reduced mobility, we should recommend dorsiflexion and plantar flexion exercises. These specific exercises, in addition to pumping blood at rest, help to maintain or improve the flexibility of the ankle joint, which is essential for the correct functioning of the plantar and calf muscle pumps during walking [6].

The main purpose of compressing a leg is to increase venous and lymphatic return flow. The effects of compression therapy are not limited to oedema reduction, but also affect tissue regeneration. Therefore, compression therapy is not only focused on the decongestive phase, but also on the maintenance treatment of phlebedema and phlebolymphoedema, as well as on the prevention of ulcer recurrence [7].

Regarding local treatment, the primary goal is to promote an optimal microenvironment for healing, with adequate control of inflammation, exudate, removal of denatured tissue and stimulation of granulation and epithelialisation. With regard to the available scientific evidence on the actual usefulness of the different types of dressings in different clinical situations, there is a lack of high quality studies. It should be clear that the most effective treatment for excessive exudate in any leg wound is not any dressing, but reduction of oedema [8]. Corticosteroids, both topical and systemic, may help to reduce inflammation, specially in the perilesional skin [9].

Skin grafting and negative pressure therapy may enhance healing in hard-to-heal wounds [10].

The frequency of dressing changes will depend essentially on the evolution of the wound. The limit of this spacing is not established, as it will be determined by the control of exudate, pain, odour, itching and the maintenance of the dressing or bandage in place. Ideally, dressing changes should be spaced as far apart as possible if the wound is progressing well. Moreover, those wounds that are having a good evolution may not need cleansing or debridement in each dressing change.

In this chapter you will find real life cases with both diagnosis and treatment pearls that are not always found in guidelines but, without a doubt, will be very helpful in your clinical practice.

For an adequate management, both diagnostic and therapeutic, of venous leg ulcers, it is important to be trained to:

- Know the cutaneous changes associated with chronic venous insufficiency and understand their prognostic significance
- Perform a peripheral pulse examination and the ankle-brachial index, since it is essential to rule out an associated arterial component to the wound.
- Rule out other etiologies of leg ulcers that can simulate a venous ulcer.
- Remember that leg wounds, especially in the elderly, are not usually due to an isolated cause.
- Remember that early compression therapy is key in venous leg ulcers
- Understand the necessity of a referral for assessment, diagnosis and possible treatment by a vascular surgeon.
- Understand the benefits of corticosteroids in inflammatory skin lesions, their potencies, excipients and routes of administration.
- Know the characteristics and indications of the different commercially available compression systems. Bandages should be used until complete healing and afterwards, to prevent recurrence, compression stocking or compression wraps should be used. The technique of putting these devices should also be learned.
- Know the debridement techniques and the different antimicrobial products, without forgetting that the best anti-inflammatory, debridement and antimicrobial treatment is the compressive therapy.

- Understand and know in which indications and how to apply negative pressure wound therapy. It is also important to know the devices marketed.
- Know the technique and follow-up of punch grafting. The punch grafting technique is a thin total skin graft, like mesh grafts, but it does not need to be performed in the operating room and is very efficient. In the follow-up it is important to have previously seen photos of cases to understand the types of coloration that we can find and that the most important thing is not to manipulate the wound.

Case 3.1. When Adapted Compression Therapy is not Enough

Introduction

Chronic wounds are due mainly to vascular causes. Treatment of chronic wounds depends on their aetiology, but the healing process is influenced by many other factors. The case below is about a patient with a venous ulcer with a torpid evolution.

Case Report

We present a 70-year-old woman who consulted for 3-year duration chronic ulcers. As personal history, she presented arterial hypertension, dyslipidemia and grade II obesity (BMI 37). She had been treated with sclerotherapy for varicose veins in both legs. She lived alone, walked without any aid and was independent for all basic activities. The patient had been admitted in hospital repeatedly to receive parenteral antibiotic therapy due to isolation from the wound bed of methicillin-resistant *Staphylococcus aureus*, multidrug-resistant *Pseudomonas aeruginosa,* and *Proteus mirabilis*, without clinical signs of infection. She was treated with systemic ceftriaxone, ceftazidime, and cloxacillin. On physical examination, she had ulcers in both legs. Distal pulses were palpable. The wound on the left leg was larger, up to 7 cm in diameter. Abundant adherent sloughy tissue stood out in the wound bed. She did not present associated cellulitis or other signs of infection. Both legs showed ochre dermatitis, corona phlebectatic corona and varicose veins, that is, signs of chronic venous insufficiency (Fig. 3.1). Both pedal and posterior tibial pulses were palpable.

Adapted compression therapy was started in both lower limbs in combination with sequential punch grafting sessions every 4 weeks. The ulcer on the right leg healed quickly, but the wound on the left leg had a recalcitrant progression, requiring multiple sessions of punch grafting. During its follow-up, the wound presented excessive granulation tissue, which was biopsied to rule out overgranulation due to neoplasia (Fig. 3.2).

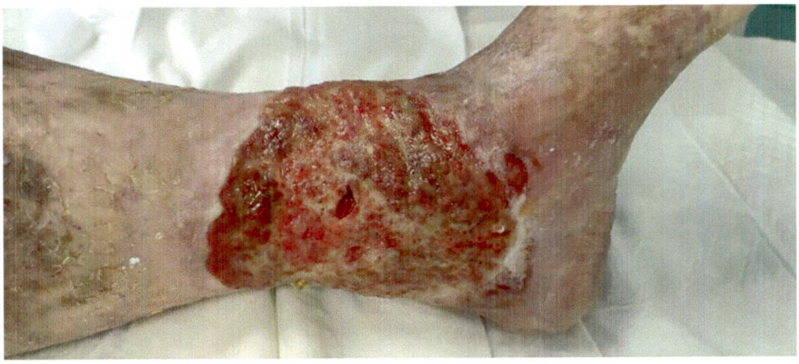

Fig. 3.1 Initial clinical presentation of the left leg wound

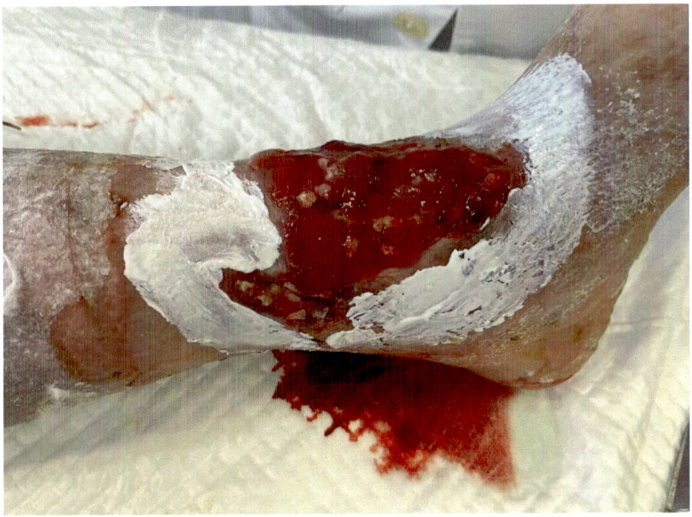

Fig. 3.2 Overgranulation after several sessions of punch grafting

Granulation tissue was reduced after treatment with topical corticosteroids in occlusion. After 3 years of treatment, the wounds continue to progressively reduce and the pain has disappeared.

Discussion

Venous leg ulcer is the most common type of leg ulceration and it is a significant clinical problem, affecting approximately 1% of the population and 3% of people over 80 years of age in Western countries [11]. Among the predisposing factors, it should be highlighted chronic venous insufficiency, female sex, inactivity and obesity, which were all present in our patient.

The abuse of antibiotic treatment without the presence of signs of infection is unfortunately a widespread reality, as it does not take into account that the diagnosis of infection is clinical, not microbiological.

Regarding the therapeutic options, compression therapy is considered the fundamental key of the etiological treatment of venous leg ulcers, even if endovenous flux ablation should always be considered to treat directly the endovenous hypertension [7, 12, 13]. The application of autologous punch grafting may also accelerate the healing of venous leg ulcers. Even if the bed is not in perfect conditions and the grafts do not succeed to get attached to the wound bed, growth factors and cells are produced to promote epithelialization and reduce inflammation [14]. Sometimes several punch grafting sessions must be performed to achieve complete epithelialization, a treatment that is very well accepted by the patient [15].

However, this case illustrates situations that we can frequently find in our clinical practice, such as patients who do not perform physical exercise, who do not consider losing weight or who do not have family support to encourage them to avoid prolonged sitting or standing. In these cases, it is very likely that the progression of the wound will not be as expected despite the prescription of compression therapy in the lower limbs. For this reason, it is essential to address the patient as a whole, including the social sphere, which in many patients has a great impact on healing [16].

As a summary, it must be assumed that if the factors that are stagnating the wound are not being modified, good results cannot be expected, even with advanced therapeutic strategies, such as skin grafting.

Case 3.2. The Challenge of Ulcerated Atrophie Blanche

Case Report

We present a 54-year-old man, who works as a schoolteacher, with a medical-surgical history of dyslipidemia, deep vein thrombosis with pulmonary thromboembolism and saphenectomy, under treatment with acenocoumarol and atorvastatin. He presented with a recurrence of venous ulcer in the internal supramalleolar region of his right leg of one month duration. According to the patient, the would had worsened despite adequate compression therapy.

Physical examination revealed an ulcer of approximately 2 × 1 cm with intense atrophie blanche in the perilesional skin (Fig. 3.3a, b). Distal pulses were present.

Despite the small size of the wound, taking into account the intense pain (8/10 on the VAS pain scale) and the underlying white atrophy, it was decided to perform punch grafting on an out-patient basis.

The donor site was the anterolateral aspect of the left thigh. After tumescent lidocaine injection to the donor site, the thin split-thickness skin grafts were obtained with a surgical blade and placed on the wound bed. The grafted ulcer was covered with a interface dressing and an alginate dressing and a multi-component compression bandage were used. The donor site was covered with an alginate

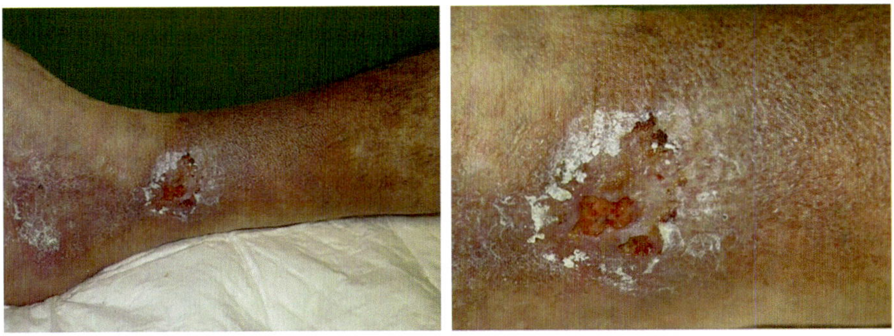

(a) (b)

Fig. 3.3 a Venous ulcer with atrophie blanche in the perilesional skin. b Close-up figure

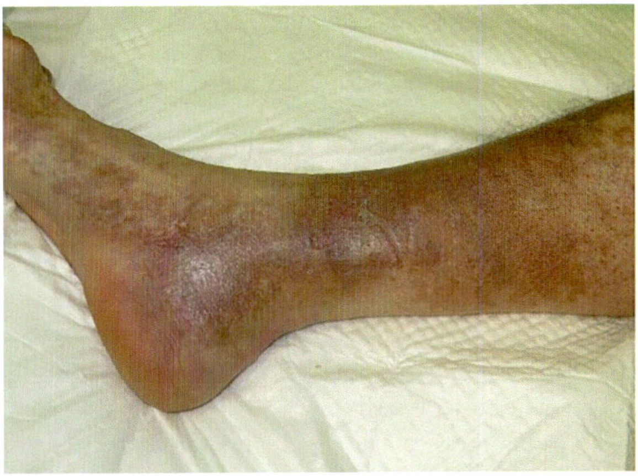

Fig. 3.4 Complete epithelialization 5 weeks after punch grafting

sheet and gauze as a secondary dressing. Absolute rest was recommended for one week. The first dressing change occurred 7 days after the surgical procedure and frequency of subsequent dressing changes ranged from 7 to 14 days. Pain was promptly reduced, and complete epithelialization was achieved 5 weeks later (Fig. 3.4).

Recommendations after complete healing were daily use of moisturizers, elevated legs during rest and 34–46 mm Hg compression stockings.

Discussion

Venous ulcers appearing on a leg with atrophie blanche are characteristically painful and more resistant to treatment [17].

The pathophysiology of atrophie blanche is not exactly known, but it is usually associated with the alteration of the microcirculation, and a typical clinical sign of the post-thrombotic syndrome. The authors who have histologically studied these lesions initially describe occlusions of the small vessels of superficial dermis with fibrinous microthrombi, hyalinization and wall thickening and, in lesions of longer evolution, dermal sclerosis and epidermal atrophy [18].

Therefore, all the diseases that produce this type of decrease in microcirculatory flow can trigger tissue infarcts and the consequent scar areas which we call white atrophy. Chronic venous insufficiency is one of these diseases and, in fact, the one most commonly associated with white atrophy [18, 19].

However, it may appear secondarily to other disorders involving coagulation disorders (such as hypercoagulability states, collagen disorders, alteration of fibrinolysis) and even in a primary presentation. All of these primary and secondary causes of atrophie blanche would be included within the entity known as livedoid vasculopathy, a type of occlusive vasculopathy without associated vasculitis. In many patients with white atrophy and a diagnosis of livedoid vasculopathy, we also find chronic venous insufficiency. Livedoid vasculopathy usually affects middle-aged women and presents with painful purpuric papules, typically on the dorsum of the feet and inframalleolar region, progressing to ulcers and areas of atrophie blanche [19]. Therefore, in cases of atrophie blanche without associated chronic venous insufficiency, we should perform both lab tests to exclude thrombophilia and biopsy of the edge of the ulcerated lesions [18, 19].

The treatment of atrophie blanche will be that of the associated disease and the objective will be, mainly, to avoid the progression of the lesions. In cases of chronic venous insufficiency, the control of venous hypertension is essential, with anti-edema measures, compression therapy and, if significant venous reflux is present, endovenous treatment (sclerotherapy or thermal ablation techniques) [19, 20]. Compression therapy must be adapted to the patient's tolerance, as these lesions can be very painful.

To promote the closure of ulcers that appear in the context of atrophie blanche, as in this case, skin grafts are a good alternative, with a rapid decrease in pain due to their analgesic effect [14, 17].

Case 3.3. Recurrence is a Sign of Poor Prognosis

Case Report

A 58-year-old man was referred to our Wound Center for a recurrent non-healing venous leg ulcer. He had a history of hypertension, obesity non-alcoholic fatty liver disease and hyperuricemia with gout arthritis. His regular treatment was omeprazol, valsartan/hydrochlorothiazide and allopurinol. The vascular surgeon excluded significant venous reflux to be treated with endovenous techniques. Clinical examination revealed an extensive superficial ulcer in the internal distal aspect of his right leg, measuring 14.5×9 cm. The wound edges were undermined, exhibiting erythema and inflammation, with granulation and sloughy tissue in the wound bed.

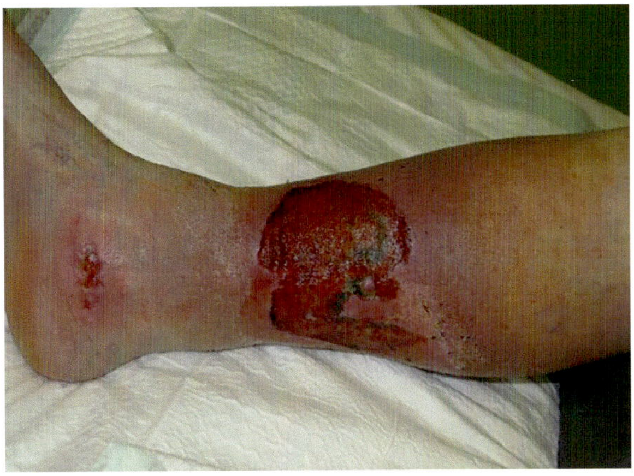

Fig. 3.5 Initial clinical presentation of the wound showing an extensive ulcer that affects the internal distal third of the leg

He also showed intense eczema and phlebolymphedema in both legs. He presented no signs of infection (Fig. 3.5).

Distal pulses were palpable. The lesion was diagnosed as a venous leg ulcer (CEAP classification stage C6). He was treated with topical corticosteroids mixed with moisturizing cream on the whole leg, topical corticosteroids mixed with zinc oxide cream on the wound edges and zinc oxide lotion in the wound bed. Then, the wound was covered with alginate dressing and Unna Boot bandage as compression therapy. Moreover, he received one month of systemic corticosteroids (prednisone 30 mg/day) in order to reduce inflammation. Dressing and bandage changes were performed monthly. Two weeks later, an important improvement was observed, with eczema reduction and control of inflammation at the edges. Reduction of pain was also observed.

One month later, punch grafting was performed in an outpatient basis with the aim of decreasing wound extension and depth. Complete bed rest at home and anti-edema measures was recommended and Enoxaparin 40 mg per day was prescribed for thromboprophylaxis.

In the first follow-up visit (day 15 after punch grafting), complete graft attachment was achieved with progressive contraction of the ulcer in the following weeks. Wound healing protocol in the follow-up visits included the application of topical zinc oxide, alginate dressings, and compression therapy avoiding cleansing in each dressing change. Complete epithelization was obtained three months after the referral (Fig. 3.6).

Daily use of emollients and compression wraps were recommended to protect the skin barrier and prevent recurrences.

Discussion

Venous leg ulcer is the most common type of leg ulceration and it is a significant clinical problem, affecting approximately 1% of the population and 3% of

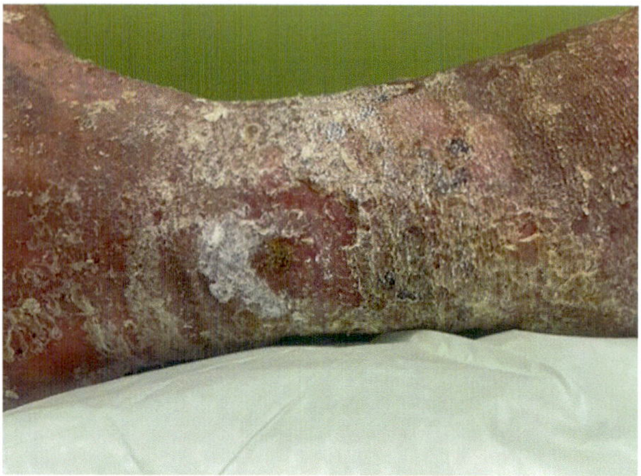

Fig. 3.6 Complete epithelization within five weeks after punch grafting

people over 80 years of age in developed countries [11]. A venous ulcer constitutes the most advanced stage of chronic venous insufficiency, that is, the result of poorly controlled venous hypertension. The subsequent decreasing in microcirculatory flow, age, deterioration of calf muscle pump, contribute to recurrent lesions resistant to treatment. Other predisposing factors, such us female sex and obesity are also associated with the development of venous ulcers [7].

The cornerstone of treatment of venous leg ulcers is an accurate aetiological treatment [21]. Compression therapy, adapted to the patient's acceptance and needs, is key. Moreover, anti-edema measures and, if venous reflux is present, or endovenous treatment (sclerotherapy or thermal ablation techniques) can help to control venous hypertension [21].

The application of autologous punch grafts has also been shown to accelerate the healing of venous wounds with progressive contraction of the ulcer and pain reduction due to their analgesic effect. Even if the wound bed does not present with perfect conditions and the grafts do not get attached to the wound bed, molecular mediators are produced that promote epithelialization and reduce inflammation. Sometimes several punch grafting sessions must be performed to achieve complete epithelialization, a treatment that is very well accepted by the patient [14].

This case demonstrates the importance of an appropriate aetiologic treatment for a venous leg ulcer with compression therapy, the benefit of adding corticosteroid treatment to decrease inflammation and punch-grafting to promote epithelialization.

Despite the fact that there are few studies about the benefit of corticosteroid therapy in wound healing, both topical and oral corticosteroids may be interesting to reduce excessive inflammation associated to venous hypertension and consequently accelerate good healing [9, 22].

Punch grafting is a simple and traditional technique to promote the closure of ulcers that appear in the context of chronic venous insufficiency. Basic wound treatment and simple surgical techniques can provide the best results in healing wounds and alleviate patient's pain.

Case 3.4. When Compression Therapy is not Enough and Advanced Treatments Are Needed

Introduction

Chronic venous insufficiency is the most common vascular disease, with 48.5% of prevalence and increasing with age. It is more common in women and has peak incidence between 40 and 49 years in women and 70–79 years in men [23].

The appearance of ulcers is the most advanced stage of chronic venous disease and it presents high morbidity rates [24]. Ulcers of venous etiology account for 70–90% of lower limb ulcers and are an important socio-health problem due to their high frequency and high impact on the quality of life of patients [25]. Its comprehensive assessment should include a detailed clinical history, risk factors, eating habits, genetic factors, work activity, general physical examination and clinical examination of the wound, with assessment of pain if present, and a doppler ultrasound. However, an early assessment by a vascular surgeon is not feasible in all health care systems. Pain care should be a priority in patients with chronic ulcers. In addition to the usual pain killers, irrigation with sevoflurane and punch grafting are two procedures that have proven useful in analgesic control in chronic and hard to heal ulcers [14, 26].

Case Report

An 52-year-old female patient as presented to our unit with a 4-year history of lower left leg nonhealing ulcers. She had a history of high blood pressure, obesity, chronic kidney disease, chronic venous insufficiency diagnosed with doppler ultrasound and contact allergy to balsam of Peru, colophony and isothiazolinone. The wounds were in the external and internal malleolus of the left leg, up to 9.5 cm in diameter the largest ulcer (Fig. 3.7a).

She had preserved pulses and cutaneous signs of chronic venous insufficiency. She had very intense and disabling pain (EVA 8/10) despite oral analgesia and the local pain prevented proper cleaning of the wounds, the use of cream analgesics and even made it difficult to use compression therapy due to intense pain in the ankle crease. The patient was offered off-label treatment with topical sevoflurane to improve pain. The corresponding informed consent was obtained. After three sevoflurane irrigations twice weekly, a notable improvement in pain was achieved (EVA 2/10) and a remarkable additional improvement in the wound bed was obtained (Fig. 3.7b).

After the third irrigation two punch graft sessions were done one on each side (Fig. 3.8a).

The autologous grafts were obtained from the anterior thigh. The procedure was very well accepted by the patient, total pain control was achieved, and

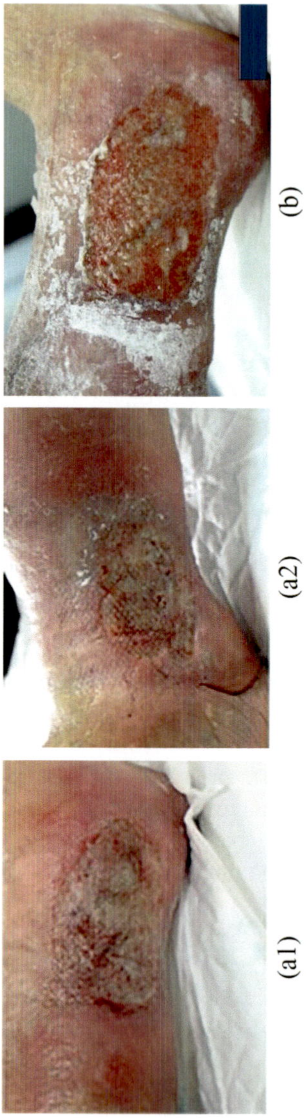

Fig. 3.7 a Lower extremity venous ulcers before treatment (a1. internal malleolus; a2. external malleolus). b Wound aspect after two irrigations of sevoflurane

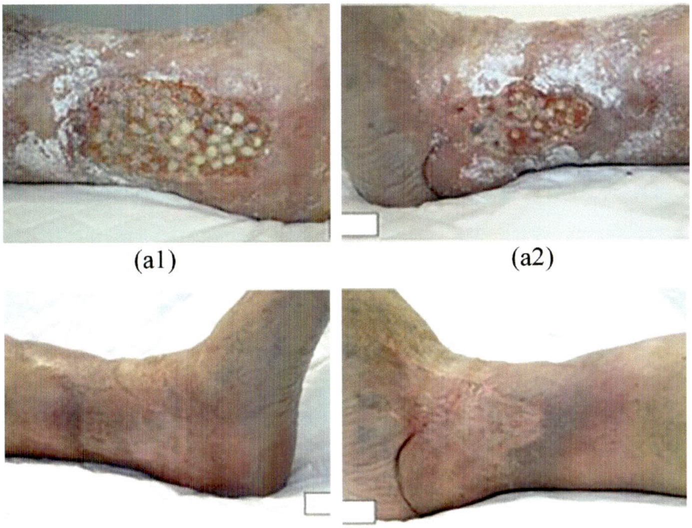

Fig. 3.8 a Clinical aspect 10 days after coverage of the ulcers with punch grafting (8a1. internal malleolus; a2. external malleolus). b Complete epithelialization after 2 months (8b1. internal malleolus; b2. external malleolus)

complete epithelialization of the lesions was achieved 2 months after the procedure (Fig. 3.8b). To prevent recurrences, compressive therapy with an adjustable medical compression system was started.

Discussion

The key of venous ulcer treatment is the control of venous hypertension with early therapeutic compression [27] and, if possible and indicated, venous reflux ablation after assessment by a vascular surgeon (not needed in this case). The pain associated with venous ulcers can be very disabling and the reduction in quality of life for patients is difficult to measure [28]. Moreover, it can impair adherence to compression therapy. Sevoflurane is an inhalational anaesthetic agent that has demonstrated off-label analgesic action when it is irrigated on painful chronic ulcers [29, 30]. In addition to reducing pain, it could improve the wound bed due to its bacteriostatic action and its ability to promote neovascularization [14, 29, 30]. Although the studies published in the literature are mostly isolated cases or short series, the results are promising. Punch grafting is another procedure with analgesic effect, which also promotes wound epithelialization [27]. The benefit of the combination of therapeutic compression, sevoflurane irrigation and punch grafting has also been described in arteriolopathic ulcers [31].

Finally and regarding this patient, in patients with chronic ulcers it should be remembered that the wet and occluded environment together with the damaged skin barrier are predisposing factors for contact sensitization, so potentially sensitising substances should be avoided as much as possible [32].

Case 3.5. The Complex Post-thrombotic Syndrome

Case Presentation

A 54-year-old male presented to the Wound Care Department for recurrent, long-standing ulcers on his left lower extremity. The patient had been diagnosed with post-thrombotic syndrome several years before following deep venous thrombosis, which had occurred in the context of pneumonia. Additionally, he had HIV infection, a history of recurrent venous leg ulcers in both legs, pulmonary embolism, bilateral saphenectomy. His current treatment regimen included acenocoumarol, antiretroviral therapy and analgesics for pain management. A left iliac vein stent had been implanted five years prior without success and no other treatments were viable. The thrombophilia study performed showed no alterations of interest.

Physical examination revealed two oval-shaped imprecisely defined, painful ulcers on the distal third of the inner aspect of his left leg measuring 2.9 × 1.8 cm, respectively 3.3 × 2.4 cm, encompassed by eczematous and hyperpigmentation changes (Fig. 3.9). Distal pulses were palpable.

Granulation tissue was found at the wound bed and wound edges were undermined. Furthermore, he presented an 1.4 × 0.9 cm sized ulcer situated on the dorsal face of his left foot (Fig. 3.10), in the context of phlebo-lymfoedema with verrucous skin changes.

No signs of infection were observed. A diagnosis of recurrent post-thrombotic venous leg ulcers was established on clinical grounds. Punch-grafting was proposed, but the patient initially refused due to the inability to maintain bed rest after the procedure for work reasons. Consequently, the treatment plan consisted in zinc oxide cream on the wound edges along with zinc oxide lotion and alginate dressing on the wound beds. Also, compression therapy with multi-component system

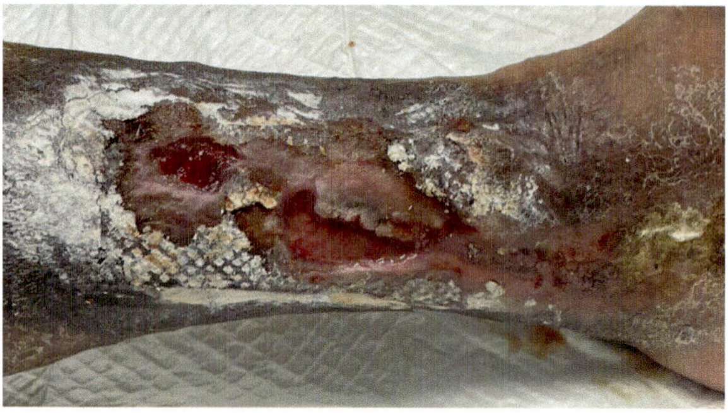

Fig. 3.9 Two ulcers located on the distal third of the inner aspect of the left leg

Fig. 3.10 Third ulcer situated on the dorsal face of his left foot

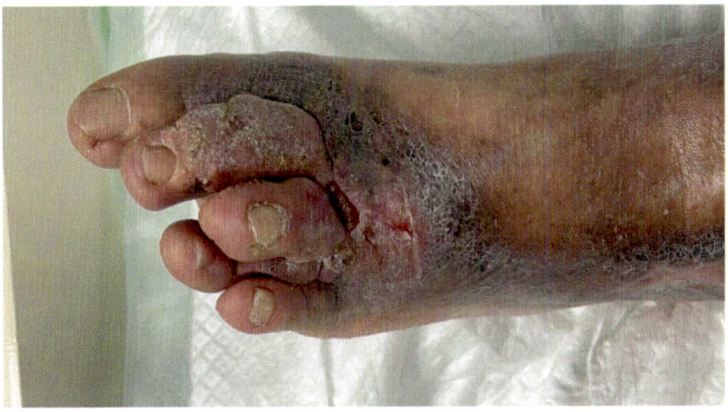

Fig. 3.11 Complete epithelialization of the ulcers with scab formation

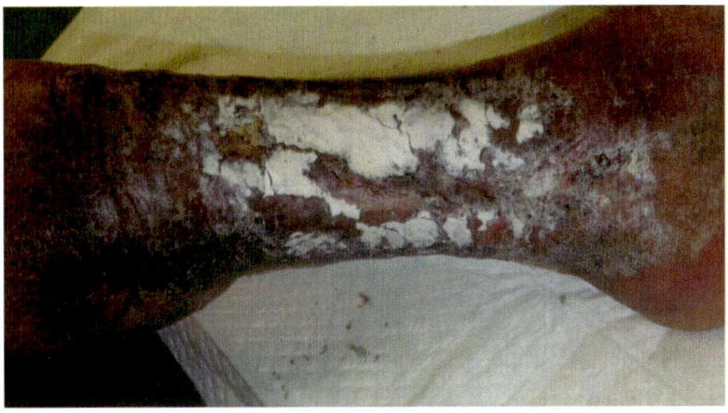

was applied. The initial follow-up visit occurred two weeks later, with subsequent appointments scheduled weekly or every two weeks for ongoing assessment and continuation of the same treatment protocol. During dressing changes no cleansing was performed. Reduction in the size of the wounds and pain relief was seen. After four months, punch-grafting in an outpatient setting was conducted. The donor site was the anterolateral region of the left thigh. Alginate sheets covered the grafted ulcer and a multi-component compression bandage was applied. In the next weekly follow-up visits, the management of the wounds consisted in zinc oxide lotion, alginate sheets and compression therapy without any cleansing or debridement. Complete epithelialization was achieved one month after the procedure (Figs. 3.11 and 3.12).

Discussion

Thrombotic events are occurring among patients with HIV despite their relatively young ages. Advanced HIV disease is a risk factor for development of thromboses, possibly due to an increased inflammatory state or the presence of concurrent comorbidities such as infections [33].

Post-thrombotic syndrome (PTS) represents a commonly encountered complication that affects up to half of the patients diagnosed with deep vein thrombosis

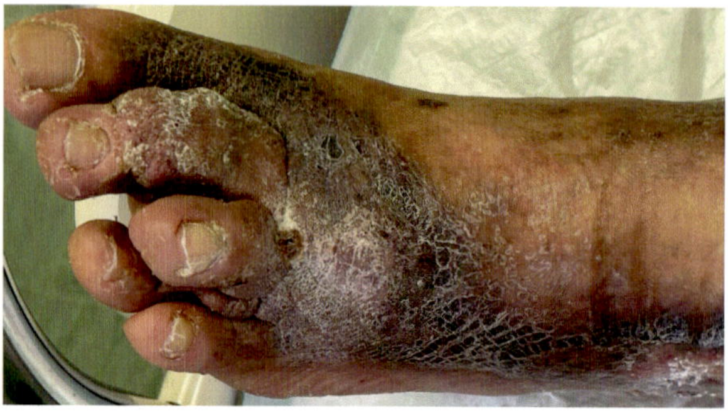

Fig. 3.12 Complete epithelialization of the ulcers with scab formation

with a significant impact on their quality of life [34]. The most frequent symptoms are mild and consist of pain, pruritus, swelling and a sensation of heaviness in the affected limb. Even if there is no objective diagnostic test to define PTS, it is recommended the use of the Villalta scale (VS) as a standard in the clinical setting to diagnose PTS because of its practicality, good interrater reliability, and external validity [35].

However, leg ulcers, though rare, represent a severe manifestation of this syndrome [34]. The appearance of post-thrombotic syndrome is firstly associated with high venous pressure resulting from defective valves or blockage of the blood flow due to deep vein thrombosis [36]. The main treatment options include compression therapy, medication and lifestyle changes with surgical and endovascular procedures such as deep venous stenting being considered for suitable patients [37]. The post-thrombotic ulcers may be recalcitrant and unresponsive to conventional therapy [2]. While the stenting procedure may appear as a promising therapeutic option, its clinical outcomes aren't always successful, as evidenced in this case presentation.

In accordance with the CEAP classification, the patient's ulcers correspond to class C6r indicating recurrent disease. Venous leg ulcers that recur are challenging to heal due to their development in areas with significant scar tissue [2].

Consequently, cutaneous changes secondary to post-thrombotic syndrome, mostly associated to tissue sclerosis secondary to inflammation due to venous hypertension, represent a challenging barrier for wound healing and advanced treatments such as punch-grafting should be considered.

Case 3.6. Pretibial Venous Leg Ulcer

Case Report

A 48-year-old woman, who worked as a cook, was referred to our Wound Center for a painful ulcer located on her left leg, which had been progressing over a period of two months. She was under follow-up at her Primary Care Center with unsatisfactory outcomes. As part of her medical history, she had chronic

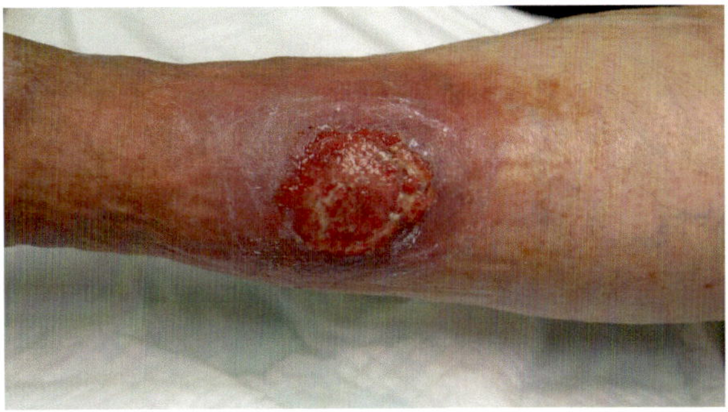

Fig. 3.13 Ulceration located in the left medial pretibial region observed at initial consultation

deep venous insufficiency in the lower extremities, with varicose veins involving the territory of the internal and anterior saphenous veins without indication of endovenous ablation by the vascular surgeon, an episode of deep venous thrombosis treated with heparin, obesity (BMI 35) and smoking habit. The patient had been evaluated for thrombophilia ten years ago, revealing an elevated factor VIII level. Her regular treatment was acenocoumarol, sulodexide, ebastine, pregabalin, as well as several analgesics since the onset of the ulcer. In the clinical examination, she presented signs of chronic venous insufficiency with ochre dermatitis and edema in both lower limbs, predominantly on the left side, with palpable dorsalis pedis pulses. An ulcer measuring 6 cm in maximum diameter was present in the medial pretibial region of the left lower extremity, with superficial sloughy tissue, erythematous edges and perilesional erythema, being painful to palpation (Fig. 3.13). She presented with palpable pulses.

Diagnosis was consistent with venous leg ulcer (CEAP classification stage 6). The patient was managed applying zinc oxide paste to the wound edges and zinc oxide lotion to the wound bed. Subsequently, the wound was dressed with alginate and a two-layer compression bandage. Punch grafting was performed a week later, covered with alginate dressing and two layers of zinc oxide bandage (Unna boot). Bed rest and anti-edema measures at home were recommended, and enoxaparin 40 mg per day was prescribed as thromboprophylaxis.

At the follow-up appointment on day 14 after grafting, complete graft attachment was observed (Fig. 3.14).

Subsequent visits involved a wound healing regimen comprising topical zinc oxide application, alginate dressings, and the application of an Unna Boot bandage as compression therapy, with avoidance of cleansing at each dressing change.

In the ensuing weeks, the ulcer gradually contracted, achieving full epithelialization two months post-referral (Fig. 3.15). The patient was discharged with daily use of compression stockings and anti-edema measures, without subsequent recurrences.

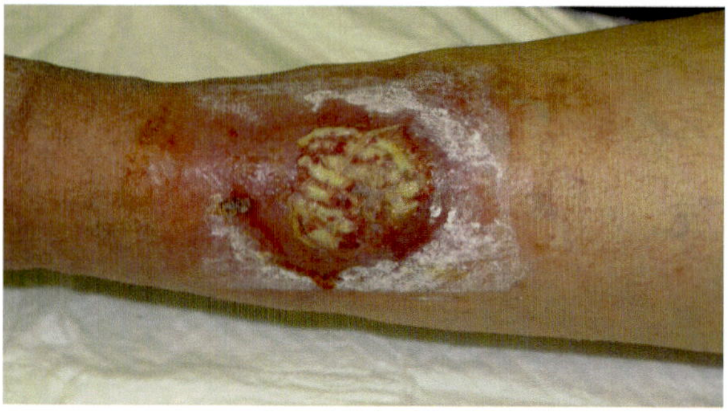

Fig. 3.14 Appearance of the ulcer at the initial 14-day follow-up visit after punch grafting

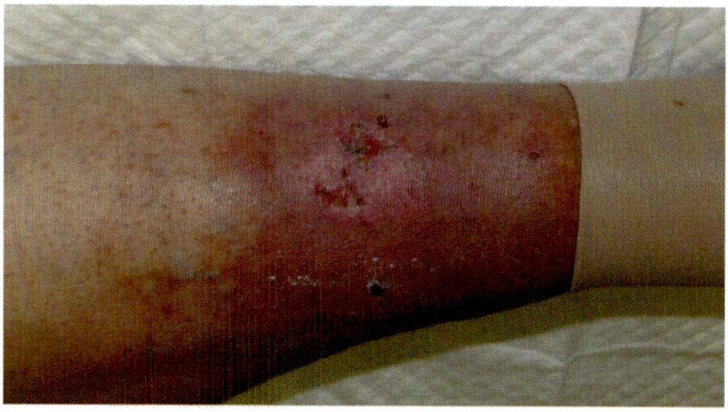

Fig. 3.15 Reepithelialization at seven weeks post punch grafting

Discussion

Venous pathologies in the context of leg ulcers are effectively assessed by Doppler ultrasound. It is the first-line non-invasive test in case of a suspected venous leg ulcer. The examination allows to visualise the deep and superficial venous system and the perforating veins of the lower limbs. Doppler ultrasound examination can be divided into three parts—deep vein assessment and deep venous thrombosis protocol; reflux testing in deep and superficial systems; perforating vein study. The venous valve function and presence of reflux can be evaluated by measuring the retrograde flow in the veins by squeezing the calf muscle and observing the brief backward flow [38].

Deep Venous thrombosis in certain cases can be caused by inherited thrombophilia or antiphospholipid syndrome. Clinical clues for thrombophilia are venous thrombotic events (VTE) at a young age (< 50 years), especially unprovoked or in association with weak provoking factors (oral contraceptives, minor surgery, immobility); strong family history of VTE at a young age; recurrent VTE, especially at a young age; VTE in unusual sites such as cerebral or splanchnic veins. In case of clinical suspicion of clotting disorders, the following tests should be performed:, protein C, protein S, antithrombin, prothrombin gene mutation, Factor V Leiden, myeloproliferative neoplasms, lupus anticoagulant and anticardiolipin antibody [39].

When treating leg ulcers, several prognostic factors should be considered. A recent study [40] has found that negative predictive factors are ulcer size greater than 8.25 cm^2, as in our case, underlying chronic venous disease for more than 20 years, multiple comorbidities, ulcer depth, presence of unpleasant smell and ulcer location other than medial ankle area, as it was observed in this case.

Punch grafting can be considered as a therapeutic option for hard-to-heal wounds. It has overall low costs due to the autologous nature of the grafted material. Thin slices of epidermis down to papillary dermis are being taken from the donor site, usually the upper thigh, and placed on the ulcer bed. The donor site dressing change (commonly alginate sheets) is spaced out as much as possible to achieve complete epithelialization. The ulcer is covered with alginate or an interface dressing. Multicomponent compression therapy is applied. Such a method has shown complete epithelialization even in ulcers previously resistant to therapy [41].

Compression therapy is key in the treatment of venous leg ulcers. It is a gradual external layer of compression that ensures the reversal of the main pathophysiological factor of venous ulceration—ambulatory venous hypertension. Compression therapy can be performed by short-stretch bandages, multicomponent compression systems, compression stockings or wraps. The recommended pressure around the ankle should be 40 mmHg. Compression systems should be adapted to the patient and applied by trained professionals to avoid possible complications of poor bandage application [42]. In contrast to previous long lists of absolute and relative contraindications for compression therapy, recent expert consensus agrees on two main contraindications: severe peripheral artery disease and severe heart failure [43].

In addition to medical treatments, there are certain lifestyle changes that can benefit ulcer healing, such as smoking cessation, nutritional changes, adequate pain management, exercise and leg elevation during rest. For leg elevation patients are advised to keep the legs at 10–30° and above heart level. On the contrary, high leg compression with leg elevation was associated with worse clinical outcomes [44]. Patients should be advised on appropriate techniques, considering the type of compression they are receiving. Lifestyle changes require a multidisciplinary approach, including motivational interviews [44]. Often, they are hard to be achieved and implemented. In this clinical case no lifestyle changes were made.

Case 3.7. Some Venous Leg Ulcers Do not Need Cleansing or Debridement

Case Report

A 73 year old woman came to our wound clinic with a recurrence of a venous ulcer on the inner side of the left leg of two months of evolution. The previous episode had been in the same location 2 years earlier. Her medical history included arterial

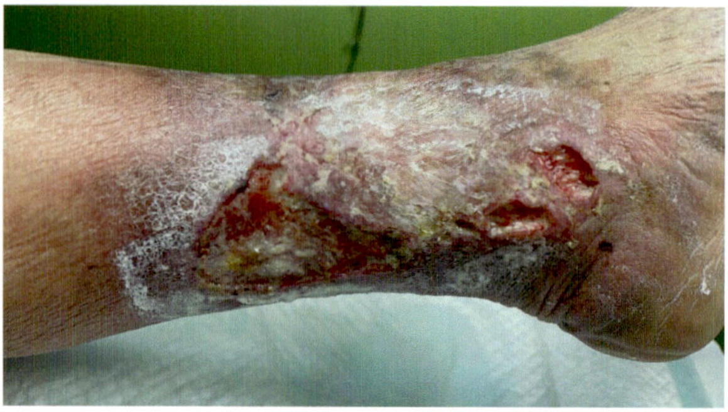

Fig. 3.16 Venous leg ulcer on the inner aspect of her left leg

hypertension and saphenectomy in her left leg 20 years before, without present significant venous reflux.

The ulcer had undermined edges, adherent slough to the wound and no signs of infection. The leg presents ochre dermatitis (hyperpigmentation due extravasation of erythrocytes, hemosiderin-laden macrophages and melanin deposits), atrophie blanche and lipodermatosclerosis in the context of her chronic venous insufficiency (Fig. 3.16).

The diagnosis of venous ulcer recurrence (CEAP6r) was established and without cleansing or debridement of the bed, it was covered with a fiber dressing and multicomponent bandage. The first dressing change was performed 15 days later, with wound contraction and absence of pain (Fig. 3.17).

The same treatment was repeated, without cleansing or debridement and, on the follow-up visit 2 weeks later, there was complete epithelialization with scab formation, at which time compression wraps were prescribed to prevent recurrence (Fig. 3.18).

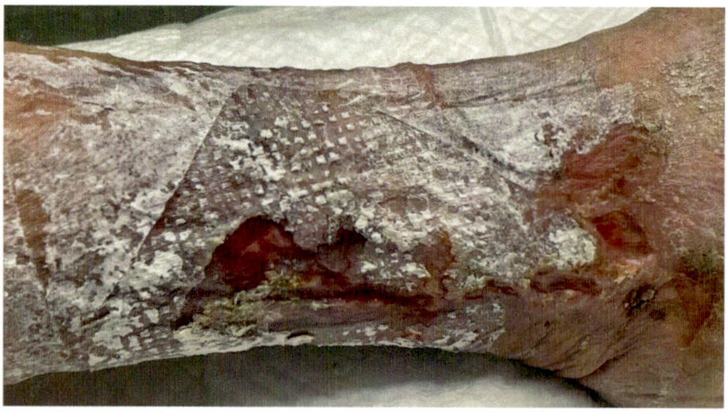

Fig. 3.17 Great improvement evidenced at the first dressing change 15 days later

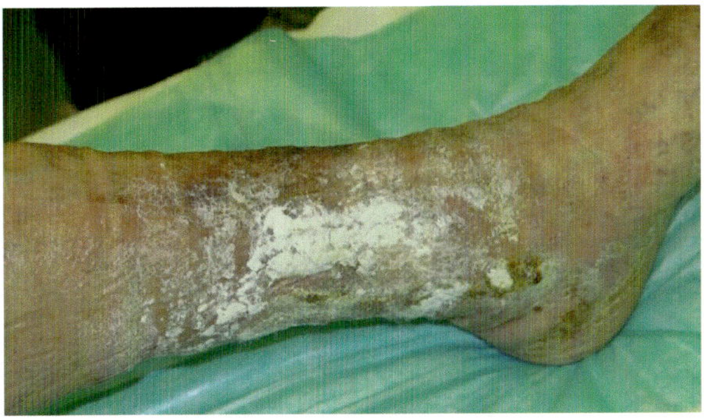

Fig. 3.18 Complete epithelialization one month after initial visit

Discussion

Venous leg ulcer is the most common type of leg wound and the one for which there are more treatment protocols endorsed by scientific societies [8].

While compression therapy has the highest degree of evidence and recommendation (1A) for venous ulceration, it is not clear what is the best wound bed management strategy, including optimal frequency of dressings. In fact, although most expert consensus and clinical guidelines recommend that every dressing change should be followed by cleansing and debridement of the wound bed, the available evidence does not support the need for such a protocol [45].

Each dressing change is an opportunity to promote, with cleansing and debridement, the removal of what is hindering healing (excess exudate with proinflammatory cytokines, non-viable tissue, bacterial load). However, any manipulation of the wound bed will also have an impact on the cells and growth factors that are promoting wound closure.

Wounds exudate in wounds that are having a good progression is a source of cells and growth factors that promote healing. Therefore, in these cases, frequent and/or aggressive washing with friction should be avoided, as we can interrupt the formation of new tissue.

In the absence of denatured tissue or signs of infection in the wound bed, the practice of routinely cleansing a wound during dressing changes is nothing more than a ritual and may actually delay healing [46].

Therefore, when faced with a venous ulcer, the most important thing is to focus on adequate treatment of the cause (compression therapy adapted to the individual and assess the possibility of interventional treatment of reflux), encourage physical exercise and elevation of the legs during rest. Consequently, compression therapy should be initiated early in case of recurrence, as in this case, and a vascular surgeon should verify if significant reflux is present.

These anti-edema measures will, by themselves, be the best anti-gravity, anti-inflammatory, antimicrobial and debridement treatment for venous ulcers.

Therefore, if the ulcer is progressing well, the ideal is the maximum spacing of dressing changes that allows, as long as the bandage stays in place and exudate is controlled. Moreover, during dressing changes, the microenvironment of the ulcer should be altered as little as possible so as not to damage the neoformed tissue.

Case 3.8. Comprehensive Management of Lower Leg Ulcers in a Morbidly Obese Patient

Case Description and Medical History

A 55-year old female, known with class III obesity (morbid obesity), BMI 44.08, presented in the Dermatology clinic in September 2022 for the appearance of several ulcers affecting the lower legs, bilaterally. Lesions had been present for more than 3 years, each of them appearing after minor local trauma and the lesions had gradually increased in size and depth. The patient was previously consulted several times by the general practitioner who recommended the use of local creams for epithelization, with no further investigations. She is working in an office, which demands a prolonged sitting position, with no regular walking throughout the day. It was decided on the patient admission to the hospital, for further investigations and initiation of wound management.

Clinical Findings

At the time of the first clinical examination, the patient had significant bilateral lower extremities edema and swelling. The skin was thickened, with a shiny, tight appearance, and felt warm to the touch. On the antero-lateral aspect of the left lower leg, there was an ulceration measuring 20 cm × 15 cm, covered with adherent yellow deposits and necrotic areas, surrounded by an erythematous plaque, indurated, warm to the touch (Fig. 3.19a). On the anterior aspect of the right lower leg, the wound was 6 cm × 5 cm and square in shape with a peri-wound area of erythema previously treated with topical hydrocortisone (Fig. 3.19b).

The tissue surrounding the erythema was healthy. Tortuous and dilated veins noted in the greater saphenous vein territory along the medial side, up to above the knee level was noticed. All the peripheral pulses were palpable normally bilaterally.

Diagnostic Assessment

The bilateral Doppler ultrasound assessment revealed mild reflux in the left great saphenous vein without significant varicosities in its side branches. In the right great saphenous vein, moderate reflux was noted, with prominent varicosities in the side branches. The femoral, popliteal, posterior tibial, and small saphenous veins were within normal limits, showing no evidence of reflux.

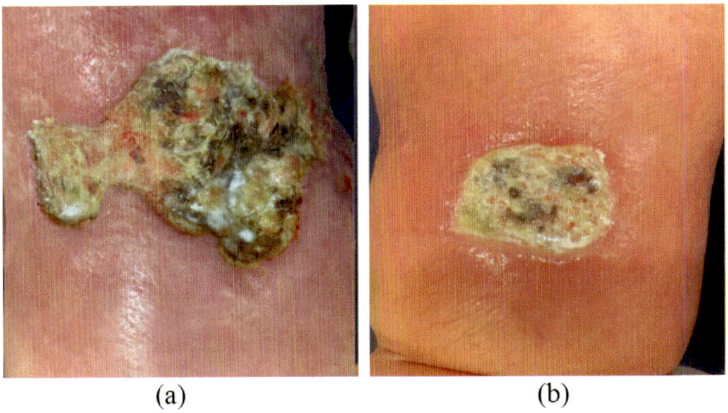

Fig. 3.19 Aspect of the wounds during the first consultation. a Wound of the left lower limb. b Wound of the right lower leg

Routine blood evaluations including hemogram and blood sugar levels were within normal ranges, although the blood sugar level was close to the upper limit. Considering also the association of obesity, it was decided to be evaluated by a specialist in metabolic and nutritional diseases, to discuss an individualised nutritional plan for losing weight.

Due to the associated pain, malodor, purulent exudate, periwound skin changes (erythema, heat, swelling), wounds were considered to be infected, and a swab was collected from the wound bed tissue, to identify the bacteria involved in the wound infection. Bacteriological examination revealed the presence of *Pseudomonas aeruginosa* and *Escherichia coli,* both with sensitivity to ceftriaxone.

Therapeutic Interventions

Therapeutic interventions for this patient included the combination of compression therapy, cleansing of debris from the wound, debridement, infection treatment, special dressings, and nutritional plan for weight control. Compression therapy was started in both lower limbs, initially with a low degree of compression (17–22 mmHg), followed by a higher degree (28–30 mmHg) after 2 months. This strategy promoted treatment adherence.

The wound was cleansed using a chlorhexidine solution, with jet lavage, every other day for the first 2 weeks of treatment. In this way we managed to remove the wound debris, soften the necrotic tissue, reduce the bacterial burden and reduce the malodor. Wound cleansing was combined with mechanical debridement, performed by a specialised nurse and aiming to create an optimal wound-healing environment by producing a well vascularized, stable wound bed with optimal exudate. For the control of wound infection, it was decided to use a systemic antibiotic recommended Intravenous ceftriaxone was recommended for 10 days. Considering wounds' depth and associated level of wounds' exudation, during the first 2 weeks, it was decided to use local absorbent dressings (alginates) to manage the moisture of the wounds. This treatment regime combining wound cleansing, mechanical debridement, dressings and compression therapy was performed every other day until hospital discharge. After these two weeks, the erythema was reduced at the wound margins, the level of exudate decreased, and the wound bed had less slough. Granulation tissue could be seen at the wound margins and under the slough.

After one month, when the wound infection was controlled and the level of exudate decreased significantly, it was decided the use of hydrocolloid dressings for wound management, to promote the formation of granulation tissue. All the local therapies were combined during the whole period with lymphatic drainage sessions, 3 times per week in the first month and reduced to once per week afterwards.

Follow-Up and Outcome

The patient was evaluated periodically, every month after leaving the hospital, until present. Significant wound improvement was noticed 2 months after starting with the treatment plan (Fig. 3.20a, b), showing signs of granulation and epithelialization in both wounds.

Currently, the wound on the right lower leg is completely healed while the one on the left lower limb is closed in a proportion of 60% (Fig. 3.21a, b).

During the last visit, the patient also reported a lifestyle change, combining a more balanced diet with an increased level of daily physical effort, which also determined a weight reduction of 15 kg in a 6 month period.

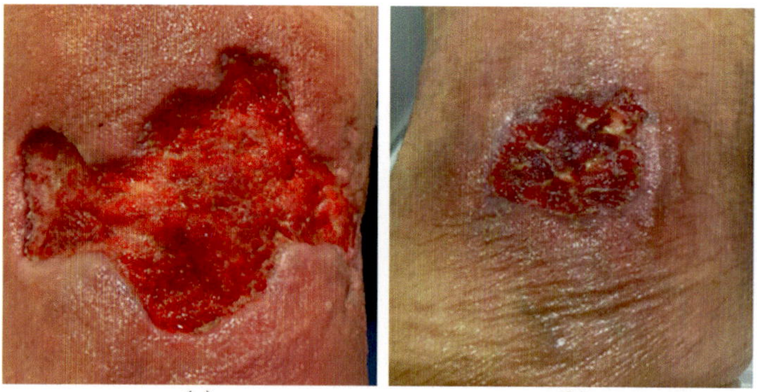

(a) (b)

Fig. 3.20 Aspect of the wounds after 2 months of wound management (a. before; b. after 2 months)

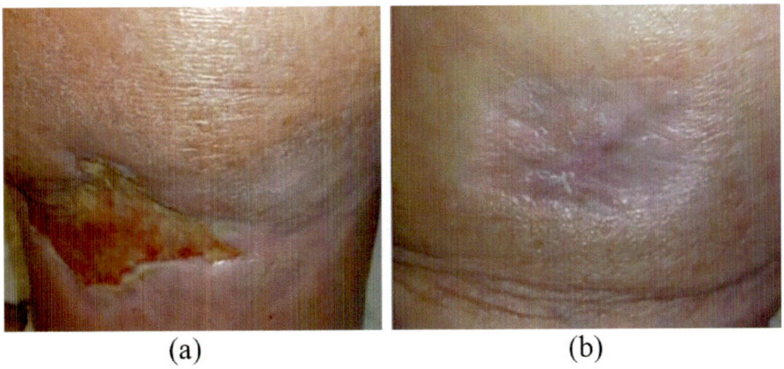

Fig. 3.21 Present aspect of the wounds (after 6 months of therapy) (a. right lower leg; b. left lower leg)

Discussion

The presented case of lower leg ulcers in a morbidly obese patient highlights the importance of a comprehensive diagnostic approach and a multidisciplinary treatment plan. Class III obesity, characterised by a body mass index (BMI) above 40, is a known risk factor for various comorbidities, including venous insufficiency, impaired wound healing, and chronic inflammation [47, 48]. Obesity-related changes in adipose tissue function and inflammation contribute to the development of insulin resistance, dyslipidemia, and chronic inflammation, leading to further metabolic and cardiovascular complications [49].

In addition to pain and discomfort, chronic wounds are associated with prolonged hospitalisation, increased healthcare costs, and a higher risk of complications. Therefore, an individualised nutritional plan for weight control, as well as management of comorbidities, is essential for optimal wound healing.

Venous insufficiency is a common cause of lower extremity ulcers, particularly in obese patients, and the presented case was no exception. Venous reflux and valvular insufficiency lead to increased hydrostatic pressure, which causes tissue damage and ulcer formation [50]. However, recent literature supports the fact that centripetal obesity results in both structural and hemodynamic changes in the lower limb veins, leading to venous ulcers, even in the absence of significant venous reflux [51]. This underscores the multifactorial nature of venous ulcer development in obese patients. Centripetal obesity results in both structural and hemodynamic changes in the lower limb veins.

In this particular case, the patient exhibited venous reflux, which contributed to ulcer formation. Despite the presence of reflux, the decision was made not to directly treat it at this stage. This decision was influenced by the patient's morbid obesity, which can complicate and delay wound healing. Addressing the patient's obesity through nutritional and lifestyle interventions was prioritised to improve overall vascular health and enhance the effectiveness of subsequent treatments for venous reflux.

The presence of *Pseudomonas aeruginosa* and *Escherichia coli*, as identified in our patient's wound swab, is common in chronic wounds and diagnosis of infection represents a challenging aspect of wound management. As in this case, infection delays wound healing, and it is associated with increased morbidity and healthcare costs [52].

The management of chronic wounds is complex and requires a comprehensive approach that addresses the underlying causes of the wound, such as poor nutrition, impaired mobility, and comorbidities. In this case, the patient received a multidisciplinary treatment plan that included wound cleaning, debridement, compression therapy, and systemic antibiotic therapy. Finally, lifestyle changes, including an individualised nutritional plan and increased physical activity, are essential for long-term wound healing and prevention of recurrent ulcers. The importance of a multidisciplinary approach to manage comorbidities and promote lifestyle changes is crucial for long-term wound healing success.

In conclusion, the successful management of chronic wounds requires involvement of different healthcare representatives who can address the underlying causes of the wound and promote healing. Effective wound management strategies must include a comprehensive assessment of the patient's comorbidities, nutritional status, and lifestyle factors. A multidisciplinary team approach that includes wound care specialists, nutritionists, physical therapists, and psychologists is crucial in the management of chronic wounds.

References

1. JJ Bergan GW Schmid-Schönbein PD Smith AN Nicolaides MR Boisseau B Eklof 2006 Chronic venous disease N Engl J Med 355 5 488 498
2. Lurie F, Passman M, Meisner M, et al. The 2020 update of the CEAP classification system and reporting standards J Vasc Surg Venous Lymphat Disord. 2020;8(3):342–52.
3. N Piller 2009 Phlebolymphoedema/chronic venous lymphatic insufficiency: an introduction to strategies for detection, differentiation and treatment Phlebology 24 51 55
4. J Kerr D Devane J Ivory C Weller G Gethin 2020 Effectiveness of implementation strategies for venous leg ulcer guidelines: a systematic review J Tissue Viability 29 161 168
5. MS Gohel F Heatley X Liu 2018 A randomized trial of early endovenous ablation in venous ulceration N Engl J Med 378 22 2105 2114
6. Qiu Y, Osadnik CR, Team V, Weller CD. Effects of physical activity as an adjunct treatment on healing outcomes and recurrence of venous leg ulcers: a scoping review. Wound Repair Regen. 2022;30(2):172–85.
7. E Conde Montero N Serra Perrucho DP Cueva de la 2020 Theory and practice of compression therapy for treating and preventing venous ulcers Actas Dermo-Sifiliogr (Engl Ed). 111 10 829 834
8. Isoherranen K, Montero EC, Atkin L, Collier M, Høgh A, Ivory JD, KirketerpMøller K, Meaume S, Ryan H, Stuermer EK, Tiplica GS, Probst S. Lower leg ulcer diagnosis & principles of treatment. Including recommendations for comprehensive assessment and referral pathways. J Wound Manage. 2023;24(2 Sup1):s1–76.
9. D Hofman K Moore R Cooper M Eagle S Cooper 2007 Use of topical corticosteroids on chronic leg ulcers J Wound Care 16 5 227 230
10. C Horn A Fierro JC Lantis Ii 2023 Use of negative pressure wound therapy for the treatment of venous leg ulcers Wounds 35 6 117 125

11. Franks PJ, Barker J, Collier M, Gethin G, Haesler E, Jawien A, et al. Management of patients with venous leg ulcers: challenges and current best practice. J Wound Care. 1 de junio de 2016;25(Sup6):S1–67.
12. Patton D, Avsar P, Sayeh A, Budri A, O'Connor T, Walsh S, et al. A meta-review of the impact of compression therapy on venous leg ulcer healing. Int Wound J. febrero de 2023;20(2):430–47.
13. T Paranhos CSB Paiva FCI Cardoso PP Apolinário RCM Rodrigues HC Oliveira 2021 Systematic review and meta-analysis of the efficacy of Unna boot in the treatment of venous leg ulcers Wound Rep Reg. mayo de 29 3 443 451
14. Conde-Montero E, de Farias Khayat Y, Pérez Jerónimo L, Vázquez AP, Marín LR, Guisado S, et al. Punch grafting for pain reduction in hard-to-heal ulcers. J Wound Care. 2 de marzo de 2020;29(3):194–7.
15. J Navarro Pascual E Conde-Montero K Díez Madueño A Peral Vázquez DP Cueva de la GA Abad 2023 Topical sevoflurane and early and sequential seal grafts in atherosclerotic ulcers: a case series MPJ Multi Pain J 1 2
16. Atkin L, Bućko Z, Montero EC, Cutting K, Moffatt C, Probst A, et al. Implementing TIMERS: the race against hard-to-heal wounds. J Wound Care. 1 de marzo de 2019;28(Sup3a):S1–50.
17. A Orbea Sopeña ME Conde 2023 Punch grafting for the treatment of ulcerated atrophie blanche Phlebology 38 10 695 697
18. Alavi A, Hafner J, Dutz JP, Mayer D, Sibbald RG, Criado PR, Senet P, CallenJP, Phillips TJ, Romanelli M, Kirsner RS. Atrophie blanche: is it associated with venous disease or livedoid vasculopathy? Adv Skin Wound Care. 2014;27(11):518–24; quiz 525–6.
19. E McVittie S Holloway 2015 Aetiology and management of atrophie blanche in chronic venous insufficiency Br J Community Nurs 20 Suppl 12 S8 S13
20. C Montfrans van MGR Maeseneer De 2019 Atrophie Blanche (C4b) Can be reversible after targeted treatment Eur J Vasc Endovasc Surg 58 3 435
21. C Wittens AH Davies N Bækgaard R Broholm A Cavezzi S Chastanet 2015 Editor's choice—management of chronic venous disease: clinical practice guidelines of the European society for vascular surgery (ESVS) Eur J Vasc Endovasc Surg Off J Eur Soc Vasc Surg 49 6 678 737
22. DC Bosanquet A Rangaraj AJ Richards A Riddell VM Saravolac KG Harding 2013 Topical steroids for chronic wounds displaying abnormal inflammation Ann R Coll Surg Engl 95 4 291 296
23. JM Ramírez Torres J Caballer Rodilla M Frías Vargas O García Vallejo GI Gil 2022 Chronic venous disease in the new times Venocheck Proposal Semergen 48 344 355
24. Green J, Jester R, McKinley R, Pooler A. The impact of chronic venous leg ulcers: a systematic review. J Wound Care. 2014;23:601–12.
25. AH Davies 2019 The seriousness of chronic venous disease: a review of real-world evidence Adv Ther 36 Suppl 1 5 12
26. P Amores Valenciano A Navarro Carrillo MA Romero Cebrián M Gerónimo-Pardo 2018 Topical sevoflurane for rescue analgesia in refractory pain due to chronic venous ulcers Emergencias 30 138
27. Isoherranen K, O'Brien JJ, Barker J, Dissemond J, Hafner J, Jemec GBE, et al. Atypical wounds. Best clinical practice and challenges. J Wound Care. 2019;28(Sup6):S1-S92.
28. L Leren E Johansen H Eide RS Falk LK Juvet TM Ljoså 2020 Pain in persons with chronic venous leg ulcers: a systematic review and meta-analysis Int Wound J 17 2 466 484
29. A Imbernón C Blázquez A Puebla M Churruca A Lobato M Martínez 2016 Chronic venous ulcer treatment with topical sevoflurane Int Wound J 13 1060 1062
30. F Dámaso Fernández-Ginés M Cortiñas Sáenz H Mateo-Carrasco AN Aranda de E Navarro Muñoz R Rodríguez Carmona 2017 Efficacy and safety of topical sevoflurane in the treatment of chronic skin ulcers Am J Health Syst Pharm 74 e176 e182
31. Navarro Pascual J, Conde-Montero E, Díez Madueño K, Peral Vázquez A, de la Cueva Dobao P, Abad Gurumeta A. Topical sevoflurane and early and sequential punch grafting in arteriolosclerotic leg ulcers: a case series. Multi Pain J. 2023:1.

32. A Massimiliano D'Erme M Iannone V Dini M Romanelli 2016 Contact dermatitis in patients with chronic leg ulcers: a common and neglected problem: a review 2000–2015 J Wound Care 25 Suppl 9 S23 S29
33. NF Crum-Cianflone J Weekes M Bavaro 2008 Review: thromboses among HIV-infected patients during the highly active antiretroviral therapy era AIDS Patient Care STDS 22 10 771 778
34. NJ Mouawad 2022 Chronic venous ulcer resolution and post-thrombotic syndrome improvement after percutaneous mechanical thrombectomy of a 42-year-old deep vein thrombosis J Vasc Surg Cases Innov Tech 8 2 196 200 https://doi.org/10.1016/j.jvscit.2022.03.001
35. MW Polak J Siudut K Plens A Undas 2019 Prothrombotic clot properties can predict venous ulcers in patients following deep vein thrombosis: a cohort study J Thromb Thrombolysis 48 4 603 609 https://doi.org/10.1007/s11239-019-01914-w
36. AM Ferreira J Oliveira-Pinto L Duarte-Gamas A Coelho A Mansilha 2021 Mid-term patency of iliac venous stenting for post-thrombotic syndrome Int Angiol 40 3 196 205 https://doi.org/10.23736/S0392-9590.21.04659-9
37. R Chen R Feng S Jiang G Chang Z Hu C Yao B Jia S Wang S Wang 2022 Stent patency rates and prognostic factors of endovascular intervention for iliofemoral vein occlusion in post-thrombotic syndrome BMC Surg 22 1 269 https://doi.org/10.1186/s12893-022-01714-9
38. . Srisuwan T. Ultrasound use in diagnosis and management of venous leg ulcer. Int J Lower Extremity Wounds 2020;19(4):305–14.
39. Connors J (2017) Thrombophilia testing and venous thrombosis. New-England Med Rev J. 2017
40. Mościcka P, Szewczyk MT, Cwajda-Białasik J, Jawień A. The role of compression therapy in venous leg ulcers. Adv Clin Exp Med. 2019;28(6):847–852. https://doi.org/10.17219/acem/78768
41. Conde-Montero E. Association of autologous punch grafting, TLC-NOSF dressing and multi-type compression therapy to rapidly achieve wound closure in hard-to-heal venous leg ulcers. JMV-J de Médecine Vasculaire. 2020:45(6):316–25.
42. Evaluation of factors affecting the healing process of venous ulcers: a 12-week longitudinal study, Paulina Mościcka Ph.D, Wound Repair and Regeneration; 2023.
43. E Rabe H Partsch J Hafner 2018 Indications for medical compression stockings in venous and lymphatic disorders: an evidence-based consensus statement Phlebology 33 3 163 184
44. Heinen MM, Achterberg TV, Reimer WSO, Kerkhof PCMVD, Laat ED. Venous leg ulcer patients: a review of the literature on lifestyleand pain-related interventions. J Clin Nurs 13:355–66. https://doi.org/10.1046/j.1365-2702.2003.00887.x
45. Gethin G, Cowman S, Kolbach DN. Debridement for venous leg ulcers. Cochrane Database Syst Rev. 2015;2015(9):CD008599.
46. Brown A (2018) When is wound cleansing necessary and what solution should be used? Nursing Times [online]; 114:9, 42–45.
47. CJ Lavie RV Milani HO Ventura S Obesity 2009 Obesity and cardiovascular disease: risk factor, paradox, and impact of weight loss J Am Coll Cardiol 53 21 1925 1932
48. A Hruby FB Hu 2015 The epidemiology of obesity: a big picture Pharmacoeconomics 33 7 673 689
49. GS Hotamisligil 2006 Inflammation and metabolic disorders Nature 444 7121 860 867
50. E Rabe F Pannier 2012 Clinical, aetiological, anatomical and pathological classification (CEAP): gold standard and limits Phlebolymphology. 19 3 123 128
51. Langan EA, Wienandt M, Bayer A, Ellebrecht L, Kahle B (2023) Effect of obesity on venous blood flow in the lower limbs. JDDG: J der Deutschen Dermatologischen Gesellschaft. 21(6):622–629
52. C Lindholm R Searle 2016 Wound management for the 21st century: combining effectiveness and efficiency Int Wound J 13 5 15

4 Look at the Foot but Focus on the Patient: A Collection of Complex Cases of Diabetic Foot Syndrome

Elisabetta Iacopi, Francesco Giangreco, Tommaso Belcari, Martina Capobianco, Lea Contartese, Alessio Faranda, Vittorio Malquori, Benedetta Migliorucci, and Alberto Piaggesi

Abstract

The Diabetic Foot Syndrome (DFS) is a chronic relapsing/remitting disease affecting more than 3 million patients in Europe, exposing them to a risk of lower extremity amputations and death which has been estimated 20 times higher than the general population. The real prevalence and severity of DFS has so far largely been underestimated and its systemic aspects neglected. We profit of the occasion of presenting a series of DFS cases of ours, to display the complexity and the severity of DFS, which ranges from local hyperacute presentation to systemic chronic multiorgan decompensation, with the aim of adequately depict the real extent of this terrible disease for the benefit of our patients and their doctors.

Keywords

Diabetic Foot • Chronic limb-threatening ischemia • Heart failure • Multidisciplinary approach • Negative pressure therapy

Abbreviations

CLTI	Chronic limb-threatening ischemia
CT	Computed tomography
DF	Diabetic foot
DFS	Diabetic foot syndrome
EBUS	Endo-bronchial ultrasound-guided

E. Iacopi (✉) · F. Giangreco · T. Belcari · M. Capobianco · L. Contartese · A. Faranda · V. Malquori · B. Migliorucci · A. Piaggesi
Diabetic Foot Section—Department of Medicine, Pisa University Hospital, Pisa, Italy
e-mail: elisabettaiacopi@gmail.com

G.-S.Tiplica and K. Isoherranen (eds.), *Wound Healing*,
https://doi.org/10.1007/978-3-031-84579-6_4

GAD	Glutamic acid decarboxylase
GP	General practitioner
IA2	Isoform 2 of tyrosine phosphatase antibodies
MR	Magnetic resonance
NT-proBNP	N-terminal portion of precursor of Brain natriuretic peptide
PET	Positron emission tomography
SGLT2	Sodium glucose cotransporter 2
TMA	Trans metatarsal amputation

Introduction

The International Diabetes Federation estimated that the number of patients who presents a diabetic foot (DF) episode every year ranges from 9.1 to 26.1 million [1, 2]. Among diabetes complications DF is associated with the highest levels of morbidity and mortality [3]. DF is still now the most frequent cause of lower limb amputation and the risk of death in five years in a patient with a DF ulcer is 2.5 times higher compared to a patient without ulcers and remains two times higher after ten years of follow up [4].

At variance from what was thought for decades, we are now aware that diabetic foot is not an acute episodic disease but rather a relapsing remitting disease in which, after the complete healing of an ulcer, the recurrence rate is 40% within one year, 65% within three years and 80% ten years after the first episode [5]. After each acute episode, the health status of the patient progressively worsens, rendering him even more prone to recurrences. Recently this new point of view has been synthesized with the term "Diabetic Foot Syndrome" (DFS), a clinical definition which includes both local and systemic aspects of DF and its chronic progressive evolution [6].

DFS represents not only the most invalidating complication of diabetes, but also a marker of severity for diabetes and its related comorbidities [7]. DFS patients represent the paradigmatic example of a high complexity patient: they are typically affected by a series of comorbidities and chronic complications [8]. Furthermore, their clinical status is so fragile that each change, therapy or procedure can expose them to an increased clinical risk, with often dramatic consequences [9]. Many of these conditions subtly develop, being asymptomatic for years. It is therefore a frequent finding that cardiac, renal, hepatic or other comorbidities are diagnosed during an admission for DFS [10]. Moreover, DFS patients undergoing to treatment or procedures are particularly prone to develop complications, because of their delicate compensation [11]. For this reason, in the last decades, it has been developed the concept of *multidisciplinary team* approach [12]. DFS specialists were, and still now are, aware that a such a complex syndrome could not be managed by a single specialist but needed a multidisciplinary team composed by many different competences integrated to treat these patients [13]. This approach has demonstrated to be able to improve the clinical chances of these patients' reducing amputation and mortality [14]. We selected from the cases followed at our department those that could best demonstrate the complexity of patients with diabetic foot, the severity of the condition and the need for multidisciplinary management coordinated with other specialists. We also sought to focus attention on the insidious nature of the condition and its tendency to recur. Indeed, the diabetic foot represents not only a particularly burdensome condition for the patient but also and especially a marker of risk and complexity of the overall clinical status.

For an adequate management of diabetic foot ulcers is mandatory to be trained to:

- Know the relationship between diabetes and lower limb complications
- Understand that diabetic foot is not only an ulcer in the foot
- Recognize the course of diabetic foot pathology characterized by recurrence and progressivity
- Execute adequately physical assessment and objectivation
- Perform proper staging and stratification of cases
- Be aware of the need for a prompt referral of more severe patients
- Recognize the importance of multidisciplinary team as the only option for managing diabetic foot
- Know revascularization modalities and the main indications for the different modalities
- Know and implement infection control methods
- Enforce offloading modalities and educate patients on compliance with them
- Distinguish local treatment techniques and adapt them to different clinical cases
- Know the need for close follow-up with frequent reassessment and careful surveillance

Case 4.1. The Sudden Worsening

A 67-year-old gentleman was followed for more than 10 years in our DF clinic. He had type 2 diabetes mellitus since 1996, complicated by laser-treated retinopathy in right eye and chronic ischemic heart disease treated by coronary angioplasty in 2017, and still characterized by occasional angina episodes with no more indications to revascularization procedures. Accordingly, he also developed chronic limb-threatening ischemia (CLTI). He underwent, in the last years, to multiple bilateral percutaneous angioplasties and to partial calcanectomy in the right foot and amputation of II left and I right toes because of osteomyelitis and gangrene, respectively.

He came at our attention on 4th August for occurrence of new lesions, bilaterally but more severe at right limb: plantar ulcer at the base of the first metatarsal with ulcerative infected lesion of the anterior, medial and posterior surfaces of the ipsilateral leg (Fig. 4.1a). At the contralateral limb he had only superficial lesions with no signs of infection. The patient was immediately admitted, it was sampled for cultural exams and promptly started empirical parenteral antibiotic treatment. The lab exams showed an only slight increase of phlogistic indexes but no signs of infection. The ultrasound assessment highlighted a worsening in an already compromised arterial district and indications for revascularization were given, the patient underwent angioplasty of the posterior tibial and lateral plantar artery of the right foot. He underwent surgical debridement to control local infection (Fig. 4.1b). The cardiological evaluation, that had not been performed for two years, confirmed the severity of heart involvement, revealing a dilated left ventricle with severe global systolic dysfunction. We adapted therefore antidiabetic therapy introducing dulaglutide and dapagliflozin trying to ensure better cardiovascular protection.

At discharge, the local conditions were fairly good, with good control of local signs of infection subsequent to surgical debridement. According to the bacterial culture performed, diagnosis for Methicillin sensitive *Staphylococcus aureus* was made and therapy with amoxicillin/clavulanate was prescribed.

Three weeks later, at first DF clinic control the patient showed a severe worsening of the infection of the right lower limb with erythema extending to the knee, wide adherent eschars, abundant exudation, despite prosecution of antibiotic therapy. The duplex scanning confirmed the patency of the angioplasty performed during the recent admission so, as an attempt of limb salvage, the patient was again hospitalized. An MR-scan excluded the presence of osteomyelitis confirming the location of the infection only at the soft tissue level. Therefore the patient underwent a new surgical debridement and intravenous antibiotic treatment. During

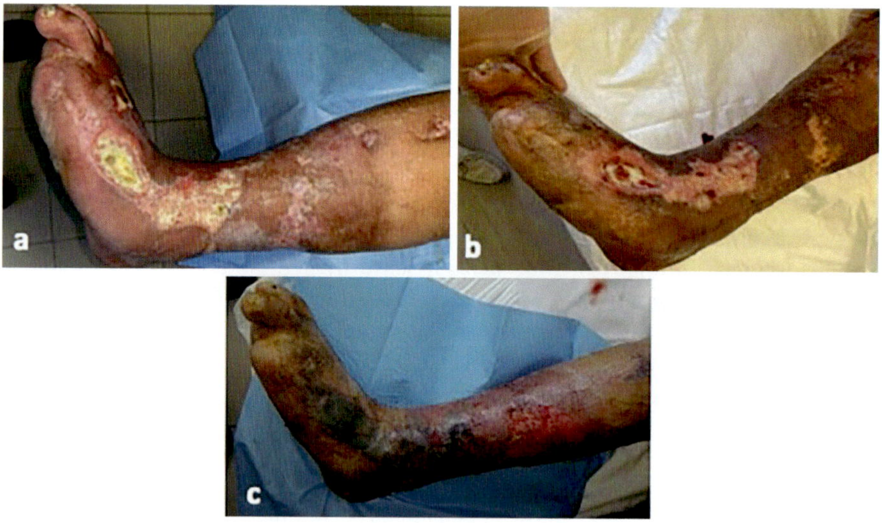

Fig. 4.1 a Local state of the lesion at first admission; b: local state after surgical procedure of debridement; c: new worsening observed at new control

hospitalization we could observe a slow but evident improvement of local conditions and so the patient was dismissed with the indication to continue systemic antibiotic therapy under control of the GP.

At the next follow up we observed a new worsening, probably due to too tight bandages (Fig. 4.1c). For this reason, we admitted the patient for a new debridement. During pre-operative cardiological evaluation, congestive heart failure with reduced ejection fraction and widespread hypokinesia were noted. The cardiologist did not pose any indication to a coronary evaluation but rather to change diuretic and vasoactive therapies: furosemide, mannitol and metolazone were enhanced also in consideration of the slight worsening of creatinine values and of the edema component of venous origin affecting the lower limbs. Despite this, the patient continued to present persistent dyspnea. Therefore, we performed a CT-scan of the chest which excluded the presence of pulmonary embolism but described a pseudo-nodular formation in the anterior segment of the right upper lobe. As the patient was considered "unfit", the pneumologist considered that no further diagnostic investigations were deemed appropriate. The patient also presented dullness at abdominal percussion associated with tenderness: an ultrasound of the abdomen showed abundant ascitic effusion mainly in the peri-splenic area and at the decline level. Hepatological consultancy did not indicate percutaneous drainage also in consideration of the normal values of liver enzymes and preserved hepatic synthesis. Once stabilized the heart status, the patient underwent a new eschar-ectomy and debridement with pressure hydrosurgery to decrease the bacterial load. As soon as possible, the patient was discharged. He died unhealed after less than a month for acute pulmonary oedema.

Case 4.2. The Long Pathway to Limb Salvage

In the mid of January 2022, a 65 years-old man arrived at our attention, affected by diabetes mellitus for 30 years complicated only by laser-treated retinopathy. He had voluntarily resigned from a hospital in the south of Italy and traveled alone by train for 900 km to our clinic, where he showed up unexpectedly and was visited as an urgent case. He presented gangrene of III and IV toes and necrotizing fasciitis on medial and lateral compartment of dorsum of the foot extended to the lateral surface of the leg (Fig. 4.2a). He had fever and severe asthenia. The urgent blood tests showed a marked glycometabolic decompensation, with marked leukocytosis and significant increase in inflammatory indexes.

The patient was carried to the operating room within one hour from presentation to undergo urgent fasciotomy, amputation of III and IV toes of the right foot and debridement of the lesion through hydrosurgery to reduce the bacterial load (Fig. 4.2b). Immediately after sampling for culture, empiric antibiotic therapy with piperacillin/tazobactam and daptomycin was started and then adapted according to the results of cultural exams. Since the first postoperative day, we observed a gradual and constant reduction of indexes of inflammation. The vascular ultrasound study showed stenosis in the femoral district but at leg level its reliability

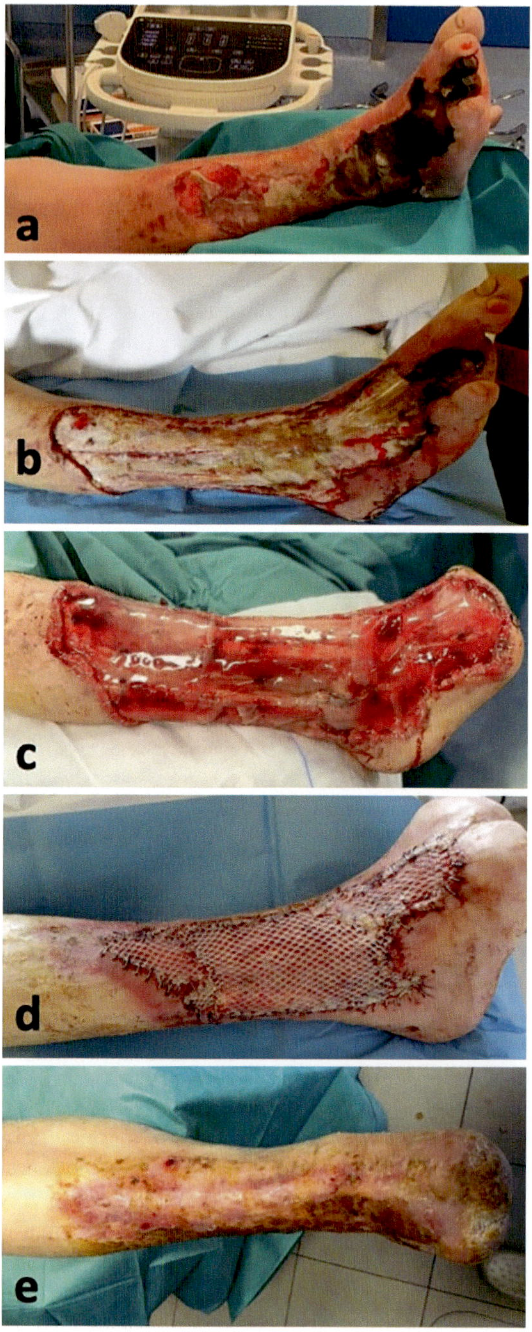

Fig. 4.2 a Clinical presentation at first access of the patient; b: local state after first urgent debridement; c: local state after new surgical debridement and implant of dermal substitute graft; d: local state after autologous graft; e: complete healing

appeared to be severely limited by the extensive loss of substance. It was therefore scheduled for an angiographic exam of the right lower limb which showed haemodynamic stenosis at the level of both tibial vessels and plantar circulation. The interventional radiologist then proceeded to endoluminal revascularization of the anterior tibial artery, posterior tibial artery, lateral plantar artery and plantar arch with vascular remodeling and improvement of the foot circulation. During hospitalization, despite the successful outcome of the revascularization procedure, due to persistence of ischemic suffering at the level of the distal tissues, it was necessary to proceed with transmetatarsal amputation. Then the patient underwent a cycle of negative pressure therapy associated with the installation of poly-hexamethyl-biguanide solution.

For the high values of the cholestasis and hypoalbuminemia markers, an ultrasound of the complete abdomen and a CT of the abdomen with contrast and hepatological consultations were performed with subsequent diagnosis of chronic liver disease with steatosis imprint on a dysmetabolic etiology, with suspected initial cirrhosis.

After discharge the patient started a regular follow up in our DF clinic. First controls showed dehiscence of transmetatarsal amputation with tendon exposure and some areas partially covered by eschars. The patient performed an MR-scan which excluded the presence of osteomyelitis but showed the persistence of diffuse thickening of the soft tissues on the lateral side of foot and leg with obliteration of the subcutaneous adipose tissue and edema of the muscle bellies. He was therefore newly admitted to a new surgical debridement, followed by grafting of dermal substitute (Fig. 4.2c). In this occasion a duplex scan confirmed the patency of angioplasties performed. During hospitalization, despite having already undergone a full course of anti-COVID vaccination, the patient resulted positive for the Delta variant of the virus, for which he was transferred to the Infectious Diseases Unit until remission. He remains almost completely asymptomatic during all the hospitalization.

He continues the regular follow up in DF clinic and in November, in consideration of the good local evolution, it was scheduled a new admission during which underwent autologous skin grafting (Fig. 4.2d).

At the following DF clinic control, three weeks after the autologous skin graft surgery, the graft had completely integrated and the lesion was almost completely re-epithelialized (Fig. 4.2e).

Case 4.3. Diabetes, the Foot and the Heart

In October 2021, a 86-year-old female patient, arrived to our outpatient DF clinic for a right foot abscess originating from dehiscent V metatarsal ray amputation, extended dorsally and associated to partial gangrene of the ipsilateral first toe (Fig. 4.3a). The continuous wave doppler analysis allowed us to sample only the dorsalis pedis artery. The patient was immediately hospitalized. In the patient's medical history we found type 2 diabetes mellitus for more than 10 years complicated by ischemic cardiopathy, treated with angioplasty, and chronic heart failure, atrial fibrillation, hypertension and dyslipidemia. Since 2020, she suffered from multiple episodes of lower limb ulceration for which she underwent bilateral endovascular revascularization and amputation of V right toe and partial amputation of II right toe.

The duplex scanning performed at admission showed regular patency of femoral-popliteal vessels while below the knee the flow was reduced by vascular calcification but sufficient, in the opinion of vascular surgeon, confirmed by a $TcP0_2$ of 41 mmHg, to allow surgical wound healing. The patient underwent a transmetatarsal amputation of the right foot. In post-operative days, despite a reduction of the phlogistic indexes, the stump showed a wide dehiscence in the central region and signs of ischemic suffering. We performed then an angio-CT scan to study the iliac vessels and we found a reduction in flow velocity starting from the abdominal sub renal aorta associated with the almost complete sparing of femoral vessels and a severe infra-popliteal involvement characterized by proximal obstruction of posterior tibial and peroneal arteries and absence of plantar arteries. The cardiologic revaluation by hemodynamic showed a severe worsening of the cardiac kinesis with evidence of aortic valve stenosis and mitral sclerosis determining moderate insufficiency and dilation of the right heart chambers with moderate tricuspid insufficiency and pulmonary hypertension. The patient underwent coronary percutaneous angioplasty with implantation of medicated stents on right coronary and anterior interventricular arteries. The cardiac function showed a significant improvement in postoperative days and therefore the patient was newly admitted after 4 weeks from coronary intervention to be submitted to a surgical revision of the TMA. At the moment of the new admission, the patient complained of fatigue and dyspnea: chest X-ray showed pleural effusion at the right lung base and enlarged cardiac shadow. The cardiological evaluation confirmed the presence of severe aortic stenosis complicated by congestive heart failure. After execution

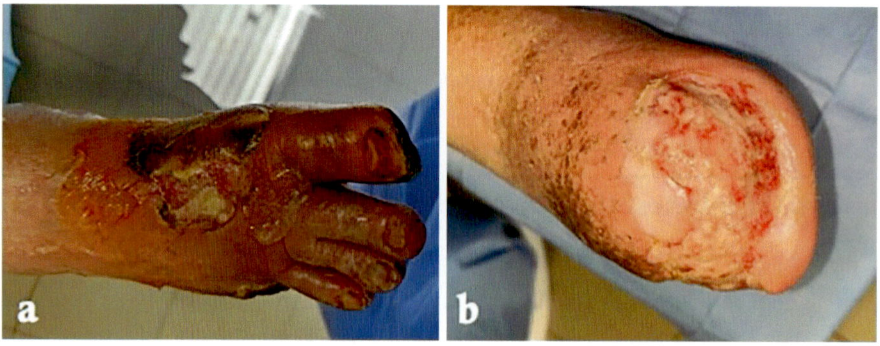

Fig. 4.3 a Clinical presentation of the case; b: last visit performed: permanent non healing ulcer

of angio-CT to study thoraco-abdominal aorta the patient underwent the implantation of a biological aortic valve prosthesis by percutaneous transfemoral route. Patient showed a severe fluid and electrolyte imbalance which was adequately supplemented and a state of anemia for which she was transfused. Subsequent telemetric electrocardiographic monitoring was regular. After the stabilization of cardiac status, a new surgical debridement and a dermal substitute grafting was performed.

During the following months, the patient's cardiac follow up showed persistent stability with a good hemodynamic compensation.

The patient also continued her regular follow up at DF clinic: the ultrasound controls showed partial restenosis of angioplasties performed but the cardiac status contraindicated neither new vascular interventional procedures nor alternative therapies such as prostanoids. We activated a protocol of active surveillance with periodic regular assessment and the patient did not show further episodes of infection or pain. Despite this, the post-surgical lesion in the stump did not heal. In Fig. 4.3b is reported the local status at the last visit performed.

Case 4.4. Transplant and Comorbidities

In May 2022 arrived to our attention a 50 years old male affected by type 1 diabetes since he was 6 years old, complicated by diabetic retinopathy, ischemic cardiomyopathy treated with percutaneous coronary angioplasty in 2008 and 2020 respectively, for the impossibility to perform aorto-coronary by-pass with a severe reduction of left ventricular function and widespread hypokinesia which required Cardioverter Defibrillator implant.

The patient developed from end stage renal disease treated with peritoneal dialysis and in May 2018 with Kidney transplantation from cadaver, subsequently evolute to functional exhaustion, for a Polyomavirus BK nephropathy with initial interstitial fibrosis, and therefore treated again with peritoneal dialysis.

At the beginning of 2021, during controls for a new renal transplant, the patient performed a vascular surgery evaluation for severe peripheral arteriopathy associated with a partial gangrene of the first toe of left foot (Fig. 4.4a). The Angio-CT scan performed showed, in addition to the stenosis of previous kidney graft vessels, multiple steno-obstructions from the common iliac arteries to the foot vessels. The patient was then admitted to the Vascular Surgery Department and there underwent multiple angioplasties of the left iliac axis. After revascularization the patient came to our attention, and we performed amputation of the I toe of the left foot (Fig. 4.4b). Few days after discharge the patient came back to our DF clinic for fever and pain: we observed necrosis on the stump of the amputation with abscess on plantar side and local and systemic signs of infection (Fig. 4.4c). The patient was immediately hospitalized and started antibiotic intravenous therapy. At admission we observed an increase of inflammatory indexes, neutrophilic leukocytosis

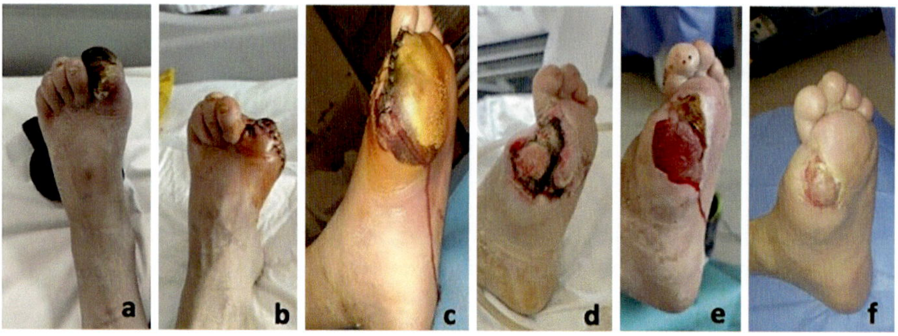

Fig. 4.4 a Clinical status at our first evaluation; b: clinical status after first surgical procedure of first toe amputation; c: abscess on first toe amputation; d: wound after surgical debridement; e: after 4 weeks of negative pressure associated to instillation of polihexametilbiguanide; f: last visit performed: the lesion is almost healed

and a fall in hemoglobin values for which we performed a blood transfusion. The vascular re-evaluation showed no worsening, with patency of angioplasties and therefore the patient underwent immediately to drainage of abscess with osteotomy of first metatarsal head. The surgical wound, left open to heal for secondary intent, was treated with a cycle of negative pressure therapy associated with installation of polihexametil-biguanide (Fig. 4.4d). After 5 days the patient was discharged, continuing negative pressure at home; all blood exams at discharge completely normalized.

At first outpatient control, two weeks later, transcutaneous oxygen tension showed on left lower limb good level at malleolar region (65.4 mmHg) but sharp reduction at inter-metatarsal level with severe hypoxic ischemia (pO2 14.5 mmHg). In agreement with the nephrologists and cardio-angiologists the patient was newly admitted and treated with infusion of prostanoids at increasing concentration for a total duration of 6 h infusion per day for a total of five days, with a brisk recover from the critical status ($TcP0_2$ 27 mmHg).

After discharge, the patient continued domiciliary negative pressure for four weeks with newly-produced granulation tissue and the complete coverage of the bone stump (Fig. 4.4e). After one month he showed markedly improved values in oxygen tension at inter-metatarsal level (pO2 41.7 mmHg). The patient attended regularly controls every two weeks and local dressing with gauze impregnated of sucrose octasulfate. Progresses were soon observed: the lesion became non exudating, superficialized and granulating. In Fig. 4.4ef is reported the local state at the last visit, in advanced healing status.

Case 4.5. The Weight of Interfering Pathologies

In December 2021, a patient known and followed in our DF clinic, a 52 years old male, arrived at scheduled visit with a new lesion on the plantar surface of the left foot, complicated by the presence of a phlegmon (Fig. 4.5a). The patient was affected by morbid obesity complicated by type 2 diabetes for 15 years. In 2019 he had been admitted for fasciitis of the right forefoot treated by trans metatarsal amputation, and septic osteoarthritis of III-IV metatarsophalangeal joint of left foot, treated with osteo-arthrectomy, bilaterally in absence of arterial vascular disease, although not critical. Since then, he had been followed up regularly at our outpatient clinic with no recurrences until the moment we are reporting. During these years he had deeply changed his life habits achieving a weight loss of about 65 kg.

The patient was immediately hospitalized and treated with drainage of the purulent collection on the plantar surface of the foot with immediate reduction of inflammatory indexes and local sign of infection. After the urgent procedure the patient was evaluated with ultrasound duplex scanning, which did not show signs of CLTI, and X-ray of the foot (Fig. 4.5b), which showed results of previous intervention with lateral deviation of forefoot and osteomyelitis on II ray. The patient underwent transmetatarsal amputation (Fig. 4.5c) with no periprocedural complications and complete normalization of inflammatory indexes.

At admission, as per pre-operative procedural evaluation, the patient was subjected to chest x-ray which documented a pulmonary thickening in the right perilary region. The pneumologist required a CT-scan of the thorax which showed "*diffuse and confluent lymph node involvement mediastinal, prevascular, right and left paratracheal, subcarinal and bilateral hilar, with associated right ilo-peril-interstitial parenchymal involvement, and coexistence of lymph nodes in the coeliac, interporto-caval, intercaval-aortic, retro-caval and left para-aortic areas*". For the

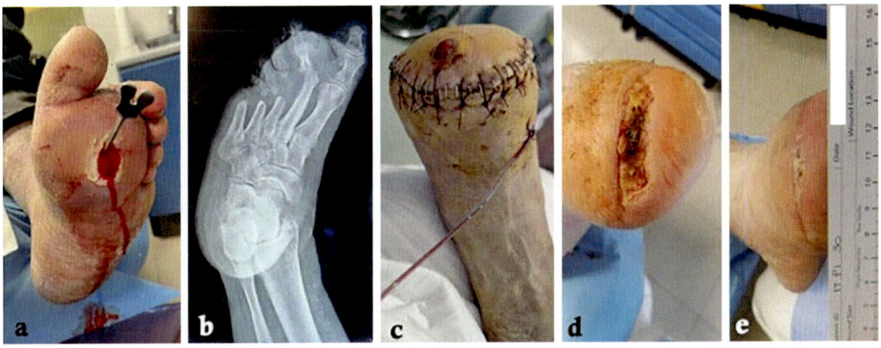

Fig. 4.5 a Clinical case at first presentation of new lesion on left foot; b: plain X ray of left foot; c: first postoperative day after transmetatarsal amputation; d: first outpatient visit: minimal signs of suffering on lateral side of flap juxtaposition; e: complete re-epithelialization

diagnostic suspicion of sarcoidosis, the patient underwent bronchoscopy with bronchoalveolar lavage and lymph node needle aspiration to exclude neoplasms of a lymphoproliferative or primary pulmonary type. Being the results not conclusive, the specialist posed an indication to an endo-bronchial ultrasound-guided (EBUS) bronchoscopy with transbronchial needle aspiration. Meanwhile, the patient performed a spirometric examination and bronchoalveolar diffusion which diagnosed a possible restrictive deficit. The EBUS bronchoscopy performed after discharge confirmed the diagnosis of sarcoidosis for which the patient started a regular pneumological follow up, still ongoing.

After discharge, regarding the foot the patient underwent to a regular outpatient follow up, showing initially minimal signs of suffering on lateral side of flap juxtaposition (Fig. 4.5d), completely resolved in few weeks with local dressing with vaseline gauzes and management, until reaching the complete re-epithelialization (Fig. 4.5e).

Case 4.6. What Should Be Done Versus What Can Be Done

In November 2021, a male patient came to our attention and was referred from another Hospital. He was 52 years old, affected by type 2 diabetes mellitus for 15 years, obese, affected by ischemic cardiopathy complicated by heart failure and permanent atrial fibrillation, ischemic encephalopathy, chronic kidney disease and hypertension. A few weeks before our evaluation, the patient had observed the occurrence of lesions on IV and V toes, lateral margin and calcaneal region of the left foot. The lesions had been treated with local dressing and no revascularization was suggested. The patient was referred to the vascular surgery unit of our hospital for a second opinion. The colleagues immediately hospitalized the patient. At admission he had gangrene of IV and V toes associated with lesions on the lateral margin and in the calcaneal region of the left foot (Fig. 4.6a). The systemic assessment showed a septic state with marked neutrophilic leukocytosis, an increase in inflammation indexes and a deterioration of renal function. He was therefore immediately treated with urgent trans-metatarsal amputation. From the first postoperative days, the suffering of the stump, due to a reduced blood perfusion, became evident (Fig. 4.6b). The need for a revascularization procedure, in the perspective of a risk/benefit evaluation was discussed both with interventional radiologists and nephrologists. In order to adequately weigh the risks, we performed an ultrasound scan of the abdomen which did not sort hepatic problems but rather confirmed the presence of mold stones on the right kidney. The patient had to be considered functionally as a monokidney with a consequent complication of his therapeutic pathway. We carried out a further collegial evaluation with a nephrologist, interventional radiologist and urologist who indicated, in consideration of persistent fever despite intensified antibiotic therapy, the possibility of positioning a percutaneous urinary shunt. The required CT-scan of the urothelial system (Fig. 4.6c) and PET confirmed the mold stone on the right kidney and excluded hypercaptation areas. The colleagues, in consideration of resolution of the septic state and of multiple comorbidities, decided not to position the shunt, re-evaluating the option in the future in case of recurrence. The patient was fully and extensively informed on the risk of the revascularization procedure, in particular about the possible worsening of renal function or need for dialysis treatment after the contrast medium injection. After his consent the patient underwent endovascular revascularization of femoro-popliteal axis, tibio-peroneal trunk, all the three leg vessels and foot vessels, as reported in Fig. 4.6d. As expected after the procedure, the patient's renal function worsened. A careful follow-up, with strict monitoring of both renal and cardiac functions, alongside with a reset of pharmacological therapy allowed a slow but constant restoration of normal renal values in the following days. At this point the foot was revised, and a dermal substitute was grafted (Fig. 4.6e).

At discharge the lesion was improving, all bone stumps were completely covered, and glycemic, renal and cardiac compensations were achieved and maintained. The patient is continuing his regular follow up on outpatient DF clinic.

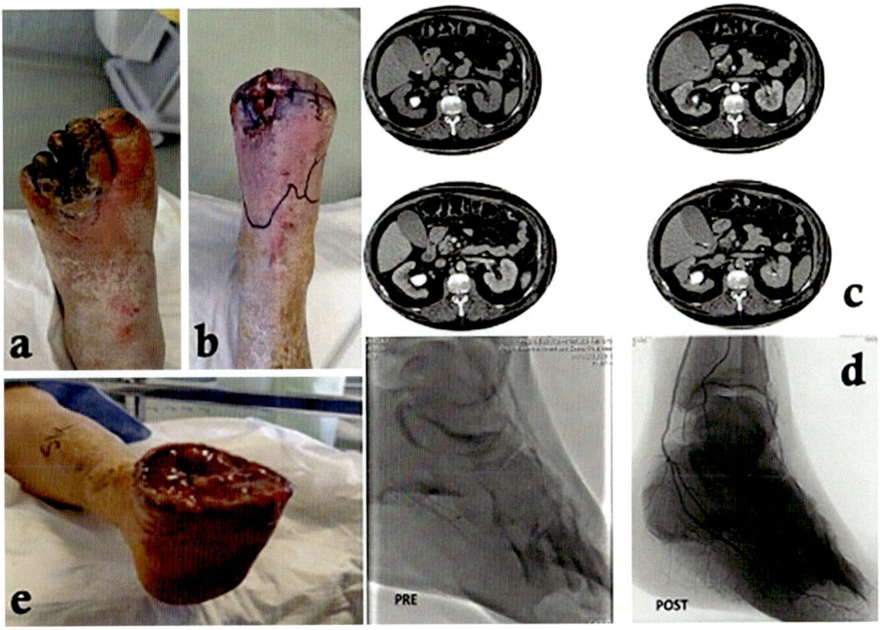

Fig. 4.6 a Clinical presentation at admission; b: in post-operative days: suffering of the stump; c: CT-scan of urothelial system; d: endovascular revascularization images; e: revision of the amputation stump

Case 4.7. DFU as a First Clinical Manifestation of Diabetes

At the end of March 2022 came to our attention a 63-year-old man, affected only by hypertension with no other known health problems and with a negative family history for diabetes and positive for only lung cancer. Because of the appearance of swelling in the dorsum of right foot, he consulted his family doctor, who started oral antibiotics and prescribed blood tests, with consequent diagnosis of diabetes mellitus. After a few days, for the worsening of the local condition and the appearance of necrosis of the right II and III toes, the patient went to the Urgency Department of a hospital near to our Center, and we were asked for an urgent consultation. The patient was hemodynamically stable, blood test showed a severe glycometabolic disturbance (HbA1c 93 mmol/mol) with only a moderate increase of inflammatory indexes. He had an abscess of the dorsum of right foot and necrosis of II and III toes (Fig. 4.7a). Duplex scanning excluded the presence of arterial stenosis and superficial and deep venous thrombosis.

During objective examination at admission, we observed swelling, oedema (the circumference was approximately 9 cm greater than the contralateral) and erythema in the anterior and lateral surfaces of the left thigh, not previously reported. The patient did not remember previous trauma in the affected region. The patient underwent immediately an MR-scan with findings of multiple abscesses collections in close communication in the upper thigh. He was therefore brought to the operating room, where fasciotomy was done, with the drainage of copious amounts of pus. Negative pressure was then applied, associated with installation of poli-hexametil-biguanide antiseptic solution. At the same time systemic antibiotic therapy, hydration, insulin and electrolytes were initiated.

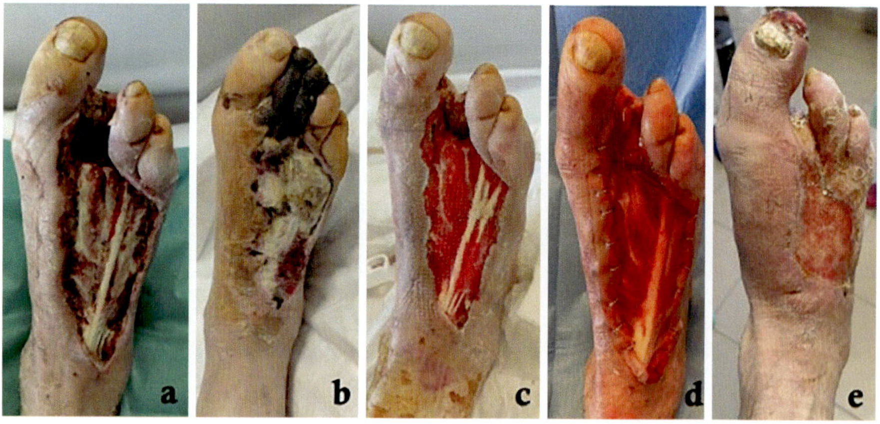

Fig. 4.7 a Clinical presentation at first access; b: clinical status after surgical debridement; c: clinical status after 4 weeks of negative pressure; d: new surgical debridement and dermal graft; e: last outpatient visit and advanced healing status

Once stabilized, the patient underwent surgical revision and amputation of II and III toes, also in this case the surgical wound was left open to heal by secondary intent, assisted by negative pressure (Fig. 4.7b).

On the third day post-surgery, despite systemic antibacterial therapy, oedema and erythema appeared again, and therefore the patient was submitted to MR scan that showed an evolution of the abscess towards gluteus muscles. The patient was therefore operated again with further drainage. Immediately after the procedure inflammatory indexes showed a reduction. But we were unfortunately far from resolution: the level of phlogistic indexes returned to grow and, in fact, the thigh showed a recurrence of pain and edema with increased texture. The ultrasound showed presence of purulent collection in the organization phase, located laterally to the vastus intermedius muscle, stretching the trochanteric bursa and reaching up to the passage between the gluteal muscles. The patient underwent a new fasciotomy with extension of the surgical wound, evacuation of serum-blood material and repositioning of negative pressure. As in previous procedures deep cultural exams were performed to adapt antibiotic therapy to bacterial species. On the 5th postoperative day, the orthopedic surgeons cleaned again the wound and sutured it. The subsequent CT-scan showed no further signs of bleeding.

Meanwhile, the right foot showed a progressive improvement with 4 weeks of negative pressure (Fig. 4.7c) and before the discharge the patient underwent further debridement and dermal substitute graft (Fig. 4.7d).

During hospitalization we performed a characterization of diabetes type and chronic complications: antibodies against GAD and IA2 were negative and basal C-peptide value showed a nice insulin reserve (1.62 ng/ml). We were therefore able to discontinue insulin therapy, introduced at diagnosis, and prescribe metformin and SGLT2 inhibitor for the detection of microalbuminuria.

After discharge the patient began a regular follow up at DF clinic, during which we observed a gradual but continuous improvement. During this follow up we applied three times a graft of fish skin to enhance healing speed. In Fig. 4.7e it is reported the clinical status at the last visit performed.

Case 4.8. Finding Solutions for No-Option Patients

In October 2021 an 88-year-old non-smoker man presented at our attention complaining of diabetic foot lesions associated with rest pain. He was affected by type 2 diabetes for about 20 years, ischemic cardiomyopathy treated with coronary angioplasty and implant of biventricular defibrillator, peripheral arterial disease treated in 2020 with percutaneous angioplasty of right lower limb, chronic kidney disease, chronic obstructive pulmonary disease and hypertension. At objectivation we observed bilateral acrocyanosis, more severe on the right foot, bilateral calcaneal lesions and, on the right foot, apical necrosis of first, second and fourth toes (Fig. 4.8a). Ultrasound assessment of the right lower limb confirmed the patency of femoral vessels (revascularized in another hospital) and showed multiple stenosis in tibio-peroneal trunk and peroneal and posterior tibial arteries with

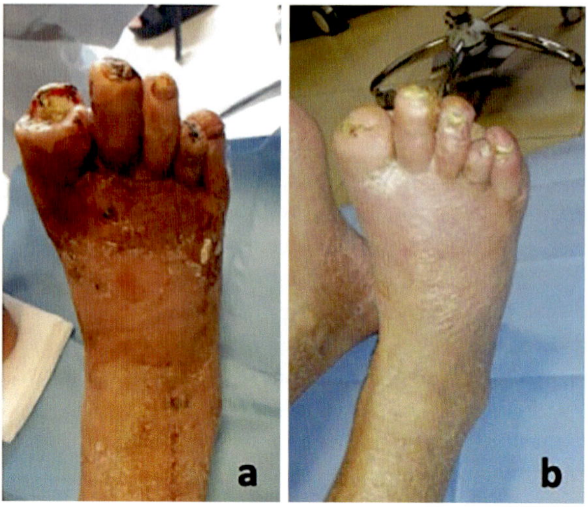

Fig. 4.8 a Patient at first visit: apical parcel gangrene of first, second and fourth toes; b After third cycle of monocytes. Complete healing

obstruction of anterior tibial one. On the left side the vascular tree was similar, but less severe. The patient was then hospitalized, and a new percutaneous transluminal angioplasty was planned for the day after: angioplasties of femoral-popliteal axis, tibio-peroneal trunk and anterior tibial artery were performed, while posterior tibial artery remained obstructed. On the second day post-revascularization, the patient underwent a partial amputation of II and IV toes. Trans-cutaneous oxygen tension after the procedures was 41.9 mmHg on the right and 46.2 mmHg on the left foot. The patient was discharged two days after with no complication and stable from a systemic point of view.

Few days after discharge the patient accessed the DF clinic for persistence of significant pain at rest, not responding to painkillers and worsening in supine position. Locally, we observed dehiscence of surgical wounds and occurrence of a new apical lesion of the second toe of the right foot. Trans-cutaneous oxygen tension at this moment was severely reduced bilaterally: 10.6 mmHg on the right and 26.0 mmHg on the left foot, while duplex scanning showed the partial restenosis of tibio-peroneal trunk and anterior tibial artery. The patient was then re-evaluated collegially by diabetologist, vascular surgeon and cardio-angiologist that excluded the possibility of new vascular procedures for high operative risks or for intravenous prostanoid administration for the risk of cardiological decompensation. We decided therefore to treat patients with implants of peripheral blood mononuclear cells. According to the published procedure, peripheral blood mononuclear cells population was prepared by means of a filtration system applied to total nuclear cells derived from peripheral blood [15]. After preparation the mononuclear cells population was divided in 0.25 ml boluses and injected along the vascular axis, predefined under ultrasound guide [16]. The treatment scheme consists of three consecutive applications, with 1-month interval in between. The patient was immediately submitted to the first one.

He performed a surgical revision with associate drainage of new purulent collection on plantar side and installation of autologous peripheral blood mononuclear cells along the anatomical sites of obstructed vessels previously marked under echographic guidance. During the admission the patients showed an important increase of NT-proBNP and a worsening of renal function. Cardiological assessment showed a stable despite critical state and the modulation of diuretic and vasoactive therapies progressively allowed the restoration of values similar to those observed at admission. A reduction in total hemoglobin values required, in the first day post-surgery, a concentrated red blood cells transfusion. Immediately after the procedure the patient referred to a decrease in pain and an improvement of well-being.

After three weeks, the patient was newly admitted to perform the second administration. At admission we could observe a marked improvement of trans-cutaneous oximetry: on the right foot 31 mmHg basal and 44.1 with the leg declivous and on the left 41 mmHg basal, 69.7 mmHg. Also in this second case, after the surgical procedure, the patient required blood transfusion. During the blood supply patient presented chest pain with ECG-graphic alterations and increase of myocardial cytonecrosis enzymes and NT-ProBNP values. Cardiologists performed echocardiography in absence of apparent changes of heart kinesis and, in consideration of the impossibility of further myocardial revascularization procedures already defined, did not pose indication to further cardiac procedures. The values were in progressive reduction until discharge.

Three weeks later further improvement of transcutaneous oxygen values, reaching 48 mmHg on right foot and 54 mmHg on left foot, and a complete resolution of rest pain. The patient was newly admitted and a third cycle was performed. Four weeks after this last admission, at outpatient clinic follow up, the patient referred well-being and the lesions was completely healed (Fig. 4.8b).

Discussion

Diabetic foot syndrome is one of the most challenging pathologic scenarios: it could be defined both as a drama for the patient and a nightmare for the diabetologist. The clinical cases we reported showed DFS in almost all these facets. DFS itself is never the result of a single pathogenetic mechanism: it is rather the consequence of interaction among macroangiopathy, microangiopathy, neuropathy, immunopathy. Even more important, DFS is not only a complex and disabling disease, but a real marker of complexity and risk in these multiple comorbidities' patients. DFS is commonly associated with all the other complications and comorbidities and with an increased level of severity of all ancillary condition [9].

The complexity of the cases reported goes even further beyond the already dramatic conditions of DFS. These cases tell of fragile patients suffering from multiple comorbidities, almost always asymptomatic, in which each procedure or intervention can criticize a condition yet precarious. DFS is a chronic disease that, like diabetes, accompany the patient throughout all his life [17]. This chronic, remitting/relapsing evolution characterizes a patient who becomes even more brittle and so more prone to damage. The consequences at the level of the foot system of all these conditions unbalance a delicate equilibrium in which homeostasis is extremely limited: there is little room to improve the patients' conditions with procedures for limb salvaging, or therapies, because they can themselves put a patients at risk of losing the life for saving the limb [18].

The progression of DFS could be actually represented like a spiral progressing from the diagnosis of diabetes to the amputation and eventually death, increasing its width, proportionally with the increasing risk, at any acute phase episode, which in turn should be considered a marker of severity of the progression of the disease [19].

As exemplified in our case series, patients are extremely complex both from a local and systemic point of view, and each of them represents a therapeutic dilemma. Symptoms are scarce and detecting and monitoring them is the only way to drive the decision-making. Heart, kidney, blood, brain, all these organs were involved in our cases, and actively interfered in conditioning the clinical management, posing the question of how to improve the foot condition without worsening the general condition of the patient. In our cases the systemic conditions of the patients were actually in most cases not only worsened the prognosis, but also interfered with the therapeutic choices, consistently narrowing the possible pathways of care, for not risking patients' life.

Cardiac, renal and hematologic decompensation were all part of a multidimensional conundrum conjuring against the actual possibility of patients to survive to both the DFS clinical manifestations and to their possible treatments.

The evaluation of these cases is thus a good example of how complex DFS management can be and how important is an extensive evaluation and a multidisciplinary management, by an experienced team in well-organized dedicated centers [20].

Conclusions

Diabetic foot syndrome is a complex, progressive recurrent disease: its management and the related complications are by far more complex than what the common narration usually tells and deserve an experienced clinical team to be adequately managed.

The acquisition of experiences on all the possible districts involved and on the related complications is mandatory for DFS specialists, even if it is only with the implementation of a multidisciplinary integrated team that this intricate and dangerous pathology finds its only possible way of care.

References

1. Diabetes atlas. 9th ed.s: International Diabetes Federation, 2015 (http://www.diabetesatlas.org)
2. Diabetes atlas. 7th ed. Brussels: International Diabetes Federation, 2015 (http://www.diabetesatlas.org)
3. Lazzarini PA, Pacella RE, Armstrong DG and Van Netten JJ. Diabetes-related lower-extremity complications are a leading cause of the global burden of disability. Diabet Med. 2018. https://doi.org/10.1111/dme.13680
4. Walsh JW, Hoffstad OJ, Sullivan MO, Margolis DJ. Association of diabetic foot ulcer and death in a population-based cohort from the United Kingdom. Diabet Med. 2016;33:1493–8.
5. Armstrong DG, Boulton AJ, Bus SA. Diabetic foot ulcers and their recurrences. N Engl J Med. 2017;376:2367–75.
6. Piaggesi A, Apelqvist J, editors. The diabetic foot syndrome. Front diabetes. Basel, Karger; 2018.
7. Peters EJ, Armstrong DG, Lavery LA. Risk factors for recurrent diabetic foot ulcers: site matters. Diabetes Care. 2007;30(8):2077–9.
8. Wukich DK, Armstrong DG, Attinger CE, Boulton AJ, Burns PR, Frykberg RG, Hellman R, Kim PJ, Lipsky BA, Pile JC, Pinzur MS, Siminerio L. Inpatient management of diabetic foot disorders: a clinical guide. Diabetes Care. 2013;36(9):2862–71.
9. Jeffcoate WJ, Vileikyte L, Boyko EJ, Armstrong DG, Boulton AJM. Current challenges and opportunities in the prevention and management of diabetic foot ulcers. Diabetes Care. 2018;41(4):645–52.
10. Game F. Choosing life or limb. Improving survival in the multi-complex diabetic foot patient. Diabetes Metab Res Rev. 2012;28(Suppl 1):97–100.
11. Edmonds M. Body of knowledge around the diabetic foot and limb salvage. J Cardiovasc Surg (Torino). 2012;53(5):605–16.
12. Liew H, Bates M, Vas P, Rashid H, Kavarthapu V, Edmonds M, Manu C. Resource use within a multidisciplinary foot team clinic. J Wound Care. 2022;31(2):154–61.
13. Apelqvist J. The foot in perspective. Diabetes Metab Res Rev. 2008;24(Suppl 1):S110–5.
14. Scatena A, Petruzzi P, Ferrari M, Rizzo L, Cicorelli A, Berchiolli R, Goretti C, Bargellini I, Adami D, Iacopi E, Del Corso A, Cioni R, Piaggesi A. Outcomes of three years of teamwork on critical limb ischemia in patients with diabetes and foot lesions. Int J Low Extrem Wounds. 2012;11(2):113–9.
15. Spaltro G, Straino S, Gambini E, Bassetti B, Persico L, Zoli S, Zanobini M, Capogrossi MC, Spirito R, Quarti C, et al. Characterization of the Pall Celeris system as a point-of-care device for therapeutic angiogenesis. Cytotherapy. 2015;17:1302–13.
16. Scatena A, Petruzzi P, Maioli F, Lucaroni F, Ambrosone C, Ventoruzzo G, Liistro F, Tacconi D, Di Filippi M, Attempati N, Palombi L, Ercolini L, Bolognese L. Autologous peripheral blood mononuclear cells for limb salvage in diabetic foot patients with no-option critical limb ischemia. J Clin Med. 2021;10(10):2213.
17. Edmonds M, Manu C, Vas P. The current burden of diabetic foot disease. J Clin Orthop Trauma. 2021;8(17):88–93.
18. Edmonds M. Multidisciplinary care of the diabetic foot patient with infection. Int J Low Extrem Wounds. 2010;9(1):6–8.
19. Piaggesi A, Coppelli A, Goretti C, Iacopi E, Mattaliano C. Do you want to organize a multidisciplinary diabetic foot clinic? We can help. Int J Low Extrem Wounds. 2014;13(4):363–70.
20. Schaper NC, Van Netten JJ, Apelqvist J, Lipsky BA, Bakker K. International Working Group on the Diabetic Foot (IWGDF). Prevention and management of foot problems in diabetes: a summary guidance for daily practice 2015, based on the IWGDF guidance documents. Diabetes Res Clin Pract. 2017;124:84–92.

Pressure Ulcers

5

Outti Kaarela, Mihai Băilă, Gelu Onose, Henrik Nuutinen, Tiina Roine, Alina Samia Senn, and Jan Plock

Abstract

Pressure ulcers pose a significant healthcare challenge, particularly for individuals with limited mobility or those on prolonged bed rest. Early identification of at-risk patients using assessment tools like the Braden scale is vital to prevent the onset and recurrence of these ulcers. Pressure ulcers develop from prolonged pressure on areas with minimal soft tissue over bony prominences such as the sacrum, ischial tuberosity, and trochanter major. Treatment involves a thorough assessment of the ulcer's size, depth, stage, and signs of infection or ischemia, alongside considering patient factors le overall health, nutrition, mobility, and comorbidities. The primary goals of treatment are to promote wound healing, prevent further tissue breakdown, and manage infections. While conservative management is fundamental, surgical interventions (e.g. local skin flaps, muscle flaps) may be necessary for deeper wounds or complications, requiring a multidisciplinary approach for optimal outcomes. Successful reconstruction depends on the wound's stability and healing potential. Comprehensive postoperative care is critical, focusing on wound monitoring, drainage management, pain control, and nutritional optimization. Education on wound care and awareness of potential complications are essential to support patient recovery.

O. Kaarela (✉) · T. Roine
Department of Surgery, Oulu University Hospital, Oulu, Finland
e-mail: outi.kaarela@oulu.fi

M. Băilă · G. Onose
Neuromuscular Rehabilitation Clinical Department, Clinical Emergency Hospital "Bagdasar-Arseni", Bucharest, Romania

H. Nuutinen
Department of Surgery, Kuopio University Hospital, University of Eastern Finland, Kuopio, Finland

A. S. Senn · J. Plock
Department for Plastic Surgery and Hand Surgery, Cantonal Hospital Aarau, Aarau, Switzerland

G.-S.Tiplica and K. Isoherranen (eds.), *Wound Healing*,
https://doi.org/10.1007/978-3-031-84579-6_5

Keywords

Pressure ulcer • Pressure sore • Pressure wound • Operative treatment

Introduction

Pressure ulcers, also known as pressure sores, are a significant healthcare challenge, especially for those with limited mobility or prolonged bed rest. Identifying at-risk patients is crucial to prevent occurrences and recurrences. Various assessment tools, notably the Braden scale, aid in evaluating pressure injury risk.

These ulcers result from sustained pressure on areas with minimal soft tissue over bony prominences such as the sacrum, ischial tuberosity, and trochanter major. Treatment begins with thorough ulcer assessment, considering size, depth, stage, and signs of infection or ischemia. Patient factors like overall health, nutrition, mobility, and comorbidities guide treatment decisions.

Effective treatment aims at promoting wound healing, preventing further tissue breakdown, and managing infection. Debridement removes necrotic tissue to facilitate healing and reduce infection risk. While conservative management remains the cornerstone of pressure ulcer treatment, surgical intervention becomes necessary for deeper wounds or complications, requiring a multidisciplinary approach for optimal outcomes. Sometimes due to patient related issues reconstruction can never be considered.

For reconstruction of a pressure ulcer, the wound must be stable and show healing potential. Operative treatment involves removing unhealthy tissue and using local flap techniques or muscle flaps for reconstruction. Careful patient selection, surgical planning, and comprehensive postoperative care are essential for successful outcomes.

Postoperative care focuses on wound monitoring, drainage management, pain control, and optimizing nutrition. Patients with flap reconstruction require a period without weight-bearing post-surgery. Education on wound care and complication awareness supports patient recovery.

In summary, pressure ulcers present significant challenges in healthcare, particularly for immobile individuals. Early identification of at-risk patients and implementation of preventive measures are crucial. Effective treatment strategies, including surgical intervention, when necessary, aim to promote healing and improve patient outcomes. Comprehensive postoperative care and patient education are integral components of successful pressure ulcer management.

Case 5.1. Pressure Ulcer Healing Using Conservatory Interventions and Multiwave Locked System Laser

From within the spectrum of acute/ chronic wounds, with particular addressability in medical and non-medical (e.g. nursing homes) services, are to be found pressure ulcers/ injuries. These lesions frequently appear due to immobility and/ or sensory motor/ cognitive (e.g. altered consciousness) deficits and accompanied by systemic disorders and frailty [1–3].

An 83-year-old patient was admitted in a Neuromuscular Rehabilitation Clinic after a surgically treated left trochanteric fracture (osteosynthesis—fixation with gamma nail). The patient comorbidities were type II diabetes mellitus (treated with oral hypoglycemic medications), venous insufficiency and arterial hypertension. The clinical examination revealed a right buttock grade II eschar with elements of necrosis (Fig. 5.1a) and a body mass index of 41.23 (grade III obesity). The evaluation of the functional and nutritional status resulted in a Barthel Index of 20/100 points and a total score of the Mini nutritional assessment scale of 14.5 (IR = 24–30 normal nutritional status; 17–23 = at risk for malnutrition; < 17 = malnourished). The diagnosis of malnourishment was further evaluated with blood tests (Hb = 9.4 g/dL − IR = 12–16 g/dL; Prealbumin = 0.15 g/L − RI = 0.2–0.4 g/L; Albumin = 2,5 g/dL − RI = 3.4–4 g/dL, Iron = 37 mcg/dL − RI = 50–170 μg/dL, Transferrin = 208 mg/dL − RI = 173–260 mg/dL).

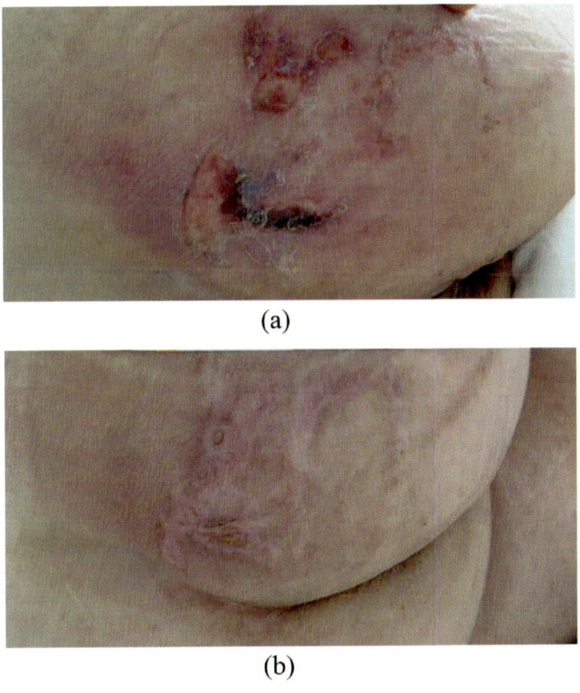

Fig. 5.1 (a) Grade II right buttock eschar. (b) Healed eschar grade II after 4 weeks

The patient followed a complex treatment consisting of rehabilitation nursing (pressure relief mattress, in-bed turning every 4–5 h), daily dressing with: antiseptic solution (based on hypochlorous acid, sodium hypochlorite) and silver sulfadiazine cream; 3 times every week for three weeks, before applying the dressings, LASER Multiwave Locked System (MLS) were performed with following parameters: 700 Hz, 2 J/cm^2, duration automatically set. The pharmacological treatment consisted of iron supplements ($\times$ 2 times), anticoagulant (enoxaparin sodium), hypoglycemic drugs and antibiotic therapy (rifaximin—for acute diarrheal disease and sulfamethoxazole/trimethoprim—for urinary tract colonization). The patient occasionally took NSAIDs (diclofenac). After 4 weeks of treatment the eschar was healed (Fig. 5.1b).

Local and/or systemic unfavorable conditions deplete the body's resources in a vicious circle, making the healing of pressure injuries particularly difficult and possibly delayed. The evolution of tissue regeneration becomes blocked/stopped by complex mechanisms of dysfunction of cells and subcellular components at the level of the wound bed: excessive inflammation and lytic activity, constant degradation of the extracellular matrix and the impossibility of new tissue formation and the impossibility of counteracting harmful bacterial flora colonization [4, 5]. The MLS LASER could prove to be an effective, non-invasive and risk-free therapeutic option that has the potential to contribute significantly to initiating/ accelerating the healing of pressure ulcers.

Case 5.2. Chronic Ischial Pressure Wound

Introduction

The patient is a 63-year-old woman. She has severe juvenile rheumatoid arthritis, type 2 diabetes mellitus, coronary artery disease and chronic atrial fibrillation. She has total endoprosthesis in both hips and knees and left elbow. During operative treatment significant medications were leflunomide, prednisolone, hydroxychloroquine and apixaban.

In 2010 a problematic rheumatoid nodule was removed from the area of left ischial tuberosity with open surgery. In 2018 and 2021 there was an acute abscess on the same area, and after 2021 the wound never healed properly with conservative treatment.

Differential Diagnosis

During 2018 to 2022 the patient's ischial wound was considered to be partly iatrogenic, due to the rheumatoid nodule removal, and partly pressure ulcer, due to the typical area. Other differential diagnosis considerations were infection of the hip endoprosthesis (but there was no sign of that in MRI) and a specific skin pathology (e.g. pyoderma gangrenosum, vasculitis). In the final debridement of the wound the excised tissue was sent to pathology and histopathological finding was chronic wound and inflammation, no histopathological findings of pyoderma gangrenosum or vasculitis as aetiology.

Treatment

The patient was evaluated for the first time in 2018 but then she was not interested in reconstructive surgery. The next evaluation was in the summer 2022, and at that point there had been an open wound on the left ischial tuberosity for 15 months. During that time there had been two major infections originating from the ischial wound. After debridement the wound bed was viable (Fig. 5.2). Otherwise the situation remained steady, and the patient was still hesitant about reconstructive surgery. There were few treatment periods (lasting 2–3 months) with negative pressure wound therapy. Periodically the wound was treated with silver-based products and care was taken to avoid maceration of surrounding tissue. During conservative treatment we made sure to optimize pressure relief, nutrition, blood glucose level and the treatment of background illnesses. During the winter 2022–2023 there were two more acute infections and at the same time the patient's ability to move independently slowly decreased. Eventually due to bilateral quadriceps tears and knee instability the patient was hardly able to stand let alone walk without significant outer support. Orthopedic surgeons considered operative treatment for the right knee and therefore it was crucial to try and fix the ischial wound.

In the fall of 2023 (Fig. 5.3), we proceeded to methylene blue assisted radical excision of the wound bed combined with reconstruction of the area with rotational

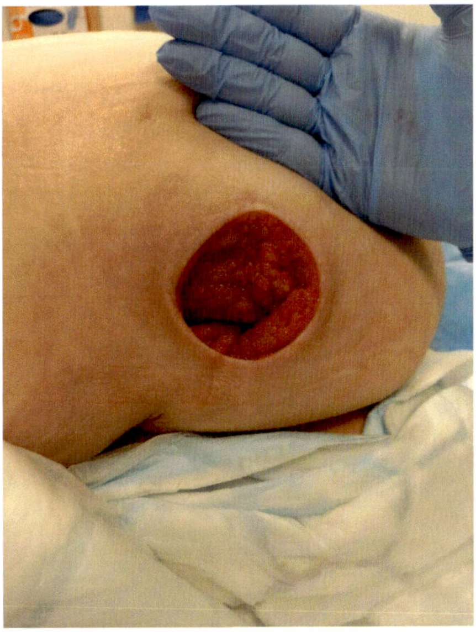

Fig. 5.2 Chronic ischial tuberosity pressure ulcer after debridement of necrotic tissue on the left

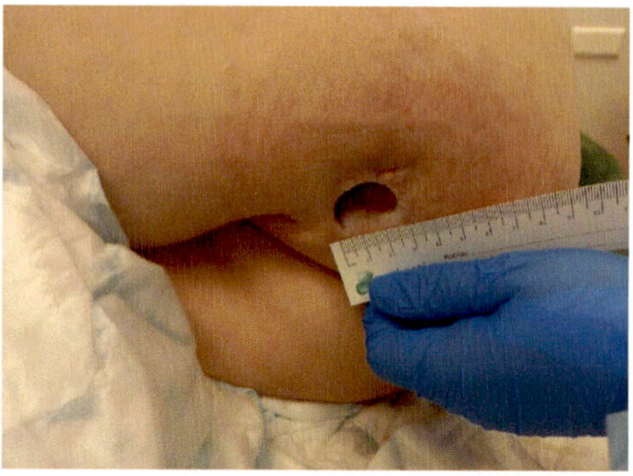

Fig. 5.3 Chronic wound on left ischial tuberosity just prior to operation on the right

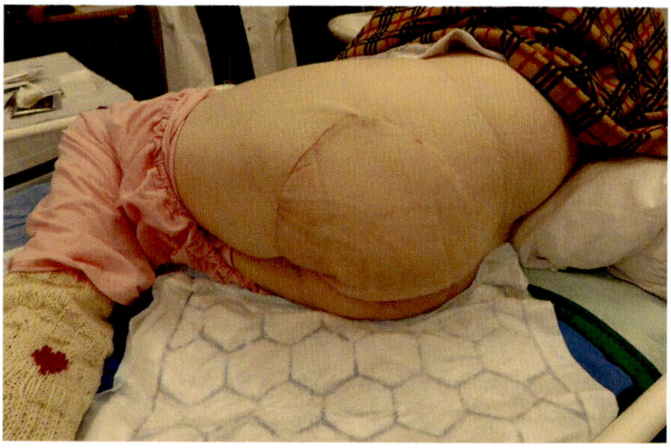

Fig. 5.4 The operated healed ischial pressure ulcerone month postoperatively

flap. A large rotation flap was designed over the left gluteal area and the defect was covered with it. The patient was forbidden to lay on her left side or sit for 6 weeks. At the 1-month postoperative control the flap and the wound had healed nicely (Fig. 5.4). At 4 months the outcome of the flap reconstruction was still good, and the patient was living without a chronic wound. Unfortunately, now the situation with the knees and atrophic leg muscles was so severe that orthopedics had to abandon all operative plans regarding the lower extremities.

Discussions

The correct timing of wound reconstruction is essential. Pressure ulcers lower the quality of life of the patients in many ways. Delayed healing leads to extended hospital stays, re-admissions and restricted rehabilitation and treatment options for other medical conditions [6].

Preoperative evaluation and patient optimizing, consisting of nutrition, pressure management, topical wound care and stabilization of background illnesses, is very important before surgical treatment. Infection management plans should also be made preoperatively since chronic wounds are always contaminated. Possibility of osteomyelitis needs to be taken care of [7].

It is shown that fascio-cutaneous flaps are equally reliable in reconstruction of pressure wounds as musculocutaneous flaps. In addition, fascio-cutaneous tissue is more susceptible to ischemia than muscle and there is no need to sacrifice a muscle (which might lead to functional impairment) [8]. In spinal injury patients it is shown that operative treatment of severe pressure ulcers leads to better quality of life [9].

The wound reconstruction in this patient was successful (of course the short follow-up period must be noted). Perhaps this patient would have benefited from earlier wound reconstruction and thus the needed orthopedic treatment would have been possible. Nevertheless, flap reconstruction cannot and should not be performed without full concordance from the patient.

Case 5.3. Negative Pressure Treatment and Flap Reconstruction of Sacral Pressure Ulcer

Introduction

A 77-year old man was driven to the hospital due to an acute stomach, the man also had tetraparesis before. As a complication of the treatment, the patient developed a pressure ulcer of the sacrum. The size of the pressure ulcer was 3 cm × 3 cm. Soft tissue necrosis was found (Fig. 5.5a).

Differential Diagnosis

The patient had a clear cause-and-effect relationship for developing the pressure ulcer. The other causes of the ulcer were not considered.

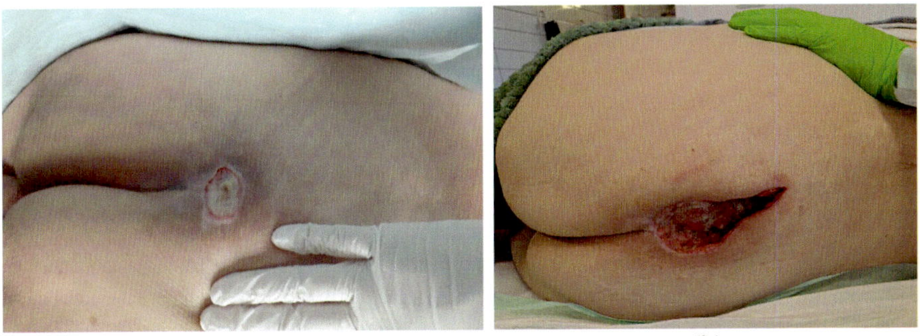

(a) (b)

Fig. 5.5 a Sacral pressure ulcer at the beginning and b after 1.5 months

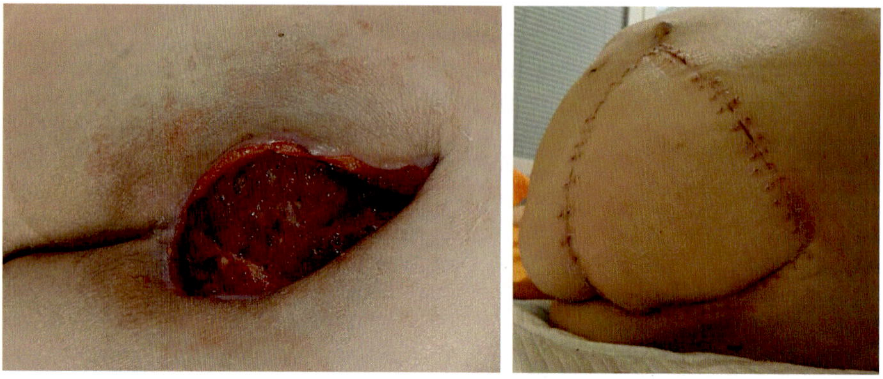

(a) (b)

Fig. 5.6 a The pressure ulcer (10 cm × 6 cm) before reconstruction and b 1.5 months after VY-flap reconstruction

Treatment

The treatment of the pressure ulcer started with conservative treatment, which included posture therapy, a pressure mattress, a protein-rich diet, and local wound treatment with medical honey. At the outpatient clinic, approximately 1.5 months after starting the local treatment, the size of the pressure ulcer was increased (10 cm × 6 cm) and as usual, the wound deepened on follow-up, and a bone contact at the bottom of the wound was suspected (Fig. 5.5b). The wound was clinically infected, and surgical debridement in the operating room was required. There was *Pseudomonas* growth on the wound, and the patient was treated intravenously with piperacillin and tazobactam while in the ward.

After the infection subsided, negative pressure wound therapy (NPWT) (125 mmHg) was started. NPWT continued for approximately for a month (Fig. 5.6a). After that, flap reconstruction was planned and was performed with VY-flap-style. About 1.5 months after surgery the operational area and flap reconstruction seemed successful (Fig. 5.6b).

Discussion

Pressure ulcers are tissue damage resulting from sustained mechanical loading on the skin and underlying tissues. They typically develop over areas subjected to prolonged pressure, shear, or friction, such as bony prominences [10]. Pathogenesis involves a complex interplay of ischemia, inflammation, and tissue necrosis, necessitating comprehensive assessment and management strategies to mitigate risk factors and optimize healing outcomes [11]. Sacral pressure ulcers are the most commonly affected site [12]. Treatment of pressure ulcers involves relieving pressure on the affected area, maintaining proper wound care to promote healing and prevent infection, ensuring adequate nutrition, addressing underlying medical conditions, considering surgical interventions if necessary, managing pain, and monitoring progress closely [3]. Negative pressure therapy may speed up the reduction of the pressure ulcer size [13]. The primary treatment for pressure ulcers is conservative. However, infection or exposure of vital structures such as a tendon, vessel, or bone may lead to surgical intervention. These are typical in deep, grade III to IV pressure ulcers [14].

Case 5.4. Pressure Ulcer Grade IV

An 80-year-old patient undergoing diagnostic procedures for diffuse myelopathy after sudden and progressive paraparesis was referred for Plastic Surgery consultation. The initial examination exhibited a 4 × 5 cm large full thickness skin necrosis with perifocal redness (Fig. 5.7). The lesion had been treated conservatively for 4 weeks with disinfection and gauze dressings. The lesion was diagnosed as grade III or IV pressure ulcer.

Conservative treatment consisted of constant pressure relief with an alternating pressure system and optimization of his nutritional status. The initial examination of the lesion showed an insubstantially infected wound environment with low to medium secretion, so a hydrofiber wound dressing (Aquacel®) was applied with local skin protection (3 M™ Cavilon™ Lolly) for the wound surrounding. When exudate levels increased and erythematous wound surrounding were observed, an iodine-based product (3 M™ Inadine™) was applied to counteract bacterial surface colonization. The dressings were changed daily. Due to a progressive wound status with high suspicion of infection of the underlying bone, broad spectrum antibiotic treatment (piperacillin/tazobactam) was started, and debridement and local defect reconstruction was planned.

Due to exhaustion of conservative treatment, surgical necrosectomy and sampling was performed. Macroscopically, the os coccyges was highly suspicious of osteomyelitis. Consecutively complete resection of the os coccyges was performed

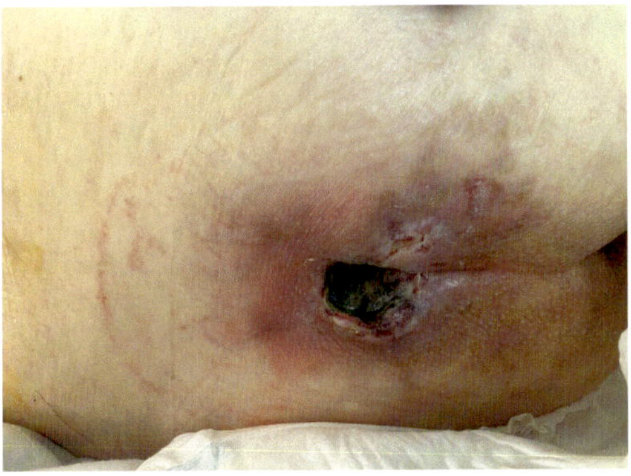

Fig. 5.7 Pressure ulcer grade III-IV, central full-thickness skin defect, perifocal erythema, no fluctuation

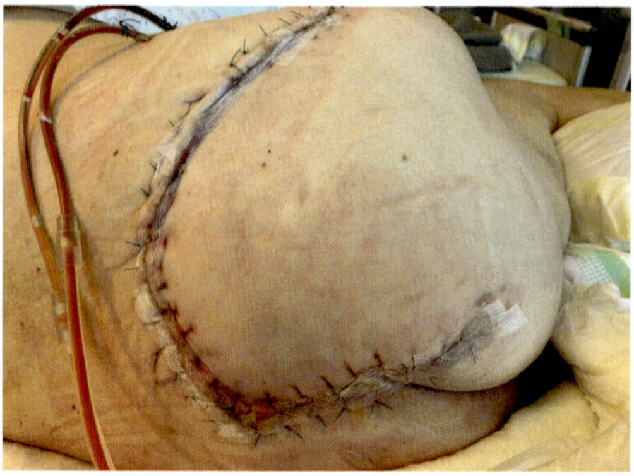

Fig. 5.8 Gluteal rotational fasciocutaneous flap. Vital flap with drainages still in place

leaving a defect size (10 × 11 cm) too large for direct closure. For a safe and reliable defect closure with exposed bone, a fasciocutaneous gluteal rotation flap was chosen (Fig. 5.8). Histopathology confirmed the diagnosis of acute osteomyelitis, biopsies from the remaining os sacrum showed it was unaffected. The patient received antibiotic regimen adjusted according to the antibiogram (ciprofloxacin and clindamycin) for 6 weeks total due to the open laying bone before surgical treatment to address an osteitis.

Following surgery, bedrest for one week with permanent decompression of the flap for 6 weeks was recommended. Sitting exercises started after 4 weeks. The healing processes showed no adverse events.

Flap surgery for pressure ulcer therapy is well established. However there is no clear evidence on timing, favorable flap selection or combination with negative wound pressure therapy so far [15].

Acknowledgements Artificial intelligence-assisted language proofreading was used (Grammarly).

References

1. HL Chen JY Cai L Du HW Shen HR Yu YP Song 2020 Incidence of pressure injury in individuals with spinal cord injury J Wound Ostomy Continence Nurs 47 3 215 223
2. Popescu C, Onose G. Current conservative approaches and novelties on pressure sores in patients needing neurorehabilitation. J Med Life. 2012;5(Spec Issue):95–101.
3. J Kottner J Cuddigan K Carville K Balzer D Berlowitz S Law 2019 Prevention and treatment of pressure ulcers/injuries: the protocol for the second update of the international clinical practice guideline 2019 J Tissue Viability 28 2 51 58
4. Wilkinson HN, Hardman MJ. Wound healing: cellular mechanisms and pathological outcomes. Open Biol. 2020;10(9).
5. Oshiro T, Popa M, B Niculae, Savu B. Laserterapie si chirurgie laser in dermatologie. Editura Național; 2000.
6. Gorecki C, Brown JM, Nelson EA, Briggs M, Schoonhoven L, Dealey C, et al.; European quality of life pressure ulcer project group. Impact of pressure ulcers on quality of life in older patients: a systematic review. J Am Geriatr Soc. 2009;57(7):1175–83. https://doi.org/10.1111/j.1532-5415.2009.02307.x. Epub 2009 May 21. PMID: 19486198.

7. J Bauer LG Phillips 2008 MOC-PSSM CME article: pressure sores Plast Reconstr Surg 121 1 Suppl 1 10
8. M Sameem M Au T Wood F Farrokhyar J Mahoney 2012 A systematic review of complication and recurrence rates of musculocutaneous, fasciocutaneous, and perforator-based flaps for treatment of pressure sores Plast Reconstr Surg 130 1 67e 77e
9. R Singh R Singh RK Rohilla R Siwach V Verma K Kaur 2010 Surgery for pressure ulcers improves general health and quality of life in patients with spinal cord injury J Spinal Cord Med 33 4 396 400
10. E Hahnel A Lichterfeld U Blume-Peytavi J Kottner 2017 The epidemiology of skin conditions in the aged: a systematic review J Tissue Viability 26 1 20 28 https://doi.org/10.1016/j.jtv.2016.04.001 Epub 2016 Apr 27 PMID: 27161662
11. B Pieper D Langemo J Cuddigan 2009 Pressure ulcer pain: a systematic literature review and national pressure ulcer advisory panel white paper Ostomy Wound Manage 55 2 16 31 PMID: 19246782
12. C Vangilder GD Macfarlane S Meyer 2008 Results of nine international pressure ulcer prevalence surveys: 1989 to 2005 Ostomy Wound Manage 54 2 40 54 PMID: 18382042
13. Shi J, Gao Y, Tian J, Li J, Xu J, Mei F, et al. Negative pressure wound therapy for treating pressure ulcers. Cochrane Database Syst Rev. 2023;5(5):CD011334. https://doi.org/10.1002/14651858.CD011334.pub3. PMID: 37232410; PMCID: PMC10218975.
14. Bosanquet DC, Wright AM, White RD, Williams IM. A review of the surgical management of heel pressure ulcers in the 21st century. Int Wound J. 2016;13(1):9–16. https://doi.org/10.1111/iwj.12416. Epub 2015 Feb 16. PMID: 25683573; PMCID: PMC7949530.
15. Norman G, Wong JK, Amin K, Dumville JC, Pramod S. Reconstructive surgery for treating pressure ulcers. Cochrane Database Syst Rev. 2022;10(10):CD012032. https://doi.org/10.1002/14651858.CD012032.pub3. PMID: 36228111; PMCID: PMC9562145.

Cutaneous Wounds in Systemic Disorders

6

Tanja Planinsek Rucigaj, Spela Suler Baglama, Vid Bajuk, Aleksandra Bergant Suhodolcan, Katarina Smuc Berger, Bor Hrvatin Stancic, Lidija Plaskan, and Eva Rauh

Abstract

Cutaneous wounds in systemic disorders pose significant challenges for physicians in terms of diagnosis and treatment. Different pathogenic causes with characteristic clinical picture needs a special tailored therapeutic approach. Chronic relapsing ulcerative wounds, including those related to venous insufficiency, neuropathy, and diabetes, account for 85% of cases. The remaining 15% are atypical wounds linked to various systemic conditions as granulomatosis with polyangiitis, Martorell leg ulcer, chronic prurigo, necrobiosis lipoidica, factitial skin ulcers to name only a few. All wounds benefit from modern dressings adapted to the wound bed and the systemic diagnosis. A multidisciplinary approach is necessary for establishing the diagnosis and optimal systemic treatment. The training requirements for systemic wounds address diagnostic and therapeutic measures and are highlighted by the European Training Requirements (ETR) of Wound Healing Multiple Joint Committee (MJC) of the European Union of Medical Specialists (UEMS).

T. P. Rucigaj (✉) · S. S. Baglama · V. Bajuk · A. B. Suhodolcan · B. H. Stancic
Dermatovenereological Clinic, University Medical Centre Ljubljana, Ljubljana, Slovenia
e-mail: t.rucigaj@gmail.com

T. P. Rucigaj
Angela Boskin Faculty of Health Care, Jesenice, Slovenia

V. Bajuk · A. B. Suhodolcan · B. H. Stancic
Faculty of Medicine, University of Ljubljana, Ljubljana, Slovenia

K. S. Berger
Dermatovenereological Outpatient Office, General Hospital Izola, Izola, Slovenia

L. Plaskan
Department of Medical Rehabilitation, General Hospital Celje, Celje, Slovenia

E. Rauh
General Hospital Novo Mesto, Novo Mesto, Slovenia

G.-S.Tiplica and K. Isoherranen (eds.), *Wound Healing*,
https://doi.org/10.1007/978-3-031-84579-6_6

Keywords

Hard-to-heal wounds • Systemic disease • Vasculitis • Granulomatosis with polyangiitis • Pyoderma gangrenosum-like ulcer • Martorell Hypertensive Ischemic Leg Ulcer (HYTILU) • Chronic prurigo • Necrobiosis lipoidica • Self-inflicted ulcers • Artefactal ulcers • Lymphoedema • Epidermolysis bullosa • Squamous cell carcinomas • ANCA • Vasculitis • Ulcer • Chronic wound • Chronic ulcer • Necrotic ulcer • Prurigo nodularis • Pruritus • Atypical wound • Wound and depressive disorder • Bizarre-shaped wounds • Erysipelas recidivans • Mixed ulcer • Marjolin ulcer

Introduction

Patients with chronic hard-to-heal wounds present specific challenges for the treating physician, both for establishing a diagnosis and treatment. Wound healing is inter-disciplinary and even inter-professional. In these approaches we have persons with different areas of expertise collaborating but they all must have a common understanding of wound healing, so that they are able to professionally talk to each other and finally find the best solution for the patient. The present chapter selects hard-to-heal cutaneous ulcers in patients with systemic disorders as a part of the wound healing European Training requirements (ETR). The clinical cases presentations include information on the different pathogenic causes of chronic wounds, clinical assessment and therapeutic concepts.

Chronic relapsing ulcerative wounds, also known as hard-to-heal wounds, persist for more than 6–8 weeks and typically affect the extremities. They are commonly linked to venous insufficiency, edema, neuropathy, impaired arterial circulation, and diabetes. Around 85% of chronic ulcers stem from these conditions. The remaining 15% are categorized as atypical wounds, which are associated with a variety of other conditions, often systemic, allergological, neurological, psychiatric/psychosomatic, mixed, or of undetermined origin. One of them is granulomatosis with polyangiitis. This is a rare pauci-immune ANCA-associated vasculitis where the diagnosis is supported by a positive biopsy, combined with a typical clinical presentation and the presence of either PR3-ANCA or myeloperoxidase (MPO)-ANCA serology. Most patients with granulomatosis with polyangiitis endure prodromal constitutional symptoms for months before the emergence of more specific symptoms. These include palpable purpura, mucocutaneous ulcers, subcutaneous nodules, ulcers resembling pyoderma gangrenosum, digital necrosis, papulo-necrotic lesions, and livedo racemosa, listed in order of decreasing frequency. The induction of remission for organ- or life-threatening Granulomatosis with polyangiitis involves a combination of glucocorticoids with either rituximab or cyclophosphamide. For non-organ- or non-life-threatening Granulomatosis with polyangiitis, the recommended combination is glucocorticoids with methotrexate, or rituximab (monotherapy). Azathioprine, methotrexate, and mycophenolate mofetil are alternatives to rituximab.

Cutaneous and other vasculitides are specific inflammations of the blood vessel wall that can happen in the skin or in any organ of the body. Vasculitis is classified based on the size of the affected vessels, which can be small, medium, or large [1]. Cutaneous vasculitis can reflect a cutaneous component of a systemic vasculitis, a skin-limited or skin-dominant expression or variant of a systemic vasculitis or be a single-organ vasculitis per se [2]. Clinical presentation of vasculitis is most commonly palpable purpura on the lower extremities. The depth of affected vessels is correlated with the type of cutaneous lesions. If small superficial vessels are involved, the lesions are urticarial plaques and papules, but relatively persistent. Involvement of vessels in the dermo-hypodermic junction or hypodermis results in ulcers, nodules, or livedo [2]. The type of inflammatory infiltrate is a key finding for the diagnosis of cutaneous vasculitis. Leukocytoclastic vasculitis is a pathophysiological process common to different causes [2]. The diagnosis of vasculitis relies on anamnesis, clinical manifestation and also on the histopathological and immunofluorescence studies [1]. Eosinophilic granulomatosis with polyangiitis (EGPA) is a rare, multi-system, inflammatory disease, belonging to the group of anti-neutrophil cytoplasmic antibody (ANCA)-associated vasculitides (AAV) [3].

On the wound bed of vasculitic wounds we often find necrosis. Another wound where we can find necrosis in the wound bed is Martorell Hypertensive Ischemic Leg Ulcer (HYTILU). This type of ulcer is a rare, progressive, disproportionately painful, necrotic ulcer on the lower extremities. Histopathological diagnostics with arteriolar calcification, subendothelial hyalinosis, and arteriolar cellularity [4], appropriate laboratory and radiological examinations, as well as direct immunofluorescence may be required in order to exclude other possible etiologies. In the differential diagnosis, care must be taken when differentiating it from pyoderma gangrenosum and necrotic vasculitis, where therapy differs greatly. 'The red lipstick sign' could be a novel clinical diagnostic feature in HYTILUs alongside purple border, livedo racemosa and necrotic/fibrinous ulcer bed [5]. Patients with Martorell ulcers need analgesics, and blood pressure regulation.

Chronic prurigo is another ulcerative condition characterized by persistent pruritus, lasting at least six weeks, and presenting with localized or generalized pruritic skin lesions, such as whitish or pinkish papules, nodules, and/or plaques [6]. Recent studies have demonstrated that the pathophysiology of pruritus involves neuroimmune interactions, opening up new therapeutic perspectives [6]. Chronic prurigo, a skin disease resistant to treatment, is managed with topical and systemic therapies, as well as phototherapy [7].

Necrobiosis lipoidica is a rare, chronic granulomatous disease of the skin that can lead to ulcerations of the skin in up to 30% [8]. Many patients with necrobiosis lipoidica also have diabetes mellitus. Early therapeutic choice for non-ulcerated necrobiosis lipoidica is usually topical treatment with a high-potency topical corticosteroid applied under occlusion and compression therapy. When ulcers occur, they heal slowly and can be difficult to treat.

Ulcers that are also difficult to treat and even more difficult to diagnose are self-inflicted ulcers—artefactal ulcers. Dermatitis artefacta (factitious skin disorder) is a rare psychocutaneous disorder that poses a complex clinical challenge to clinicians [9]. Self-inflicted lesions are most often in accessible areas as the face, mucosae and extremities, involves the hair or nails, and do not correlate with organic disease patterns [9, 10]. We have to carry out extensive diagnostics, and laboratory tests to exclude inflammatory, infectious, vascular, malignant and other reasons for wounds, which primarily excludes the diagnosis or etiology of more common, typical wounds. In this patients it is essential to focus on the psychological disorders and life stressors that have predisposed the condition with which patients satisfy a psychological need, attract attention, or evade responsibility [9, 10]. Numerous erosions and ulcers of unusual shapes in unusual places are often a sign of self-harm.

Wounds and chronic oedema are common disorders, but rarely studied together [11]. The estimated prevalence of chronic oedema is 57% in patients cared for by community nurses in the UK and 38% in hospitals in Europe [11]. Complications include cellulitis and chronic wounds. Despite this, chronic oedema with wounds remains a neglected condition [11]. When the patient is not sufficiently or incorrectly treated for the underlying disease, there may be deterioration and the formation of ulcers, such as in patients with untreated or insufficiently treated lymphedema, especially if this is accompanied by poor blood circulation, where they can also be visible at the base of the wound necrosis. In the case of untreated lymphedema, the swelling can be joined by an infection—erysipelas, which further worsens the swelling. Burian et al. found that the severity of the chronic oedema (n = 738) wounds affected 27.33% with ISL stage I, 38.67% in stage II, and 34.00% in stage III. Only 43.22% of the patient cohort with wounds had well-controlled chronic leg oedema [11]. They confirm that secondary lymphoedema has a higher association with wounds than primary lymphoedema.

Chronic wounds and chronic skin damage are risk factors for malignant skin diseases. Malignant tumors that occur in chronic wounds are more aggressive, more resistant to therapy and are also more likely to metastasize. The studies agree that a biopsy should be performed on any non-healing ulcer that is resistant to treatment. However, exactly when to opt for the procedure itself has not yet been standardized. Epidermolysis bullosa is a term for a heterogeneous group of rare skin diseases ranging from mild to life-threatening, all clinically characterized by skin and/or mucosal fragility and blistering in response to minor injury or mechanical trauma. Due to impaired skin healing and the associated chronic inflammation, Epidermolysis bullosa also represents a risk factor for skin malignancies. Squamous cell carcinomas in patients with Epidermolysis bullosa have a high likelihood of metastasis and mortality [12]. In systematic review they found that from 367 patients Squamous cell carcinomas were the most common malignancy (94.3%) with 18,8% and median survival 16.8 months [12]. In severe recessive dystrophic epidermolysis bullosa, the risk of mortality due to squamous cell carcinoma rises to 78.8% at 55 years old from 38.7% at 35 years old, and the median survival is approximately 5 years following initial squamous cell carcinoma diagnosis [13].

All chronic wounds are treated locally with modern dressings for wound treatment, depending on the tissue at wound bed of the ulcer, of course after diagnosis. A multidisciplinary approach is often necessary for establishing a diagnosis, and often also for optimal systemic treatment of chronic wounds.

The training requirements for systemic wounds address diagnostic and therapeutic measures. The trainees will be able to:

- Explain the factors that are of importance in relation to systemic wound healing and describe the stages of wound healing.
- Describe the risk factors, causative mechanisms, and essential features of the systemic wounds.
- Summarize the most important evidence-based systemic wound care recommendations.
- Outline the clinical classifications commonly used in systemic wound care and apply in practice those classifications that are relevant (e.g. CEAP classification system, SINBAD score, Nomenclature of Cutaneous Vasculitis).
- Summarize which pieces of anamnestic information and clinical findings are relevant and adapt this knowledge to interviewing and examining the patient with systemic wounds.
- Assess the patient's quality of life.
- Assess the patient's adherence to treatment.
- Outline screening for malnutrition, assess the nutritional status of the patient, and identify malnutrition.
- Assess the pain associated with a systemic wound.
- Identify the common systemic wounds.
- Identify the situations in which atypical wound should be suspected.
- Identify delayed systemic wound healing and assess its risk factors.
- Summarize the tissue effects of aging and the role of aging in tissue healing, and apply this knowledge to systemic wound care.
- Choose the appropriate laboratory and imaging studies required in the diagnostics and treatment of systemic wounds.
- Understand that treatment must be based on a diagnosis, evidence-based and patient-centered.
- Plan the treatment according to the aetiology and characteristics of the systemic wound.
- Assess the treatment options realistically and determine the appropriate treatment limitations.

Case 6.1. Granulomatosis with Polyangiitis Debut: The Pyoderma Gangrenosum-Like Ulcer

Case Presentation

A 57-year-old patient with dyslipidemia was referred to our department due to an 8-month persistent chronic umbilical ulcer, which originated from a livid patch and proved refractory to conventional treatments, including multiple rounds of oral antibiotics. Hypergranulations developed, progressing into an ulcer post-necrotomies. The patient experienced a weight loss of 5 kg, attributed to loss of appetite. One month before referral, additional symptoms manifested: severely painful gum changes, haemorrhagic discharge from the right nostril, and inflammation of the left lower eyelid. No other symptoms were reported by the patient.

Upon examination, no abnormalities were noted in general assessments. However, a notable finding was an undermined ulcer with a violaceous border in the umbilical area, measuring 4.5 × 3 cm, which was 3 cm deep, covered with little granulation and 80% of fibrin (Fig. 6.1). There was a granulation tissue on the central part of the conjunctiva of the left lower eyelid with ulceration and a purulent discharge (Fig. 6.2). Gums exhibited hypertrophy with cobblestone or strawberry-like appearance (Fig. 6.3). Additional otorhinolaryngological examination revealed the presence of necrosis accompanied by purulent and dried linings in the area of the right middle concha of the nose and anterior to it. Furthermore, distinct granulations were observed on the lower alveolar ridge.

To refine the diagnosis, various differential considerations were explored. Laboratory tests revealed elevated inflammatory parameters, with a C-reactive protein (CRP) level of 102 mg/dL, sedimentation rate (SR) of 58 mm/h, mildly increased leukocytes (11.8×10^9/L) and neutrophils (8.15×10^9/L). Bacterial swab analysis

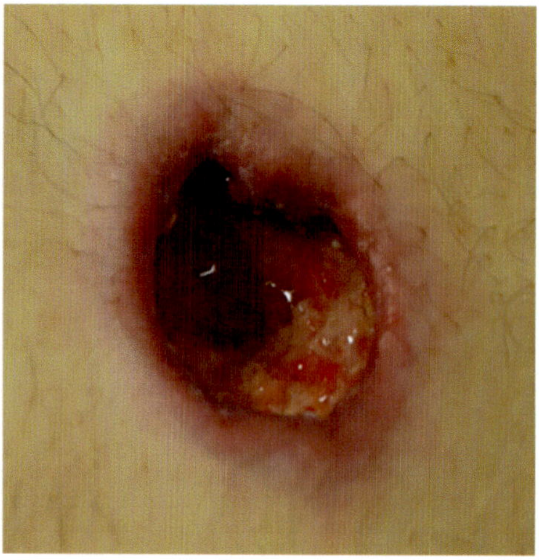

Fig. 6.1 Undermined ulcer with a violaceous border in the umbilical area, measuring 4.5 × 3 cm, 3 cm deep, featuring minimal granulation and 80% fibrin cover

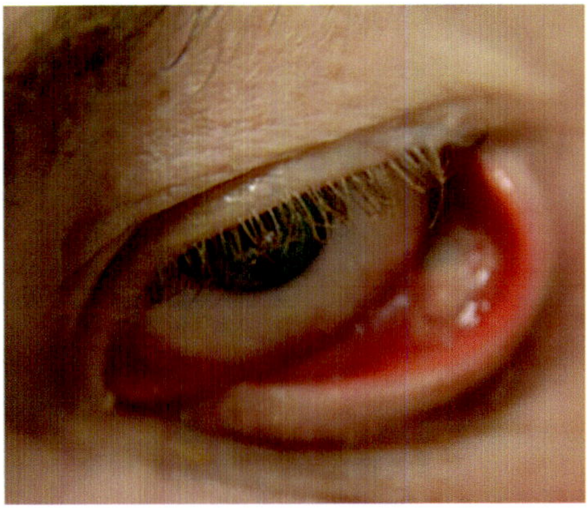

Fig. 6.2 Granulation tissue on the central part of the conjunctiva of the left lower eyelid, accompanied by ulceration and purulent discharge

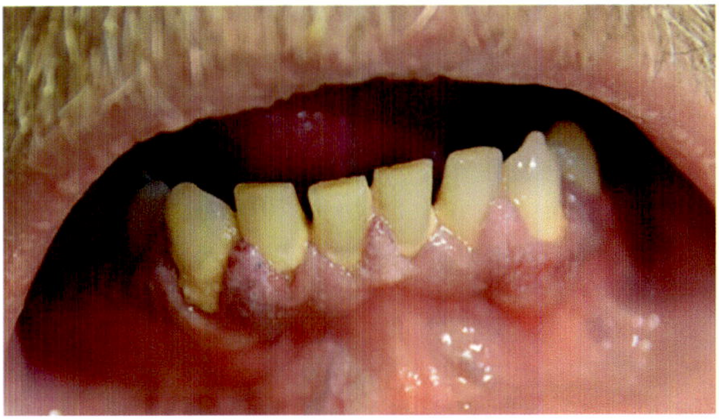

Fig. 6.3 Hypertrophy of the lower gums with a distinctive cobblestone or strawberry-like appearance

of the abdominal ulcer indicated the presence of *Pseudomonas aeruginosa*, sensitive to all antibiotics tested. However, swabs from the right nasal cavity, left lower eyelid, and oral cavity, as well as hemocultures returned negative results for both fungi and bacteria. Galactomannan and beta-D-glucan tests also yielded negative results.

Extensive biochemistry laboratory testing revealed a slight elevation in gamma-GT (2.36 μkat/L). Extensive additional tests, including indirect immunofluorescence testing for pemphigus and pemphigoid antibodies, antinuclear antibody, extractable nuclear antigen test, C3 and C4 complement, antibodies against C1q, a comprehensive tumor marker panel, lactate dehydrogenase, quantiferon test, and serology for hepatitis B virus, hepatitis C virus, and human immunodeficiency virus all reported negative results or values within the reference range. Serum protein electrophoresis demonstrated an asymmetric distribution of gamma globulin subtypes, suggesting the potential presence of immune complexes. Importantly, a positive immunoglobulin G c-antineutrophil cytoplasmic antibody (ANCA) with a titre of 1:20 and proteinase 3 (PR3) at 126 CU was detected. Chronic inflammatory bowel disease was ruled out based on a negative history, calprotectin test, and endoscopic examinations.

The orthopantomogram revealed only dental caries, which seemed inconsistent with the severe pain in the maxillary region reported by the patient. To further investigate, a CT scan of the paranasal sinuses was conducted. This revealed mucosal thickening with calcifications and extensive osteolytic changes/bone resorption in the alveolar ridge of the maxilla or the floor of the maxillary sinuses bilaterally at multiple sites. In addition, a CT scan of the abdomen was performed to assess the extent of umbilical ulceration. The results additionally showed abscess-like changes in the basal parts of the lungs and in the prostate. The patient exhibited no pulmonary or urinary tract symptoms, with negative findings in urine sediment, urine culture, and normal results in pulmonary function tests.

Several biopsies were conducted, each revealing distinct pathological findings. A biopsy from the umbilical ulceration indicated pseudoepitheliomatous hyperplasia accompanied by necrosant inflammation in the dermis. Subsequent examination unveiled vasculitis/vasculopathic changes and epithelioid granulomas. The gum biopsy exhibited polypoid changes characterized by markedly hyperplastic squamous epithelium and intense mixed chronic suppurative inflammation. Additionally, a biopsy of intranasal granulation tissue demonstrated intense mixed cellular inflammatory exudation in the subepithelial connective tissue, with mildly increased eosinophils. Individual vessels displayed fibrinoid necrosis of the wall, some of which showed initial recanalization after previous connective tissue obliteration. Staining for bacteria, fungi and mycobacteria was negative in all biopsies.

Through a thorough correlation of clinical, pathological, and serological data, the diagnosis of granulomatosis with polyangiitis (GPA) was made.

Treatment

Systemic Treatment

Following the referral, we promptly initiated 1 mg/kg prednisolone equivalent/day orally with proton pump inhibitor, calcium carbonate and vitamin D as anti-ulcer and anti-osteoporotic protection. Due to intense pain in the maxillary area, the patient required analgesia, including opioids, amitriptyline, and pregabalin, with careful titration.

Topical Treatment

Umbilical ulcer was gently cleaned every second day and covered by alginate silver dressing. The oral cavity was treated with 1% lidocaine in orabase and 0.1% triamcinolone in orabase, both administered three times a day. Additionally, the left eye underwent saline solution irrigation, followed by the application of an ointment containing a combination of dexamethasone, polymyxin B, and neomycin.

Outcome

After the initiation of therapy, CRP and SR decreased to 27 mg/dL and 29 mm/h, respectively. However, leukocytosis increased to 18.5×10^9/L, and neutrophilia rose to 14.2×10^9/L, potentially attributed to the systemic corticosteroid therapy. Upon the confirmation of a diagnosis of granulomatosis with polyangiitis, the patient was subsequently referred to the rheumatology department for additional diagnostic assessments and further treatment with rituximab. Regrettably, feedback on the efficacy of this treatment is unavailable, as the patient did not return for follow-up appointments.

Discussion

Our case report delves into the intriguing presentation of GPA in a 57-year-old patient, where the initial manifestation took an unexpected form—an umbilical pyoderma-gangrenosum-like ulcer. This rarity challenges the conventional understanding of GPA's onset, highlighting the crucial role of dermatologists in recognizing and diagnosing atypical cases to avoid diagnostic delays.

GPA is a rare pauci-immune ANCA-associated vasculitis, defined by the 2012 International Chapel Hill Consensus Conference as necrotizing granulomatous inflammation primarily affecting small- to medium-sized vessels [13]. Despite extensive research, the etiology of GPA remains unknown. The prevalence and incidence of GPA show variability across ethnic groups, likely influenced by environmental triggers, with rates ranging from 20 to 160 cases per million and 0.5 to 20 cases per million per year, respectively [14, 15]. GPA does not exhibit a significant sex predilection and typically peaks in incidence between 41 and 68 years of age [14]. A definitive diagnosis of GPA is often supported by a positive biopsy, combined with a typical clinical presentation and the presence of either PR3-ANCA or myeloperoxidase (MPO)-ANCA serology. PR3-ANCA is detected in approximately 84–85% of GPA cases, while MPO-ANCA is found in about 16% of them. It's important to note that a negative ANCA result does not rule out a diagnosis of GPA. Imaging and endoscopy are recommended for identifying organ involvement in GPA [16]. The 2022 ACR/EULAR revised and validated classification criteria for GPA, which have a sensitivity of 93% and specificity of 94%, are not appropriate for use in establishing a diagnosis of GPA [17].

Most GPA patients experience prodromal constitutional symptoms lasting for months before the onset of other specific symptoms [14]. Cutaneous involvement occurs in approximately 54% of GPA cases, yet an initial presentation of GPA, as seen in our patient, is infrequent. Cutaneous GPA can manifest as palpable purpura, mucocutaneous ulcers, subcutaneous nodules, pyoderma gangrenosum-like ulcers, digital necrosis, papulonecrotic lesions, and livedo racemosa, with decreasing frequency. Palpable purpura may serve as an indicative marker for renal involvement [18]. Our patient's case exemplifies the importance of widening the spectrum of differential diagnoses for chronic pyoderma gangrenosum-like ulcers when the imperative is to systematically exclude GPA, even in the absence of systemic symptoms and the presence of pathergy. ANCA positivity and distinct histological features serve as crucial diagnostic markers between GPA and pyoderma gangrenosum. It is essential to further differentiate GPA ulcerations from infections, connective tissue diseases, extraintestinal Crohn's disease and certain cutaneous lymphomas, underlining the significance of a meticulous diagnostic process to avoid potential misdiagnoses and ensure timely and appropriate management [19]. Additionally, GPA commonly involves the upper (85%) and lower (80%) respiratory tracts. Upper tract manifestations include sinusitis, epistaxis, nasal septal perforation, saddle nose deformity, and airway stenosis. Lung involvement can be asymptomatic or present with cough, dyspnea, chest discomfort, hemoptysis, or alveolar hemorrhage. The most common chest computed tomography findings are multiple nodules or masses, which may progress to exhibit areas of cavitation, with the potential for subsequent infection [20]. Furthermore, the kidneys are affected in up to 90% of GPA cases (2). GPA can impact the eyes in 16–78% of cases, commonly resulting in vision impairment and eye pain. Mainly associated with orbital masses and proptosis, GPA can also lead to additional changes such as episcleritis, scleritis, and ductal lacrimal obstruction [21]. In GPA patients, oral manifestations occur in 6–13%, with 50% reporting pain. Strawberry-like gingivitis is the most common presentation (61.5%), followed by rare erosive/ulcerative lesions (28.8%) and hyperplastic gingivitis/tooth mobility (25.0%) [22]. Other affected organ systems in GPA may include the nervous system, gastrointestinal tract, and cardiovascular system [14]. The manifestation of prostate involvement in GPA is infrequent and typically gives rise to symptoms such as dysuria, acute or chronic urinary retention, hematuria, or pain. Cases of asymptomatic prostate involvement, as observed in our patient, are rare [23]. In our patient we limited further investigation of pulmonary and prostate changes due to prior extensive diagnostics and confirmed GPA.

As per the 2022 EULAR recommendations, the induction of remission for organ- or life-threatening GPA involves a combination of glucocorticoids with either rituximab or cyclophosphamide. For non-organ- or non-life-threatening GPA, the recommended combination is glucocorticoids and rituximab, with methotrexate or mycophenolate mofetil considered as alternative options to rituximab. The initial dosage of oral glucocorticoids ranges from 50 to 75 mg prednisolone equivalent/day based on body weight, with a gradual reduction according to the PEXIVAS study, aiming for a dose of 5 mg prednisolone equivalent per day by four to five months. Intravenous methylprednisolone pulses, though commonly used in some institutions, lack sufficient evidence and are not recommended for routine use. The suggested duration of maintenance therapy to sustain remission of GPA is 24–48 months following the induction of remission in new-onset cases. Consideration for a longer duration is warranted in patients experiencing relapses or those at an increased risk of relapse. It's crucial to acknowledge that specific organ manifestations may necessitate targeted interventions and supportive management [16]. There are currently no recommendations for topical treatment of cutaneous GPA. Despite advancements in management, GPA remains associated with a mortality rate ranging from 12.5 to 25.7%, primarily attributed to infections [24].

To sum up, the manuscript emphasizes the need for heightened clinical awareness and a comprehensive approach to avoid overlooking GPA in its unique manifestations, advocating for collaboration between dermatologists and rheumatologists in navigating the intricacies of the atypical initial presentation of GPA as a pyoderma gangrenosum-like ulcer [25].

Case 6.2. Martorell Hypertensive Ischemic Leg Ulcer

Introduction

An 84-year-old Caucasian overweight woman presented at the Dermatologic emergency department due to an extremely painful progressive necrotic ulcers bilaterally on the lower legs. The ulcer on her right leg appeared first, 3 months prior to the visit, and the ulcer on the left leg appeared 2 months prior. Due to severe constant pain on NRS 10/10, analgesic therapy with tramadol and paracetamol was prescribed. She denied previous trauma or insect bites in the area. She has had arterial hypertension for approximately 30 years, which was poorly controlled and treated with telmisartan/hydrochlorothiazide, moxonidine and doxazosin. Her other systemic treatments included metildigoxin, trimetazidine, furosemide, atorvastatin, bisoprolol and warfarin. The physical examination revealed on her right laterodorsal leg, a relatively shallow, irregular ulcer, approximately 10 × 5 cm connecting with a tongue-like projection to a 5 × 5 cm ulcer, with 20% necrosis and 80% granulations. Above it a similar completely necrotic ulcer size 1.5 × 3 cm was observed. On the left, an equivalent smaller 3 cm ulcer with about 50% of necrosis was observed (Figs. 6.4 and 6.5). The perilesional skin was hyperemic and livedoid. Peripheral arterial pulses of the dorsalis pedis arteries were palpable bilaterally.

An ultrasound of the veins in the lower extremities revealed mild superficial venous insufficiency in the vena saphena magna. Peripheral arterial disease was ruled out, using oximetry and ankle-brachial index measurements. Extensive laboratory examinations of the blood and urine were performed, and in all likelihood excluded other ulcer etiologies. That included: complete blood count, differential blood count, sedimentation rate, C reactive protein, comprehensive metabolic panel, including serum, ionized and corrected calcium, calcium oxalate, urate, phosphate, HbA1c, homocysteine, serum protein electrophoresis, comprehensive tumor marker panel, LDH, Vitamin D, parathormone, protein S and C, antithrombin III, prothrombin time, INR, partial thromboplastin time, lupus anticoagulants, antiphospholipid antibodies, C3 and C4 complement components, HEP-2 antibodies, ENA antibodies, ANCA antibodies, anti-dsDNA, cold agglutinins, cryoglobulins and urine with sediment. In addition we performed a chest x-ray and abdominal ultrasound.

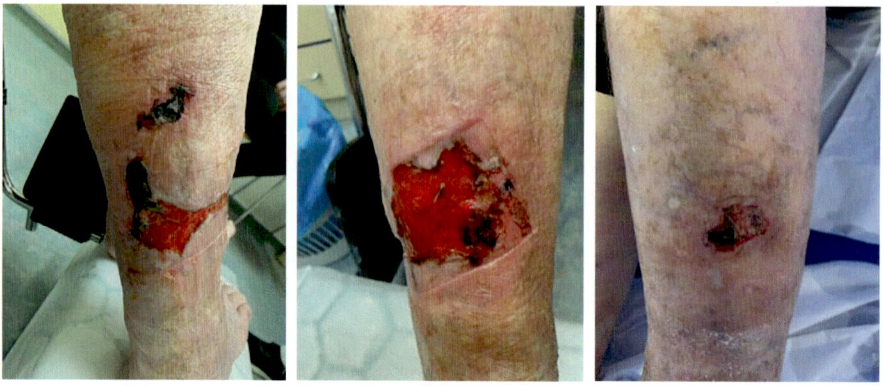

(a) (b) (c)

Fig. 6.4 Martorell HYTILU at baseline visit (**a** back; **b** front; **c** side)

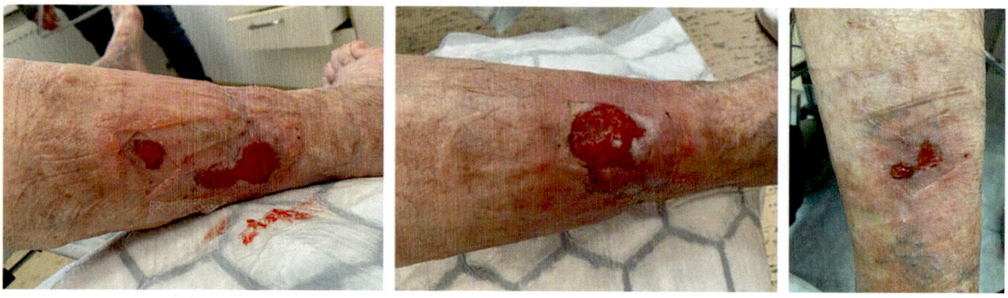

(a) (b) (c)

Fig. 6.5 6 weeks after baseline visit (**a** back; **b** front; **c** side)

Wound swabs for pathogenic bacteria were performed and revealed a mixed bacterial flora.

A punch biopsy was performed for direct immunofluorescence (DIF) and was nonspecific. A deep incisional biopsy across the ulcer and healthy skin was performed for the histopathological examination, revealing calcifications and narrowing of the lumens of larger vessels of the deep plexus, especially in the arterial system, consistent with the diagnosis of Martorell Hypertensive Ischemic Leg Ulcer (HYTILU).

Differential Diagnosis

Based on the patient history of severe pain and long standing badly controlled arterial hypertension, physical examination and localization of the ulcer, extensive laboratory examinations, vein ultrasound, oximetry, perfusion pressures, nonspecific DIF, other common and rare ulcer aetiologies were excluded, including arterial disturbance, rheumatologic, hematologic, metabolic, vaso-occlusive and coagulation disorders) as well as possible associated disease. Additionally, histopathological examination was consistent with Martorell HYTILU.

Treatment

(A) ***Ulcer***

Treatment was initiated with wound dressings at the baseline visit and included hydrogel on necrotic areas and alginate on granulations. The wound dressings were modified at every visit based on the clinical characteristics. Partial debridement was performed at every visit. Moreover, daily use compression therapy with long stretch bandages was initiated.

(B) ***Concurrent Measures***

Analgesic therapy was modified. Her arterial blood pressure was normalized, using an increased dose of doxazosin and the introduction of amlodipine.

Follow up

The patient was followed up every 1–2 weeks, based on the ulcer clinical characteristics, until sufficient healing was observed.

(C) ***Outcome***

Slow, but steady improvement of the ulcer was observed one month after the baseline visit and complete re-*epithelialization* was observed 4 months after the baseline visit (Fig. 6.6). No new ulcers have appeared for one year after the resolution. The patient's arterial pressure was well regulated.

Discussion

Martorell HYTILU is a rare, progressive, disproportionally painful, necrotic ulcer on the lower extremity with a predisposition to the lateral-dorsal part of the lower third of the tibia and the area above the Achilles tendon [26–31]. It usually begins with a livid-colored painful area that then becomes necrotic with a livid and necrotic margin [26, 32]. In the differential diagnosis, care must be taken, when differentiating it from pyoderma gangrenosum and necrotic vasculitis, where therapy differs greatly [26, 31, 33, 34]. Patients with Martorell ulcer are

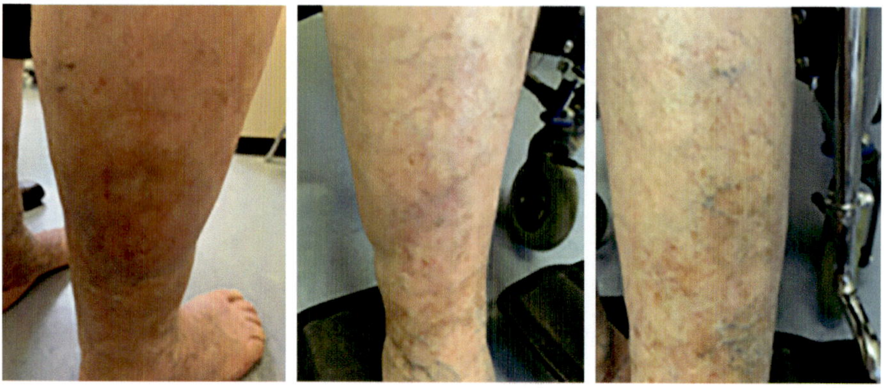

Fig. 6.6 Complete reepithelization (**a** back; **b**. front; **c** side)

usually older than 60 years, with long-standing arterial hypertension and/or diabetes mellitus type II (DM), which result in subcutaneous vessel arteriosclerosis, resulting in ischemia [26, 29]. Both comorbidities should be adequately managed [29]. Approximately half of the patients have Martorell HYTILU ulcer in the same location on the contralateral extremity either concomitantly or several months or years later [29]. Calciphylaxis (distal and proximal form) and calciphylaxis with normal renal function also have a similar clinical and histopathological picture to Martorell ulcer [26, 29, 31]. Similar risk factors are observed in all four entities, especially hypertension and diabetes [26, 29, 31].

The diagnosis of Martorell HYTILU is one of exclusion and is most likely often overlooked. A deep elliptical incisional biopsy is indicated, when clinical suspicion is high in order not to miss the specific histological findings of subcutaneous arteriolosclerosis, which include medial calcinosis, arteriolar thrombosis, narrowed vessel lumen and thickened vessel wall [31]. A superficial biopsy may miss these characteristic features.

The treatment of Martorell ulcer requires a multidisciplinary approach. Appropriate wound dressings are warranted, based on the ulcers clinical characteristics and long stretch bandages are indicated. In the initial phases, wound debridement may be required. Adequate pain management is necessary, as well as the reduction of cardiovascular risk factors, with an emphasis on blood pressure regulation, as well as adequate control of DM. Non-specific beta blockers should be discontinued in order to prevent peripheral vasoconstriction [32].

In the case of resistant disease, debridement with skin grafting, the use of vasodilators (mesoglycans, pentoxifylline), negative pressure therapy, treatment in a hyperbaric oxygen therapy, prostaglandin E and systemic antibiotic therapy can also be considered [26–39].

With the aging of the population and the high prevalence of associated cardiovascular diseases, we expect an increase in this type of ulcers. Martorell hypertensive ischemic ulcer should be considered in any severely painful shin ulcer that progresses rapidly and does not heal optimally, especially in patients older than 60 years, who have associated arterial hypertension and diabetes.

Case 6.3. Chronic Prurigo

Introduction

The 74-year-old patient had been suffering from extremely itchy changes on the skin of both shins, and occasionally also on the extensor side of the forearm, for a year before the examination in the dermatology clinic. Her GP prescribed topical gentamicin ointment and Loratadine, without significant improvement. She was treated for arterial hypertension, had a cholecystectomy, but is otherwise healthy. She had no proven allergies. She used an ACE inhibitor and Doxazosin as a regular therapy. At the first examination, erythematous prurigo papules with dried crusts were present on the pretibial sides of both shins. Individual hypo and hyperpigmentation were also present on the skin of the extensor sides of the forearms. Peripheral lymph nodes were not palpably enlarged. There were no peculiarities in the somatic status either. The laboratory results showed a slightly elevated sedimentation rate of 29, ALT 0.67, gamma GT 0.65, triglycerides 1.8, other values in the hemogram, hepatogram and lipidogram, as well as blood sugar, urea, thyroid hormones and iron were within normal limits. X-ray of chest organs was also within normal limits. Based on the anamnesis of itching lasting more than a year and the typical clinical picture, we made a diagnosis of Prurigo Chronica. Initially, we introduced betamethasone/gentamicin cream and indifferent ointment, and desloratadine, but without significant effect on itching. Therefore, at the control examination, we added therapy with hydroxyzine tablets for the evening. Betamethasone/gentamicin cream were replaced by mometasone furoate cream due to minor side effects. With this treatment, the itching subsided, new prurigo papules no longer appeared in such a severe form, for this reason, we did not add other systemic therapy to the therapy (Fig. 6.7).

Discussion

Chronic prurigo (CP) is a defined by the presence of chronic pruritus for at least 6 weeks, a history and/or signs of repeated scratching, and multiple localized or generalized pruritic skin lesions (whitish or pinkish papules, nodules and/or plaques, scratch-associated pruriginous little wounds) [6]. Prurigo papules/nodules occur either as primary lesions or as secondary lesions due to persistent scratching [40]. CP is frequently named prurigo nodularis, but that is only the main clinical aspect of chronic prurigo [6]. On the skin are present multiple, firm, flesh to pink colored nodules commonly located on the extensor surfaces of the extremities [41].

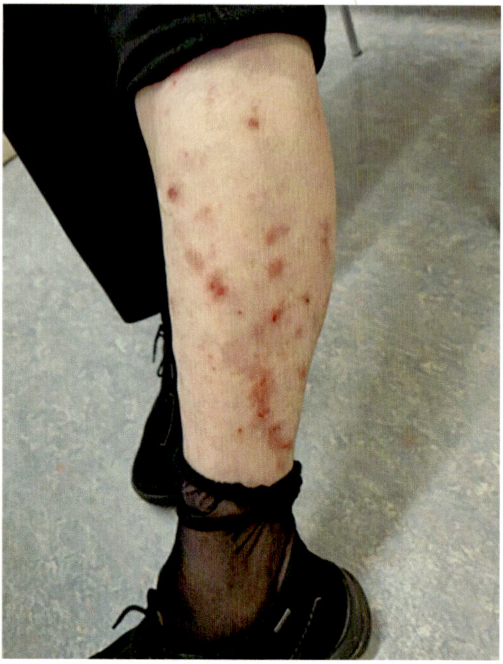

Fig. 6.7 At the end of the therapy

Etiology

CP can be of allergological, dermatological, systemic, neurological, psychiatric/psychosomatic, mixed or undetermined origin [6, 42]. The lesions may occur in any age group [41]. It is commonly associated with another disorder of cutaneous hypersensitivity such as atopic dermatitis or chronic pruritus of diverse origins [41].

The mechanisms of CP are complicated and involve the interaction of the cutaneous, immune, and nervous systems. Diverse immune cells, including eosinophils, neutrophils, T cells, macrophages, and mast cells infiltrated the lesional skin of CP, which initiated the inflammatory cytokines and pruritogens release. In addition, the interaction between the immune cells and activated peripheral sensory nerve fibers by neurotransmitters caused neuroinflammation in the skin and intractable itch. This itch-scratch vicious cycle of CP results in disease exacerbation [42].

Diagnosis

The diagnosis of CP is mainly clinical. We have to identify the cause of pruritus [41, 43] by taking a medical history, especially pruritus, medication use, comorbidities, and any psychiatric history. In addition to the typical skin lesions, the purpose of the physical examination is to detect associated skin diseases that may cause pruritus and may be the etiological factor of prurigo [43]. We also examine the mucous membranes, lymph nodes, liver, spleen and kidneys. Laboratory tests: complete and differential blood count, C-reactive protein, liver tests (AST, ALT, gGT, AP), renal retentions, lactate dehydrogenase, thyroid hormones[43]. To rule out malignancy an ultrasound examination of the lymph nodes and abdominal cavity, and a chest X-ray, are performed [43]. Histological examination and immunofluorescence are performed when we are not sure about the primary skin disease [43].

Treatment

CP is a treatment-resistant skin disease with significant physical and psychological morbidity. A whole range of general measures, pharmacological approaches and psychological therapies is often needed [41].

Available therapeutic options for CP are topical and/or intralesional corticosteroids, with topical calcineurin inhibitors and topical analgesics if necessary. We can prescribed also vitamin D derivativates. If itching persists despite topical therapy, add antihistamines, oral corticosteroids, azathioprine, cyclosporine or methotrexate. We need to add from time to time opioid modulators or antidepressants.

Recent studies indicates effectiveness of biologics: dupilumab, nemolizumab and oral Janus kinase inhibitors too. Phototherapy with UVB 311 and PUVA relives itching for some patients [6, 43].

Case 6.4. Necrobiosis Lipoidica with Ulceration

Introduction

A 55-years old woman with a history of deep vein thrombosis, arterial hypertension, hypercholesterolemia, and mild gastritis presented at Outpatient Dermatology Clinic in 2012 with skin changes on her legs that started in 1995. There was no history of diabetes mellitus. The main reason for her visit were ulcerations that appeared 2 months ago and didn't heal.

Soon after the appearance of first skin changes in 1995 the diagnosis of necrobiosis was suggested and later confirmed by histopathological examination which showed palisaded and interstitial granulomatous dermatitis in the dermis with extension into the subcutaneous tissue. Granulomas were composed of histiocytes, and multinucleated giant cells and infiltrate composed of lymphocytes, plasma cells, and scarce eosinophils was seen.

The treatment in the past consisted of topical and intralesional corticosteroids which resulted in some occasional improvement of the situation, but the disease proceeded.

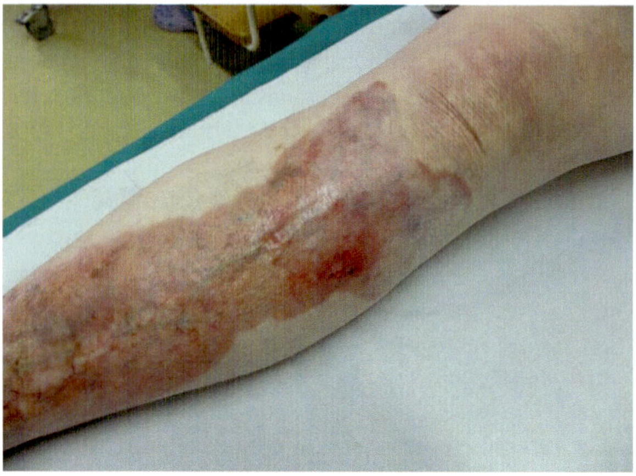

Fig. 6.8 Right leg with ulceration under the knee

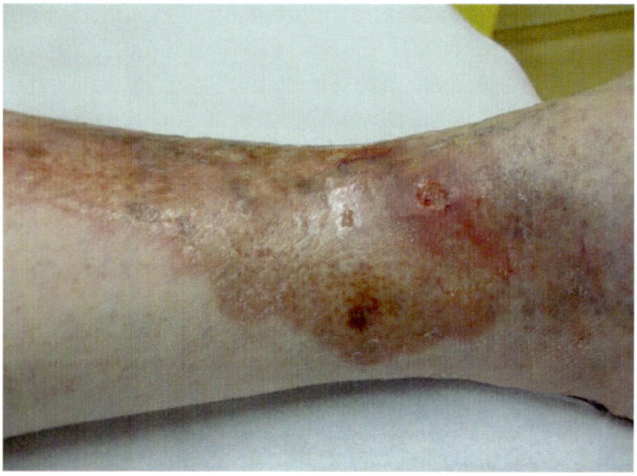

Fig. 6.9 Left leg with ulceration above the medial ankle

At the time of the visit there were typical yellow-orange plaques with atrophy and prominent telangiectasias on both pretibial areas. At the periphery some fresh lesions in the form of pink plaques were seen. There was ulceration within one of the yellow plaques on the right leg (Fig. 6.8) under the knee (15 × 7 mm) and ulceration on the medial ankle area (Fig. 6.9) of the left leg (8 × 10 mm).

Differential Diagnosis

Due to typical clinical picture and previous histopathology report other granulomatous disorders of the skin (cutaneous sarcoidosis, granuloma annulare, necrobiotic xanthogranuloma) and skin diseases with predilection for the lower legs (pigmented purpuric dermatosis, stasis dermatitis) were excluded. The duration of the disease was helpful in this case as the clinical picture was fully developed.

Treatment

Necrobiosis is a disease that is difficult to treat as there is no definitive cure. The treatment aims on management of signs and symptoms of the disease by reducing the inflammatory process and healing ulcerations.

Our patient was treated with topical and intralesional corticosteroids in the past and she refused additional application of these medications and was also reluctant to attempt systemic treatments. Topical immunomodulator tacrolimus 0.1% ointment twice daily was prescribed for the active borders of the lesions and emollient cream and avoidance of trauma were suggested. The wounds were covered by alginate dressing that was changed twice weekly. Compression therapy was started.

Two months after the introduction of the therapy the redness of the plaque borders was less prominent. The ulcerations were almost healed. The patient was then lost for follow-up and died a year later due to intracerebral hemorrhage.

Discussion

Necrobiosis lipoidica is a rare, chronic granulomatous disease of the skin that can lead to ulcerations of the skin [44–46]. The lower legs, particularly the shins, are the most common sites of involvement. Ulceration is a frequent complication, occurring in 10 to 20 percent of patients [45].

Many patients with necrobiosis lipoidica also have diabetes mellitus. Consequently, all patients with necrobiosis lipoidica without a previous history of diabetes should be evaluated for diabetes at the time of diagnosis [45, 46].

Multiple therapies have been used for necrobiotic lipoidica with unpredictable results. Early therapeutic choice for non-ulcerated necrobiosis lipoidica is usually topical treatment with a high-potency topical corticosteroid applied under occlusion and compression therapy. In case of insufficient response to this treatment, subsequent treatment is usually intralesional corticosteroid therapy.

Many other options of treatment are described including phototherapy, topical calcineurin inhibitors, biologics, immunosuppressants, JAK inhibitors and combination therapies [46, 47].

Ulceration is the most frequent complication of necrobiosis lipoidica. These ulcers frequently heal slowly, are painful and can be difficult to treat. With the aim to reduce the risk for ulceration, the patients should be encouraged to avoid trauma of the skin in affected areas [8]. Daily moisturization of atrophic areas to reduce the risk of skin breakdown is recommended.

Proper wound care is an important part of the management of ulcers in necrobiosis lipoidica. Basic principles of wound care are recommended. Wound healing is facilitated by reducing factors that may inhibit the process, such as malnutrition and lower extremity edema. Compression stockings and leg elevation are suggested in the management of lower extremity edema to promote healing [48].

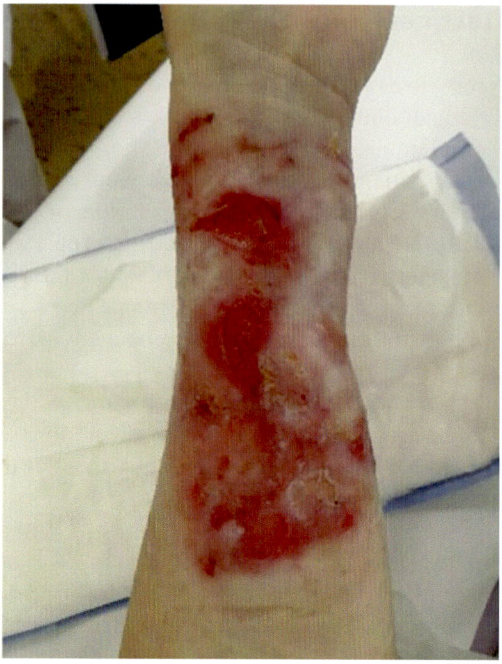

Fig. 6.10 Dermatitis artefacta (at presentation, July 2022)

Case 6.5. Dermatitis Artefacta

Introduction

A 45-year-old woman with anxiety-depressive disorder came to the dermatology department with a history of worsening ulcers on her left forearm, which had lasted for 4 years (Fig. 6.10). The wounds were initially caused by alkali damage and did not heal. She had several irregularly shaped erosions and ulcers ranging from 1 to 4 cm in a 15 cm wide scar tissue that was around the entire circumference of the middle part of her left forearm. She was treated with intralesional corticosteroid therapy and methylprednisolone with an initial dose of 32 mg, additionally she had therapy with Dapsone 50 and 100 mg daily (alternating) and 5 mg methotrexate per week. She was also treated with biological therapy with Infliximab (300 mg). Several surgical necrosectomies, skin grafts and negative pressure therapies were also performed. But the ulcers kept enlarging. New ones also appeared, even though the initial cause had long since disappeared.

Differential Diagnosis

To rule out other pathology, an MRI was performed, which showed a small skin defect distally radially, without other pathological signs. Biopsy (histology and

DIF) of the ulceration was inconclusive, showing epidermal necrosis, hypertrophic scar tissue, and mixed cellular infiltrates, without skin changes similar to pyoderma gangrenosum. Nonspecific DIF changes and a negative ANCA test spoke against vasculitis. Based on the histology, chemical dermatitis could not be excluded. She had a scintigraphy of the skeleton, there were no signs of osteomyelitis. Pemphigoid IgG antibodies were discretely positive, anti-BP 180 and μanti-BP 320 were negative, and anti-core IgG antibodies were also slightly positive. A psychiatric examination was advised, which the patient did not take, and due to the pain, an examination by an algologist was also recommended. Several tests were performed (full blood count, ANA, ENA, anti DNA, anti-cardiolipin antibodies, tumor markers, proteins, anti-beta-GPI, lupus anticoagulant, Quantiferon test, serological tests for hepatitis B and C, and an occult blood test). Only microcytic anemia (Hb 111 g/L, MCV 80.7 fl) with decreased values of iron (5.9 μmol/L) and ferritin (4 μg/L) and elevated sedimentation (48 mm/h) was found. Staphylococcus Aureus, sensitive to all tested antibiotics, was isolated from the wound swab, so she received Flucloxacillin 1 g/6 h for 10 days. Another histology of a skin sample from the ulcer and surrounding skin showed fibrosis with mixed cellular infiltrates and reactive changes that can also be seen in artifact dermatitis but are mostly present after healing. Pyoderma gangrenosum was unlikely, but not completely ruled out, due to the increased number of neutrophilic granulocytes. DIF examination was minimal and unremarkable, chest X-ray showed no past or active tuberculosis or other pathologic changes.

Treatment

After the examinations, we stopped all systemic therapy (except Iroprem) and applied only local foams with PHMB and later hydrocolloid dressings to the wounds. Compression therapy with short adhesive bandages was used. With such therapy, smaller erosions and ulcers healed, and larger ones were reduced (Fig. 6.11). Given that the ulcers healed well, and the area with the ulcers was covered with dressings all the time and the results were normal, we confirmed the suspicion of self-harm, so we did not carry out other systemic therapy (Fig. 6.12). All ulcers healed within 12 days. We confronted the patient with the fact that she inflicted these wounds on herself, at which she was outraged. In a conversation with the patient, we found out that she is the owner of a small business that was financially unstable, so she was the recipient of financial assistance from various state services. Psychiatric evaluation and treatment were again recommended.

Discussion

In patients with bizarre-shaped wounds on atypical but easily accessible spots and do not answer to the correct therapy, we need to take a thorough medical history and run a set of laboratory tests to exclude inflammatory, infectious, vascular,

Fig. 6.11 Dermatitis artefacta (one week after presentation)

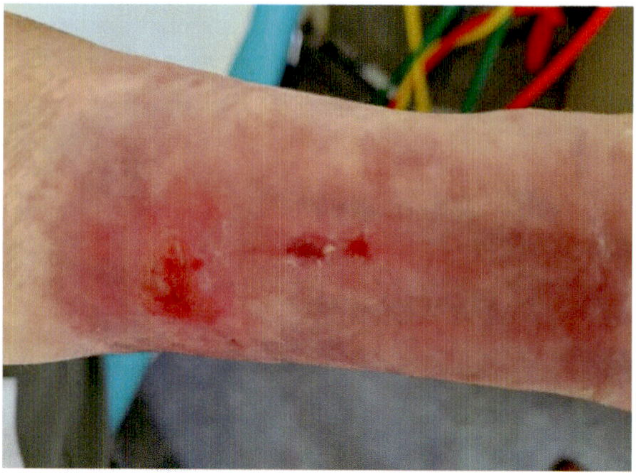

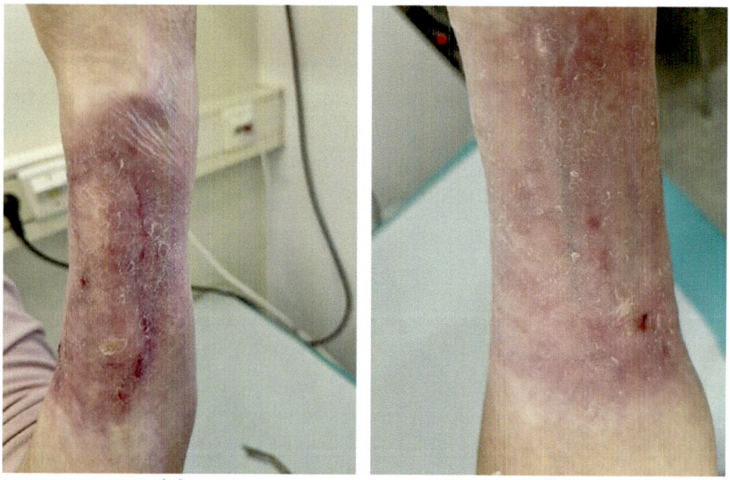

(a) (b)

Fig. 6.12 Dermatitis artefacta on the left forearm (at the end of the treatment: **a** posterior aspect; **b** anterior aspect)

malignant and other reasons for wounds. If all the results are inconclusive, we must consider an artefacta [9, 49, 50]. The most important thing is to create a trusting relationship and to offer psychiatric counseling.

Various psychiatric diseases, financial or other personal problems can lead to artefactal ulcers. Chronic wounds can heal slower also in patients with depression [51, 52].

Case 6.6. Stage III Lymphedema with Ulcer After Erysipelas Recidivans in Patients with Decreased Blood Flow

Introduction

A 61-year-old patient with an ulcer on the left tibia was examined for the first time in 2017 in the Ulcer outpatient clinic because he had severe pain and swelling on the left lower extremity. He had been involved in a traffic accident a few years earlier and had sustained severe injuries to his left tibia, which were surgically treated in the trauma unit. After that, severe pain appeared. An angiography was performed, which revealed decreased blood flow to the left tibial region, which was aggravated by the scars. Due to the swelling, which was also due to the scars, bullous erysipelas occurred (Fig. 6.13). When he came for examination, there was scarring and erosion in the lower two-thirds of his swollen shin, and the skin was reddish, with partial defects in the calf. The edema was pitting and elastic, and the tibia was 4 cm wider at the knee and ankle than the right. Stemmer's sign was positive on the left side, pulses were barely palpable, ABI was 0.49, his temperature was slightly elevated. Penicillin was administered because of suspected erysipelas, and compression therapy was not possible because of low ABI values. With the antibiotics, the temperature decreased, as did the pain. Because of the short claudication, he was unable to walk longer distances. The decrease in swelling was minimal. After this episode of erysipelas, he had three more, which were also treated with penicillin. Unfortunately, he developed an allergic reaction after the fourth episode. With a new episode of erysipelas, he was treated with cephalosporins and after the sixth episode of erysipelas, he also developed an allergic reaction to the cephalosporins (Fig. 6.14). Again, he was referred to the Ulcer Outpatient Clinic with more pronounced and firmer edema of the tibia, severe pain, and an ulcer in the lower third. His case was presented to the Angiological Council, whose expert opinion was that amputation was the best solution, since compression therapy, which could prevent worsening of the edema and recurrent episodes of erysipelas, was not possible.

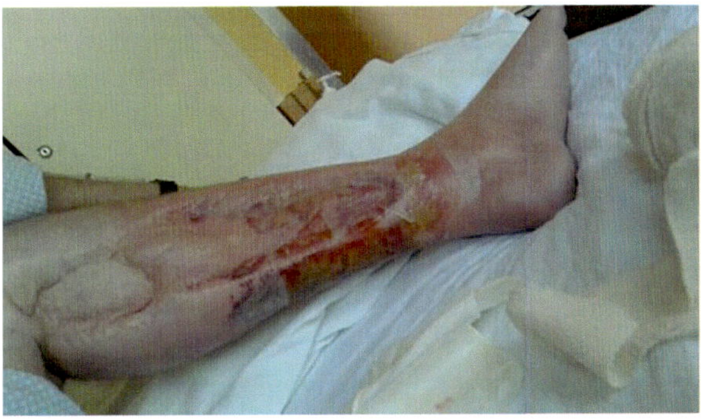

Fig. 6.13 Episode of erysipelas at presentation

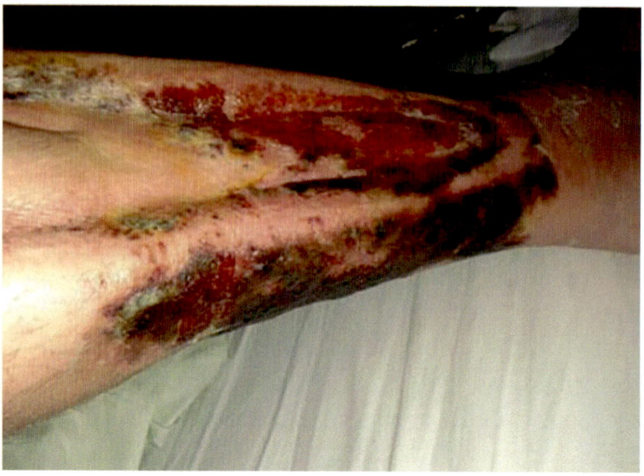

Fig. 6.14 After the sixth episode of erysipelas

Differential Diagnosis

Based on the patient's history of severe pain and poor circulation, physical examination, and localization of swelling, other common and rare etiologies of ulcers and swelling were excluded. A diagnosis of an ulcer was made as a result of recurrent erysipelas due to stage III lymphedema with reduced blood flow.

Treatment

The patient was referred to lymph node transplantation and scar reduction, which could improve circulation and reduce lymphedema (Fig. 6.15). This prevented the life-threatening erysipelas from recurring. Two lymph nodes from the left axilla were transferred to the left popliteal fossa (Fig. 6.16). After the procedure, the oedema was softer and became much smaller as the patient began to walk. Blood flow improved due to removal of scar tissue, and the ABI was postoperatively 0.71. After lymphedema was diminished with adhesive short-stretch bandages, he was prescribed medical compression garments class I because he could not tolerate stronger compression. Since limited mobility of the left shoulder occurred after the lymph node removal, he was referred to the Department of Medical Rehabilitation, where he was prescribed physiotherapy (Fig. 6.17). With supervised therapy, he regained full range of motion (Figs. 6.18 and 6.19).

Follow up

For the past six years (Fig. 6.20) he has been free of erysipelas, pain and oedema are minimal, and he is able to walk a distance of four kilometers with regular use of compression garments class I (Fig. 6.21) (EU prestandard pressure classes for compression).

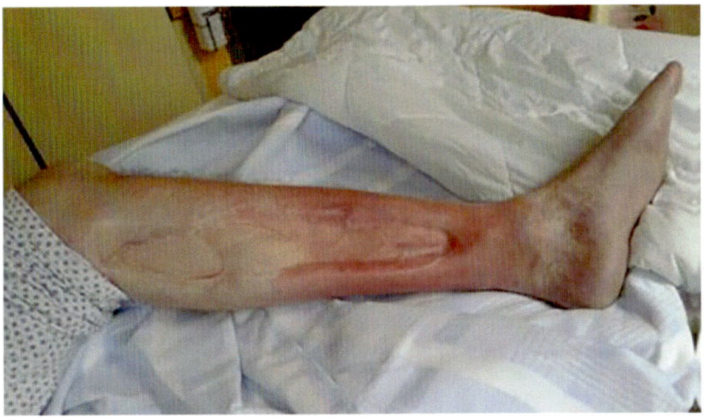

Fig. 6.15 Before lymph node transplantation

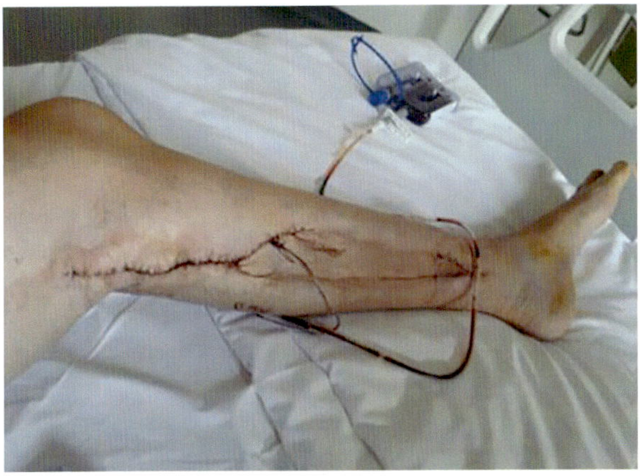

Fig. 6.16 Immediately after lymph node transplantation and surgical removal of the scars

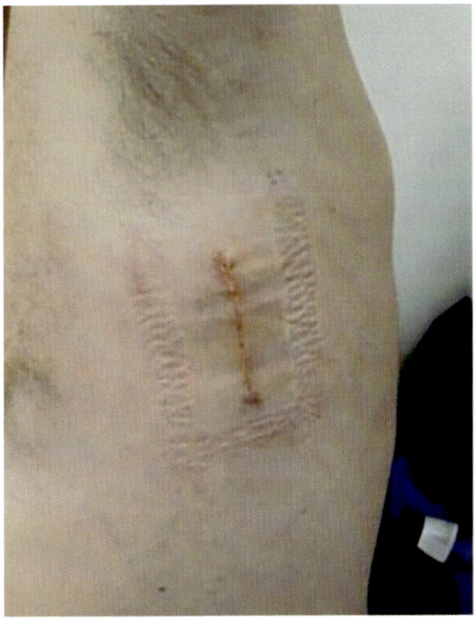

Fig. 6.17 The site of lymph nodes removal—few weeks after transplantation

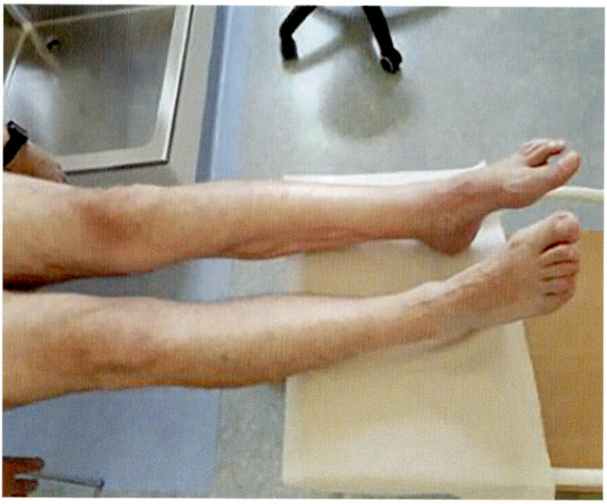

Fig. 6.18 Left leg one year after lymph node transplantation

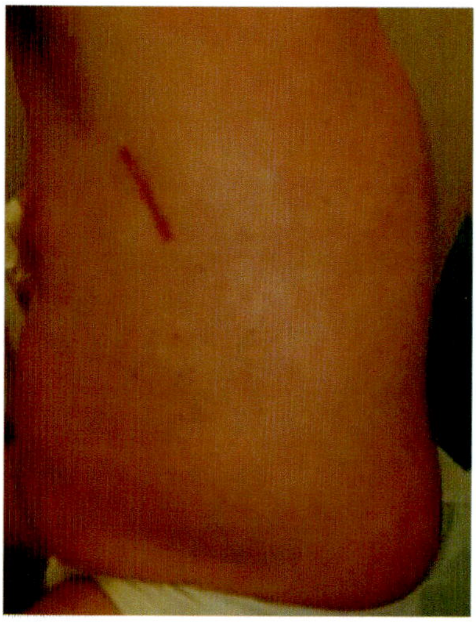

Fig. 6.19 Removal site of lymph nodes one year after transplantation

Discussion

Erysipelas and ulcers are very common in patients with lymphedema especially in stage III [53]. Besides antibiotics, compression with short-stretch bandages with zinc paste and dressings are the most important treatment in the acute phase, reducing edema and preventing the spread of infection and for ulcer healing [54–56]. Compression therapy with medical compression garments is the sustainable therapy for lymphedema, most commonly with stockings—compression III–IV, depending on the stage of lymphedema. The patient had restricted blood flow, so compression was not an option. Because of the allergic reactions he developed to the antibiotics, there was a greater risk of new ulcers and sepsis with new

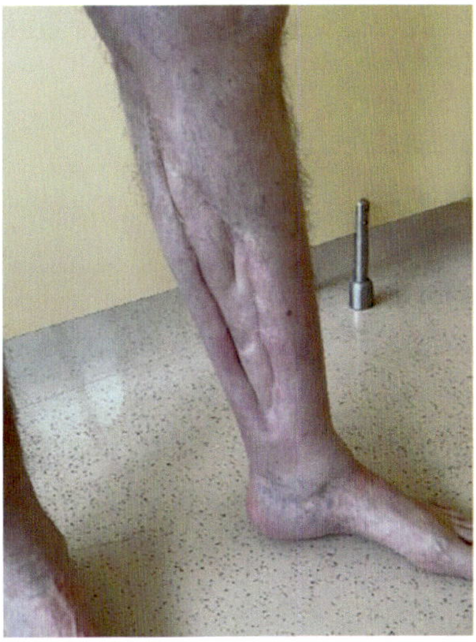

Fig. 6.20 Six years after the surgery

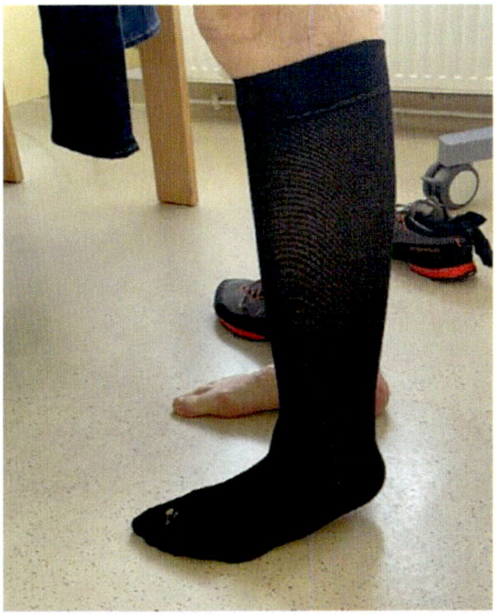

Fig. 6.21 Compression garments

erysipelas [57]. The only treatment option the angiologists and vascular surgeons saw was amputation, which the patient refused because of his active life and his own business. The dermatologists opted for lymph node transplantation; the only possible solution left that could lead to a reduction in lymphedema [58]. Additional partial excision of the scar tissue improved blood flow, which also reduced oedema and pain and minimized the possibility of erysipelas recurrence. The decision proved correct; oedema was decreased, and blood flow was improved. Only milder compression was possible, but the patient was still able to lead a normal life as he had before the accident [59]. The temporary limitation of range of motion in the left shoulder improved completely with supervised physical therapy.

Case 6.7. Epidermolysis Bullosa-Associated Squamous Cell Carcinoma Ulceration

Introduction

A 61-year-old male patient with a background of chronic venous insufficiency (CVI) and epidermolysis bullosa (EB) presented to the dermatology department with a history of worsening ulcerations on the right lower extremity that did not respond to endovenous ablation treatment. The largest ulceration was up to 15 cm wide and extended over almost the entire calf circumference. The wound was painful, of variable depth, covered mainly with granulation tissue and partly with fibrin, had a well-defined border, which was undermined in some places. Laterally there was a similar but smaller ulceration (Fig. 6.22). The foot pulses were symmetrically detectable. The right inguinal lymph nodes were significantly enlarged and tender. His EB (histologically most likely subepidermal type) presented clinically in a mild form with some blistering and erosions at sites of mechanical trauma.

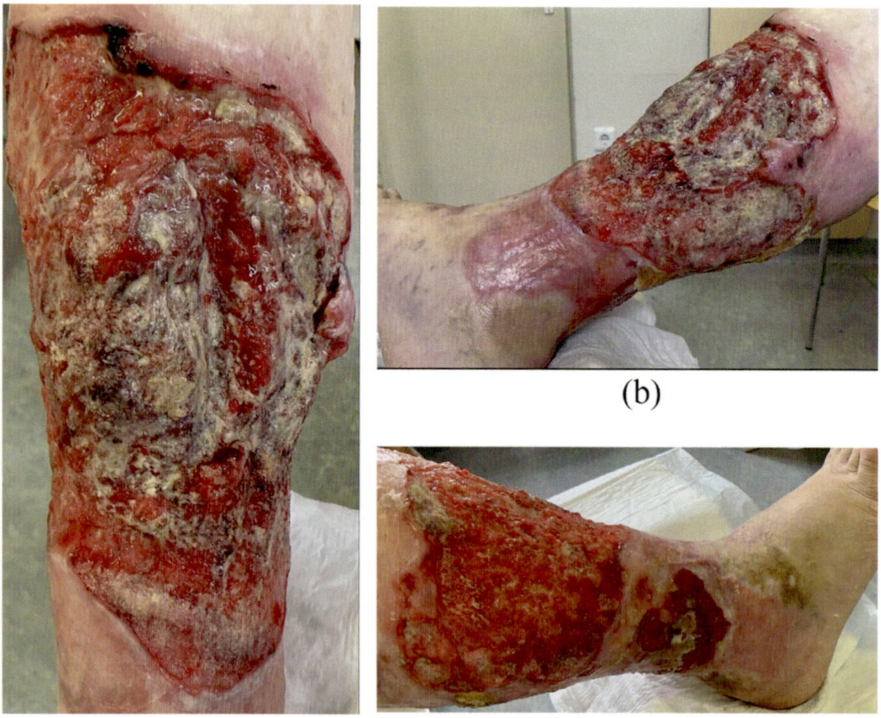

(a) (b) (c)

Fig. 6.22 Marjolin ulcer at the time of diagnosis (a. front; b. lateral side-upper image; c. medial side-lower image)

Differential Diagnosis

Based on the history and clinical findings, an arterial or venous etiology was ruled out. Other important differential diagnoses were pyoderma gangrenosum, malignancy or vasculitis. A biopsy was performed and the ulceration was histopathologically diagnosed as invasive squamous cell carcinoma (SCC) with metastases in the right inguinal lymph node (confirmed cytologically by fine needle lymph node aspiration).

Treatment

Following the diagnosis of invasive metastatic SCC, the multidisciplinary team discussed the most appropriate treatment. The decision was difficult due to the patient's concurrent EB. Several treatment options were proposed, including radiotherapy, treatment with systemic immunotherapy (cemiplimab) and leg amputation. Regular wound dressings were also performed. Due to the potential for serious side effects, it was decided not to treat with cemiplimab. Radiotherapy was not promising in view of the extent of the disease. An above-the-knee amputation was performed. Shortly afterwards, liquefaction of the metastatic inguinal lymph nodes occurred, with the sinus tract draining the necrotic contents to the skin surface (Fig. 6.23). Due to the high risk of complications, no further treatment was decided. The multidisciplinary council then opted for palliative and supportive care. The patient died a few months later.

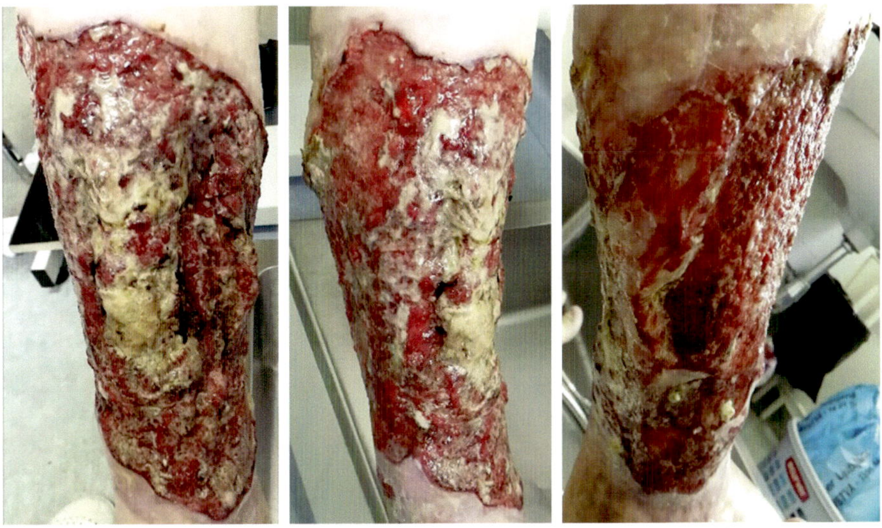

(a) (b) (c)

Fig. 6.23 Progression of the disease two months later (a. front side; b. lateral side; c. medial side)

Discussion

Chronic wounds and chronic skin damage are a risk factor for malignant skin diseases. Malignant tumors that occur in chronic wounds are more aggressive, more resistant to therapy and more likely to metastasize. This is also due to the fact that they are often not detected early enough, leading to delayed treatment [60, 61]. Another challenge in making a timely diagnosis is the interaction of several existing concomitant diseases, such as associated vascular diseases (CVI, arterial occlusive disease). The studies agree that a biopsy should be performed on any non-healing ulcer that is resistant to treatment. However, exactly when to opt for the procedure itself has not yet been standardized [62, 63].

Epidermolysis bullosa is a term for a heterogeneous group of rare skin diseases ranging from mild to life-threatening, all clinically characterized by skin and/or mucosal fragility and blistering in response to minor injury or mechanical trauma. Due to impaired skin healing and the associated chronic inflammation, EB also represents a risk factor for skin malignancies (e.g. aggressive cutaneous SCCs at lesional skin sites) which can be difficult to treat as the fragility of the skin can lead to serious complications [61]. Surgical excision is often the treatment of first choice. For locally advanced SCC, limb amputation or radiotherapy should be considered. In recent years, an increasing number of studies have investigated the use of various systemic target therapies in metastatic or locally advanced cases, such as cetuximab (epidermal growth factor receptor inhibitor) and cemiplimab (programmed cell death protein-1 inhibitor). Although the prognosis for aggressive malignancies in chronic wounds is still not promising, patients benefit from early diagnosis, a multidisciplinary approach and an individualized treatment plan that takes into account the latest reports and guidelines [64].

References

1. Shavit E, Alavi A, Sibbald RG. Vasculitis—what do we have to know? A review of literature. Int J Low Extrem Wounds. 2018;17(4):218–26. https://doi.org/10.1177/1534734618804982. Epub 2018 Dec 3 PMID: 30501545.
2. Frumholtz L, Laurent-Roussel S, Lipsker D, Terrier B. Cutaneous vasculitis: review on diagnosis and clinicopathologic correlations. Clin Rev Allergy Immunol. 2021;61(2):181–93. https://doi.org/10.1007/s12016-020-08788-4. PMID: 32378145.
3. White J, Dubey S. Eosinophilic granulomatosis with polyangiitis: a review. Autoimmun Rev. 2023;22(1):103219. https://doi.org/10.1016/j.autrev.2022.103219. Epub 2022 Oct 22. PMID: 36283646.
4. Deinsberger J, Brugger J, Tschandl P, Meier-Schiesser B, Anzengruber F, Bossart S, Tzaneva S, Petzelbauer P, Böhler K, Beltraminelli H, Hafner J, Weber B. Differentiating arteriolosclerotic ulcers of martorell from other types of leg ulcers based on vascular histomorphology. Acta Derm Venereol. 2021;101(5):adv00449.
5. Karppinen JJ, Kallio M, Lappalainen K, Lagus H, Matikainen N, Isoherranen K. Clinical characteristics of Martorell hypertensive ischaemic leg ulcer. J Wound Care. 2023;32(12):797–804. https://doi.org/10.12968/jowc.2023.32.12.797. PMID: 38060417.
6. Misery L. Chronic prurigo. Br J Dermatol. 2022;187(4):464–71.

7. Müller S, Zeidler C, Ständer S. Chronic prurigo including prurigo nodularis: new insights and treatments. Am J Clin Dermatol. 2024;25(1):15–33. https://doi.org/10.1007/s40257-023-00818-z. Epub 2023 Sep 17. PMID: 37717255; PMCID: PMC10796623.
8. Franklin C, Stoffels-Weindorf M, Hillen U, Dissemond J. Ulcerated necrobiosis lipoidica as a rare cause for chronic leg ulcers: case report series of ten patients. Int Wound J. 2015;12(5):548–54. https://doi.org/10.1111/iwj.12159. Epub 2013 Oct 7. PMID: 24119190; PMCID: PMC7950577.
9. Mukundu Nagesh N, Barlow R, Mohandas P, Gkini MA, Bewley A. Dermatitis artefacta. Clin Dermatol. 2023;41(1):10–5. https://doi.org/10.1016/j.clindermatol.2023.02.005. Epub 2023 Mar 4 PMID: 36878450.
10. Chandran V, Kurien G. Dermatitis Artefacta. 2022 Jul 12. In: StatPearls [Internet]. Treasure Island (FL): StatPearls Publishing; 2024. PMID: 28613686.
11. Burian EA, Karlsmark T, Nørregaard S, Kirketerp-Møller K, Kirsner RS, Franks PJ, Quéré I, Moffatt CJ. Wounds in chronic leg oedema. Int Wound J. 2022;19(2):411–425. https://doi.org/10.1111/iwj.13642. Epub 2021 Jul 13. PMID: 34258856; PMCID: PMC8762561.
12. Kim PJ, Abduelmula A, Mistry J, Mufti A, Sibbald RG. Characteristics and outcomes of squamous cell carcinoma and other cutaneous malignancies in epidermolysis bullosa: a systematic review. Adv Skin Wound Care. 2023;36(9):486–94. https://doi.org/10.1097/01.ASW.0000926608.29276.e9. PMID: 37098819.
13. Fine JD, Johnson LB, Weiner M, Li KP, Suchindran C. Epidermolysis bullosa and the risk of life-threatening cancers: the National EB Registry experience, 1986–2006. J Am Acad Dermatol. 2009;60(2):203–11.
14. Jennette JC, Falk RJ, Bacon PA, Basu N, Cid MC, Ferrario F, Flores-Suarez LF, Gross WL, Guillevin L, Hagen EC, Hoffman GS, Jayne DR, Kallenberg CG, Lamprecht P, Langford CA, Luqmani RA, Mahr AD, Matteson EL, Merkel PA, Ozen S, Pusey CD, Rasmussen N, Rees AJ, Scott DG, Specks U, Stone JH, Takahashi K, Watts RA. 2012 revised international chapel hill consensus conference nomenclature of vasculitides. Arthritis Rheum. 2013;65(1):1–11.
15. Grygiel-Górniak B, Limphaibool N, Perkowska K, Puszczewicz M. Clinical manifestations of granulomatosis with polyangiitis: key considerations and major features. Postgrad Med. 2018;130(7):581–96.
16. Banerjee P, Jain A, Kumar U, Senapati S. Epidemiology and genetics of granulomatosis with polyangiitis. Rheumatol Int. 2021;41(12):2069–89.
17. Hellmich B, Sanchez-Alamo B, Schirmer JH, Berti A, Blockmans D, Cid MC, Holle JU, Hollinger N, Karadag O, Kronbichler A, Little MA, Luqmani RA, Mahr A, Merkel PA, Mohammad AJ, Monti S, Mukhtyar CB, Musial J, Price-Kuehne F, Segelmark M, Teng YKO, Terrier B, Tomasson G, Vaglio A, Vassilopoulos D, Verhoeven P, Jayne D. EULAR recommendations for the management of ANCA-associated vasculitis: 2022 update. Ann Rheum Dis. 2023 Mar 16:ard-2022–223764.
18. Robson JC, Grayson PC, Ponte C, Suppiah R, Craven A, Judge A, Khalid S, Hutchings A, Watts RA, Merkel PA, Luqmani RA; DCVAS Investigators. 2022 American College of Rheumatology/European Alliance of Associations for Rheumatology classification criteria for granulomatosis with polyangiitis. Ann Rheum Dis. 2022;81(3):315–320.
19. Montero-Vilchez T, Martinez-Lopez A, Salvador-Rodriguez L, Del Carmen Ramírez-Barberena M, Tercedor-Sanchez J, Molina-Leyva A, Arias-Santiago S. Cutaneous manifestations of granulomatosis with polyangiitis: a case series study. Acta Derm Venereol. 2020;100(10):adv00150.
20. Qian J, Li J, Li J, Wang G, Zhao H. Cutaneous deep ulcerations as initial presentations of granulomatosis with polyangiitis: two case reports and differential diagnosis. Medicina (Kaunas). 2023;59(3):563.
21. Bernal-Bello D, Morales-Ortega A, Duarte-Millán MÁ, Tardío JC, Frutos-Pérez B. Lung cavitation in granulomatosis with polyangiitis: clinical implications. Clin Rheumatol. 2022;41(9):2915–6.

22. Moin KA, Yeakle MM, Parrill AM, Garofalo VA, Tsiyer AR, Bishev D, Gala D, Fogel J, Hatsis AJ, Wickas TD, Anand P, Morcos M. Ocular and orbital manifestations of granulomatosis with polyangiitis: a systematic review of published cases. Rom J Ophthalmol. 2023;67(3):214–21.
23. Labrador AJP, Valdez LHM, Marin NRG, Ibazetta KAR, Chacón JAL, Fernandez AJV, Valencia MSV, Marchant SW, Sanchez KBT, Villacrez CA. Oral granulomatosis with polyangiitis a systematic review. Clin Exp Dent Res. 2023;9(1):100–11.
24. Yatsyshyn R, Zimba O, Bahrii M, Doskaliuk B, Huryk V. Prostate involvement in granulomatosis with polyangiitis. Rheumatol Int. 2019;39(7):1269–77.
25. Grayson PC, Ponte C, Suppiah R, Robson JC, Craven A, Judge A, Khalid S, Hutchings A, Luqmani RA, Watts RA, Merkel PA; DCVAS Study Group. 2022 American College of Rheumatology/European Alliance of Associations for rheumatology classification criteria for eosinophilic granulomatosis with polyangiitis. Ann Rheum Dis. 2022;81(3):309–14.
26. Alavi A, Mayer D, Hafner J, Sibbald RG. Martorell hypertensive ischemic leg ulcer: an underdiagnosed Entity©. Adv Skin Wound Care. 2012;25(12):563–72; quiz 573–4. https://doi.org/10.1097/01.ASW.0000423442.08531.fb. PMID: 23151767.
27. Graves JW, Morris JC, Sheps SG. Martorell's hypertensive leg ulcer: case report and concise review of the literature. J Hum Hypertens. 2001;15(4):279–83. https://doi.org/10.1038/sj.jhh.1001154.PMID:11319677z.
28. Lima Pinto AP, Silva NA Jr, Osorio CT, et al. Martorell's Ulcer: diagnostic and therapeutic challenge. Case Rep Dermatol. 2015;7(2):199–206. Published 2015 Aug 5. https://doi.org/10.1159/000430884
29. Hafner J, Nobbe S, Partsch H, et al. Martorell hypertensive ischemic leg ulcer: a model of ischemic subcutaneous arteriolosclerosis. Arch Dermatol. 2010;146(9):961–8. https://doi.org/10.1001/archdermatol.2010.224.
30. Weber B, Deinsberger J, Hafner J, Beltraminelli H, Tzaneva S, Böhler K. Localization-mapping of arteriolosclerotic ulcers of Martorell using two-dimensional computational rendering reveals a predominant location on the mid-lateral lower leg. J Eur Acad Dermatol Venereol. 2020. https://doi.org/10.1111/jdv.16787.
31. Hafner J. Calciphylaxis and martorell hypertensive ischemic leg ulcer: same pattern—one pathophysiology. Dermatology. 2016;232:523–33. https://doi.org/10.1159/000448245.
32. Vuerstaek JD, Reeder SW, Henquet CJ, Neumann HA. Arteriolosclerotic ulcer of Martorell. J Eur Acad Dermatol Venereol. 2010;24(8):867–74. https://doi.org/10.1111/j.1468-3083.2009.03553.x.
33. Weenig R, Davis M, Dahl P, Su W. Skin ulcers misdiagnosed as pyoderma gangrenosum. New Eng J Med. 2002;347(18):1412–1418. https://doi.org/10.1056/NEJMoa013383.
34. Shelling ML, Federman DG, Kirsner RS. Clinical approach to atypical wounds with a new model for understanding hypertensive ulcers. Arch Dermatol. 2010;146(9):1026–9. https://doi.org/10.1001/archdermatol.2010.213.
35. Dagregorio G, Guillet G. A retrospective review of 20 hypertensive leg ulcers treated with mesh skin grafts. J Eur Acad Dermatol Venereol. 2006;20:166–9.
36. Bonfiglio B, Dipaola G, Navarra G. Two cases of hypertensive Martorell's leg ulcers. BMC Geriatr. 2010;10(Suppl 1):A44. Published 2010 May 19. https://doi.org/10.1186/1471-2318-10-S1-A44.
37. Dissemond J, Erfurt-Berge C, Goerge T, Kröger K, Funke-Lorenz C, Reich-Schupke S. Systemic therapies for leg ulcers. JDDG: Journal der Deutschen Dermatologischen Gesellschaft. 2018;16:873–890. https://doi.org/10.1111/ddg.13586.
38. Quintana-Castanedo L, Conde-Montero E, Recarte-Marín L, Peral-Vázquez A, Pérez-Jerónimo L, de la Cueva-Dobao P. Pain control with punch grafting in ulcers with underlying arteriolosclerosis. J Wound Care. 2022;31(4):356–9. https://doi.org/10.12968/jowc.2022.31.4.356. PMID: 35404703.
39. Conde-Montero E, Pérez Jerónimo L, Peral Vázquez A, RecarteMarín L, SanabriaVillarpando PE, de la Cueva DP. Early and sequential punch grafting in the spectrum of arteriolopathy ulcers in the elderly. Wounds. 2020;32(8):E38–41 PMID: 33166269.

40. Satoh T, Yoozeki H, Muota H, Tokura Y, Kabashima K, Takamori K, Shiohara T, Morita E, Aiba S, Aoyama Y, Hoshimoto T, Katayama I. 2020 guidelines fort he diagnosis and treatment of rurigo. J Dermatol. 2021;48(9):e414–31. https://doi.org/10.1111/1346-8138.16067. Epub 2021 Jul 27.
41. Mullins TB, Sharma P, Riley CA, Sonthalia S. Prurigo Nodularis. In: StatPearls [Internet]. Treasure Island (FL): StatPearls Publishing; 2023. PMID: 29083653.
42. Wong LS, Yen YT. Chronic nodular prurigo: an update on the pathogenesis and treatment. Int J Mol Sci. 2022;23(20):12390. https://doi.org/10.3390/ijms232012390.PMID:36293248; PMCID:PMC9604302.
43. Müller S, Zeidler C, Ständer S. Chronic prurigo including prurigo nodularis: new insights and treatments. Am J Clin Dermatol. 2023. https://doi.org/10.1007/s40257-023-00818-z).
44. Sibbald C, Reid S, Alavi A. Necrobiosis lipoidica. Dermatol Clin. 2015;33(3):343–60.
45. Hashemi DA, Brown-Joel ZO, Tkachenko E, Nelson CA, Noe MH, Imadojemu S, Vleugels RA, Mostaghimi A, Wanat KA, Rosenbach M. Clinical features and comorbidities of patients with necrobiosis lipoidica with or without diabetes. JAMA Dermatol. 2019;155(4):455–9.
46. Reid SD, Ladizinski B, Lee K, Baibergenova A, Alavi A. Update on necrobiosis lipoidica: a review of etiology, diagnosis, and treatment options. J Am Acad Dermatol. 2013;69(5):783–91.
47. Nihal A, Caplan AS, Rosenbach M, Damsky W, Mangold AR, Shields BE. Treatment options for necrobiosis lipoidica: a systematic review. Int J Dermatol. 2023;62(12):1529–37.
48. Nakajima T, Tanemura A, Inui S, Katayama I. Venous insufficiency in patients with necrobiosis lipoidica. J Dermatol. 2009;36(3):166–9.
49. Planinšek Ručigaj T. Diseases of the veins and arteries (leg ulcers), chronic wounds, and their treatment. In: Smoller Bruce R, editor. Atlas of dermatology, dermatopathology and venereology: inflammatory dermatoses. Cham: Springer International Publishing; 2022. Str. 1205-1331. ISBN 978-3-319-53807-5, ISBN 978-3-319-53809-9. https://link.springer.com/referenceworkentry/https://doi.org/10.1007/978-3-319-53808-2_67, https://doi.org/10.1007/978-3-319-53808-2_66.
50. Lavery MJ, Stull C, McCaw I, Anolik RB. Dermatitis artefacta. Clin Dermatol. 2018;36(6):719–22. https://doi.org/10.1016/j.clindermatol.2018.08.003. Epub 2018 Aug 16 PMID: 30446194.
51. Cole-King A, Harding KG. Psychological factors and delayed healing in chronic wounds. Psychosomat Med 2001;63(2):216–20.
52. Goldberg SR, Diegelmann RF. What makes wound chronic. Surg Clin. 2020;100(4):681–93.
53. Hay RJ, Morris-Jones R. Bacterial infections. In: Griffiths C, Barker J, Bleiker T, Chalmers R, Creamer D, editors. Rook's textbook of dermatology, 8th edn. Oxford: Wiley-Blackwell; 2016. p 26.1–26.87.
54. Planinšek Ručigaj T, Szuba A. Disorders of lymphatic vessels. In: Smoller BR, editors. Atlas of dermatology, dermatopathology and venereology: inflammatory dermatoses. Cham: Springer International Publishing; 2022. p 1333–1438. ISBN 978-3-319-53807-5, ISBN 978-3-319-53809-9.
55. Planinšek Ručigaj T, Kozak M, Slana A, Bešić N, Cokan Vujkovac A, Grmek M, Stritar A, Kecelj N. Priporočila za obravnavo bolnikov z limfedemom = Recommendations for the management of patients with lymphoedema. Zdravniški vestnik: glasilo Slovenskega zdravniškega društva. 2018; 87(7/8):393–402. ISSN 1318-0347.
56. Brindle R, Williams OM, Barton E, Featherstone P. Assessment of antibiotic treatment of cellulitis and erysipelas. A systematic review and meta-analysis. JAMA Dermatol. 2019;155(9):1033–1040. https://doi.org/10.1001/jamadermatol.2019.0884
57. Li A, Wang N, Ge L, Xin H, Li W. Risk factors of recurrent erysipelas in adult Chinese patients: a prospective cohort study. BMC Infect Dis. 2021;21:26. https://doi.org/10.1186/s12879-020-05710-3.
58. Schaverien MV, Asaad M, Selber JC, Liu J, Chen DN, Hall MS, Butler CE. Outcomes of vascularized lymph node transplantation for treatment of lymphedema. J Am Coll Surg. 2021;232(6):982–94.

59. Partsch H. Compression therapy. In: Sadick N, Khilnani N, Morrison N (eds) Practical approach to the management and treatment of venous disorders. London: Springer; 2013. https://doi.org/10.1007/978-1-4471-2891-5_17.
60. Senet P. Cutaneous cancers and chronic leg ulcers. Phlebolymphology. 2014;21(2):75–80.
61. Condorelli AG, Dellambra E, Logli E, Zambruno G, Castiglia D. Epidermolysis bullosa-associated squamous cell carcinoma: from pathogenesis to therapeutic perspectives. Int J Mol Sci. 2019;20(22):5707.
62. Senet P, Combemale P, Debure C, et al. Malignancy and chronic leg ulcers: the value of systematic wound biopsies: a prospective, multicentre, cross-sectional Study. Arch Dermatol. 2012;148(6):704–8.
63. Robson MC, Cooper DM, Aslam R, et al. Guidelines for the treatment of venous ulcers. Wound Repair Regener. 2006;14:649–62.
64. Bonamonte D, Filoni A, De Marco A, et al. Squamous cell carcinoma in patients with inherited epidermolysis bullosa: review of current literature. Cells. 2022;11(8):1365.

Wound Care in Blistering Diseases

7

Alina Suru, Mihaela Mănăilă, Klaus Fritz, and Carmen Maria Sălăvastru

Abstract

Blistering conditions manifest with fluid-filled skin lesions, vesicles, and bullae, often leading to erosions covered by crusts. These conditions encompass both inherited and acquired disorders, some frequent and other rare, some mild and other severe, possibly life endangering. Autoimmune blistering diseases can be caused by immune system dysfunction. Management aims to alleviate pain, prevent infections, and promote epithelialization, often involving immunosuppressive medications. Wound care presents challenges due to skin fragility and immunosuppressive effects of the medication, necessitating gentle cleaning, appropriate drainage techniques, and protective dressings. Topical treatments and oral care are integral, alongside pain management and infection monitoring. Stevens-Johnson syndrome and toxic epidermal necrolysis, drug-related mucocutaneous diseases, demand meticulous care to prevent epidermal detachment and infection. Inherited epidermolysis bullosa poses challenges in wound healing due to skin fragility, requiring specialized wound care approaches. Research into novel therapies, such as gene therapy, offers hope for improved management. Multidisciplinary care, nutritional support, and preventive strategies, particularly in neonates, are crucial for optimizing outcomes. Understanding the complexities of blistering conditions and tailoring management strategies are paramount in enhancing patient care and quality of life.

A. Suru (✉) · M. Mănăilă · C. M. Sălăvastru
Pediatric Dermatology Department, Colentina Clinical Hospital, Bucharest, Romania
e-mail: suru.pirvu@drd.umfcd.ro

K. Fritz
Dermatology and Laser Center, Landau in Der Pfalz, Germany

Dermatology 2, Carol Davila University of Medicine and Pharmacy, Bucharest, Romania

C. M. Sălăvastru
Carol Davila University of Medicine and Pharmacy, Bucharest, Romania

G.-S.Tiplica and K. Isoherranen (eds.), *Wound Healing*,
https://doi.org/10.1007/978-3-031-84579-6_7

Keywords

Bulla • Blister • Wound management • Dressings • Wound care • Wound healing • Blistering diseases • Pain management • Infection • Topical care

Abbreviations

KRT5	Keratin 5
LAMB3	Laminin Subunit Beta 3
PLEC	Plectin
NICU	Neonatal Intensive Care Unit
TEM	Transmission Electron Microscopy
HE	Hematoxylin -Eosin staining
DIF	Direct Immunofluorescence
EM	Erythema Multiforme
SJS	Stevens-Johnson Syndrome
TEN	Toxic Epidermal Necrolysis
LP	Lichen Planus
BLSA	Bullous Lichen Sclerosus et Atrophicus
EBA	Epidermolysis Bullosa Acquisita
BSLE	Bullous Lupus Erythematosus
PCT	Porphyria Cutanea Tarda
PV	Pemphigus Vulgaris
BSA	Body Surface Area
EB	Epidermolysis Bullosa
US	United States of America
CNS	Central Nervous System
RDEB	Recessive Dystrophic Epidermolysis Bullosa

Wound Care in Blistering Diseases

Blistering diseases are characterized by the appearance of fluid-filled skin lesions, vesicles and bullae. The roof of the blister may become detached forming an erosion that can be covered by a crust resulting from the drying of the exudation of serous fluid. Regarding the depth of the lesion, the erosion refers to a loss of epidermis, which heals without scarring. It commonly follows a blister; the ulcer refers to a loss of dermis and epidermis [1]. In partial thickness wounds the epidermis and portions of the dermis are affected, the lesions do not extend to the subcutaneous fat and the adnexal structures are preserved. In full thickness wounds, the entire dermis is involved, also the subcutaneous fat. The adnexal structures are not preserved and they cannot provide a source for reepithelization [2].

Blistering diseases can be broadly categorized into **inherited** and **acquired** conditions based on their underlying causes and origins. Blistering conditions can also be classified as **nonimmunobullous** (Table 7.1) or **immunobullous** (Table 7.2). While inherited blistering diseases originate from genetic mutations and are present from birth, acquired blistering diseases develop due to immune system dysregulation, environmental triggers, or medications.

Other vesiculobullous conditions which are encountered in special situations (e.g. coma blisters, trauma blisters) are important for the differential diagnosis (Table 7.3).

We have chosen two compelling clinical cases that presented challenges both in terms of diagnosis and treatment. The first case illustrates a rare genetic blistering disease (epidermolysis bullosa) necessitating prolonged management of the lesions (see Case 7.1), while the second case involves a common bullous disorder seldom affecting infants (bullous pemphigoid), presenting its own set of difficulties (see Case 7.2). Due to the rarity of these cases, the literature review is more extended than in other chapters.

Wound Healing ETR Correlations

For an adequate management, both diagnostic and therapeutic, of blistering diseases, it is important to be trained to:

- Know the physiology and stages of wound healing, comprehend the factors that can disrupt this process, and appreciate their prognostic significance.
- Perform a clinical examination of all the lesions and assess the patient's quality of life and pain.
- Differentiate between a normal evolving lesion and a pathological one.
- Rule out infections by considering conducting a swab test on the lesion.
- Remember that in some diseases (e.g., epidermolysis bullosa) squamous cell carcinoma can develop on chronic wounds.
- Recognize the situations in which referral to an Infectious Diseases Doctor is imperative.
- Understand the benefits of topical corticosteroids and the importance of their use in a rotational regimen.
- Know to perform the medical techniques essential for achieving a diagnosis, such as the Tzanck smear and skin biopsy.
- Know the management of bullous lesions (puncturing with a sterile needle) and remember that the blister roof must be rest intact and in place.

Table 7.1 Acquired blistering disorders—classification—nonimmunobullous (after Welsh 2009 [3])

Classification	Type	Description and treatment
Infections	**Viral** (herpes simplex, varicella zoster)	Together with the systemic agents, topical Acyclovir, 1% Penciclovir and 10% Docosanol can be used for orolabial herpes. Topical antiviral agents should be administered using a finger with intact skin Varicella in immunocompetent children can be treated symptomatically with antipyretics, antihistamines, calamine lotion, and tepid baths [4, 5]
	Bacterial (bullous impetigo, bullous erysipelas)	Mupirocin, retapamulin, and fusidic acid are the preferred treatments for impetigo For localized, uncomplicated, non-bullous impetigo, topical therapy alone is the recommended treatment. It is advised to remove crusts with soap and water before applying topical antibiotic therapy Systemic antibiotics should be prescribed for all cases of bullous impetigo and cases of non-bullous impetigo with more than five lesions, deep tissue involvement, and systemic signs of infection, lymphadenopathy or lesions in the oral cavity. Children with impetigo should uphold excellent personal hygiene practices and refrain from close contact with other children during the active outbreak. It is crucial to regularly wash hands, linens, clothes, and any affected areas that may have been in contact with infected fluids. Sores can be covered with a bandage to mitigate spread through contact. In cases of recurrent impetigo, assessment for carriage of the causative bacteria is recommended. The nasal cavity is a common reservoir, and carriers can be treated with mupirocin, applied within the nostrils [6, 7]
	Fungal (Tinea)	Bullous tinea, observed in both adults and children, frequently manifests on the feet, displaying an erythematous scaly rash accompanied by serous fluid-filled bullae. Misidentification and delays in treatment are prevalent occurrences. A wide array of potential differential diagnoses exists. Diagnostic hints encompass a unilateral and localized distribution, expanding annular scaling, concurrent onychomycosis, and an absence of response to topical corticosteroids [8] Topical antifungals are the primary treatment option for numerous patients with uncomplicated, localized cutaneous dermatophyte infections. Preventive measures encompass wearing breathable footwear and socks, utilizing antifungal or absorbent powders, regular nail clipping, and refraining from re-exposure, such as avoiding walking barefoot in locker rooms. It's important to note that old shoes frequently harbor significant numbers of infectious organisms and should either be discarded or treated with disinfectants or antifungal powders [9]
Drugs	**Bullous drug eruptions** (including phototoxic drug eruptions; major drug eruptions: EM/SJS/TEN)	Early detection and prompt diagnosis are essential for effective care because they can stop disease development and limit consequences. Specialized treatment modalities are only highly effective if initiated as soon as the disease manifests. Three pillars support therapy: early medication withdrawal or elimination, supportive therapy, and targeted therapy [10] Management in SJS/TEN is detailed in the text

(continued)

Table 7.1 (continued)

Classification	Type	Description and treatment
Vasculitis	**Bullous vasculitis**	A wide range of circumstances are included in the term cutaneous vasculitis, including skin-limited variations of systemic vasculitis, skin-only forms of single-organ vasculitis, and cutaneous presentations of systemic vasculitis Therapy is guided by the severity, mainly the presence or absence of internal organ involvement. Skin involvement in systemic diseases can often be efficiently managed with appropriate systemic treatment, though this is not always the case. Specific medication with skin-specific activity and a good risk–benefit profile are chosen in cases where the skin is the primary site of impairment. Last but not least, if skin-limited vasculitis is minimally symptomatic and self-limited, there may be no need for any treatment at all in many situations [11–13]. For limited forms of vasculitis that affect only the skin, conservative methods can promote wound healing and prevent immune complex deposition in the lower limbs. These measures include rest, elevation, and the use of compression stockings [14]. While they don't stop the development of new lesions, topical steroids and moisturizers can assist with pruritus and other localized skin complaints [15] The appearance of hemorrhagic blisters should prompt the initiation of corticosteroids (0.5–1 mg per kg body weight) [14]
Immunological	**Cellular Sweet syndrome (neutrophils)**	*Bullous variant of Sweet's syndrome* is a rare form of Sweet syndrome that exhibits clinically a bullous hemorrhagic rash and histopathologically segregated dermo-epidermal junction with dermal neutrophilic infiltrates [16, 17] The condition responds to systemic corticosteroids [16]; second-line therapies include potassium iodide, colchicine, indomethacin, dapsone, clofazimine, doxycycline and metronidazole [17, 18]. Recent case reports added Janus kinase inhibitors (baricitinib) and biological agents (adalimumab, infliximab) as treatment possibilities [17]. For bullous Sweet syndrome surgical debridement may be detrimental [19]
	Mastocytosis (mast cells)	*Bullous diffuse cutaneous mastocytosis* is characterized by blister formation and a thickening of the skin known as pachydermia [20, 21]. The hemorrhagic feature observed in some of the blisters can be linked to the release of heparin. The blisters are formed by serine proteases released by the mast cells. Histamine and other mast cell mediators can cause some patients to experience systemic symptoms, including flushing, itching, gastrointestinal distress, and even anaphylaxis Avoiding triggers is the cornerstone of treatment for bullous mastocytosis. It is important to advise parents and caregivers that certain situations, including rubbing, friction, heat exposure, abrupt temperature changes, teething, fever, and vaccinations, can exacerbate skin lesions, blisters, or anaphylaxis. The symptomatic treatment implies using topical creams and oral medications. Topical antibiotics or antiseptics are recommended in children with blistering and denuded skin areas to avoid skin infections. Topical corticosteroids aim to decrease erythema and blister formation. Topical sodium cromolyn should only be used on intact skin [20, 21]

(continued)

Table 7.1 (continued)

Classification	Type	Description and treatment
	Noncelluar Amyloidosis	*Bullous amyloidosis* is a rare cutaneous manifestation primarily of systemic amyloidosis, a condition in which abnormal proteinaceous material is formed and deposited in response to inflammatory conditions and plasma cell dyscrasias. Hemorrhagic bullae serve as a clue to the diagnosis of bullous amyloidosis Systemic amyloidosis has an unfavorable prognosis, but its morbidity and death rate can be reduced with early detection, diagnosis, and treatment of its consequences [22]
Inflammatory skin conditions	**Dyshidrotic eczema**	For *dyshidrotic eczema* the cornerstone of treatment is corticosteroids, both systemic and topical. Topical inhibitors of calcineurin might be beneficial Treatment for allergic or irritant contact dermatitis is required [23]
	Bullous lichen planus	Bullous lichen planus is a rare variant of lichen planus (LP), clinically defined by vesicular and/or bullous lesions that develop on pre-existing LP lesions or on perilesional skin as the effect of severe liquefactive degeneration of the basal layer cells Topical treatment with potent corticosteroids, but also systemic treatment with CS has been described. Based on isolated cases and random observations, further therapy options include acitretin [24], dapsone [25], mycophenolate mofetil [26], and antimalarial drugs [27, 28]. Topical tretinoin 0.025% in combination with triamcinolone 0.1% has also been successfully used for lichen planus with bullous manifestation on the lip [28, 29]
	Bullous lichen sclerosus et atrophicus (BLSA)	BLSA is also a rare occurrence in both genital and extragenital locations [30] There are reports regarding the use of corticosteroids, antimalarial drugs and doxycycline for the treatment of BLSA [31] Compared to anogenital LS, extragenital LS is usually less sensitive to topical steroids and calcineurin inhibitors, necessitating the use of additional medications; certain patients have been reported to benefit from phototherapy [30, 32]
Metabolic	**Porphyria cutanea tarda**	PCT is the most common porphyria; it is characterized by photosensitivity and skin fragility with blisters appearing on sun exposed skin (face, hand, forearms, and feet) **PCT** management is done by avoidance of precipitating factors (sun exposure, alcohol, smoking, estrogen therapy, iron overload), phlebotomy, antimalarial drugs and chelation therapy [33, 34]
	Diabetes	The management of *bullosis diabeticorum* is detailed in table 3

Table 7.2 Acquired blistering disorders—classification—immunobullous (after Welsh 2009 [3])

Classification	Type	Description and treatment
Intraepidermal blistering diseases—the Pemphigus group	– Pemphigus vulgaris (PV) – Pemphigus foliaceus – IgA pemphigus (subcorneal pustular dermatosis) – Paraneoplastic pemphigus	PV debuts with oral painful, non-healing ulcers. The cutaneous involvement is characterized by flaccid blisters that rupture and form erosions [2, 35] The main goals of topical therapy for pemphigus vulgaris are to reduce inflammation and prevent infections. For cutaneous and mucosal lesions, corticosteroids, calcineurin inhibitors, or corticosteroids plus antibiotics are typically used in combination. Low-adhesive wound dressings should be used to cover cutaneous erosive lesions. Adequate dental care and gel-containing local anesthetics are part of supportive treatment for oral lesions. Systemic corticosteroids are currently the first-line treatment for pemphigus. They are often combined with immunosuppressive drugs, such as azathioprine, mycophenolate mofetil, and the anti-CD20 monoclonal antibody rituximab, usually at initiation of treatment. For severe or refractory cases intravenous immunoglobulins or immunoadsorption can be tried [35, 36] Wound care in immunobullous disorders is detailed in the text below

(continued)

Table 7.2 (continued)

Classification	Type	Description and treatment
Subepidermal blistering diseases—the Pemphigoid group	– Bullous pemphigoid, mucous membrane cicatricial pemphigoid, herpes gestationis – Linear IgAdisease (chronic bullous disease of childhood) – Dermatitis herpetiformis	Initial lesions in BP are pruritic eczematous plaques or urticaria-like lesions. After some time patients may develop tense blisters on the initial lesions. Sterile puncture of large blisters is recommended [36] Intravenous immunoglobulin is a potentially useful alternative in severe and resistant instances. Biological medications, including rituximab, show promise in this field. Bullous pemphigoid has been treated with Omalizumab [37], and Dupilumab [38–40]
	-Epidermolysis bullosa acquisita (EBA)	For EBA, as with hereditary epidermolysis bullosa, non-adherent dressings and preventing local trauma and infection are important aspects of general care [37]
	– Bullous lupus erythematosus (BSLE)	BSLE is a rare manifestation of systemic lupus erythematosus. Dapsone is considered the first line of treatment with a good response. Immunosuppressive drugs include cyclophosphamide, azathioprine, mycophenolate mofetil, and methotrexate. Rituximab has been tried in refractory cases; Anakinra is another treatment option [41, 42]

– Know the characteristics of various types of protective dressings offered in the market and understand the proper sequence for their application. Additionally, long-term management of bullous diseases often occurs within the patient's home environment, overseen by caregivers or family members. Part of their educational regimen entails explaining the phases of gentle wound cleaning and bandaging.
– Understand the unique requirements of patients with chronic diseases, including the imperative to minimize trauma and tailor their nutrition to address any deficiencies.

Table 7.3 Other vesiculobullous diseases (after Mascaro [44])

Disorder	Description	Management
Bullosis diabeticorum	Tense blisters on acral sites (feet, lower legs, hands) in absence of trauma Asymptomatic lesions may be accompanied by a mild burning sensation [44–46]	In two to six weeks, the majority of patients see spontaneous healing of their lesions. In order to lessen discomfort and stop secondary infections, treatment consists of aspirating blisters, and using topical antiseptics or antibiotics On rare occasions, a subsequent soft tissue infection does occur and necessitates either surgical intervention or systemic antibiotics [44–46]
Coma blisters	In individuals experiencing unconsciousness or immobilization, lesions manifest at anatomical locations subjected to the highest pressure. Initially, these lesions emerge approximately 24 h subsequent to the onset of coma, presenting as blanchable erythematous patches or plaques, which subsequently evolve into violaceous plaques. Within 48–72 h following the commencement of coma, blister formation or erosions ensue at these specific sites [44, 47]	Coma-induced blisters undergo spontaneous healing within 1 to 2 weeks. In patients not experiencing coma, regular changes in posture aid in the resolution and prevention of the disorder [44, 47]
Bullous insect bite reactions	Insect bites typically present as highly itchy erythematous papules or nodules, often appearing in clusters with a frequent linear arrangement. However, variations such as vesicular and bullous reactions are not uncommon, where blisters may form centrally within papules or as bland vesiculobullae. Among insect bites, flea bites are notably prone to causing blisters, particularly on the legs, while bedbug bites can also result in bullous reactions. Certain insects like fire ants can induce pustular lesions. In individuals with hematologic malignancies, exaggerated reactions often manifest as persistent papulonodules, vesicles, bullae, and occasionally necrotic lesions [44, 48]	Treatment for most patients with bullous insect bites typically involves draining the blisters, applying topical corticosteroids, and administering systemic antihistamines. In severe cases, a brief course of systemic corticosteroids may be required. It's worth noting that while systemic corticosteroids can initially improve exaggerated reactions, lesions often reappear upon dose reduction. Dapsone has been proposed as a therapeutic alternative for these individuals Additionally, the use of protective clothing and insect repellents plays a crucial role in prevention [44, 48]

(continued)

Table 7.3 (continued)

Disorder	Description	Management
Edema blisters	Edema blisters arise in individuals experiencing an acute worsening of chronic edema, notably affecting the lower limbs, and in cases of anasarca. These tense bullae typically lack inflammation but are surrounded by edematous skin [44, 49]	Blisters resolve with the resolution of the oedema
Bullous dermatitis artefacta	Vesicles and bullae after a thermal, electrical, or chemical burn. Other substances can determine blisters as vesicants, coolants or "salt and ice"	Psychological interventions
Trauma blisters	Fracture blisters represent a relatively rare complication observed in fractures occurring in areas of the body where the skin adheres tightly to bone, such as the ankle, wrist, elbow, and foot, and where there is minimal subcutaneous fat cushioning. These blisters bear a striking resemblance to second-degree burns [44]	The management approach is subject to considerable debate. Certain authors propose maintaining blisters intact and awaiting their natural resolution before proceeding with surgical stabilization. Conversely, others advocate for early surgical intervention to prevent blister formation. In cases where blisters have already formed, some recommend incising them without consideration for their location, even if the incision would traverse a blister [50]
	Suckling blisters develop in utero in newborns in areas accessible to sucking	These blisters do not require treatment and will usually resolve within a few days to a few weeks
	Friction blisters predominantly manifest on the soles and heels, primarily due to repetitive friction such as walking or running in improperly fitting footwear. Additionally, they may arise on the palms and fingers when a repetitive action is consistently performed [44]	Friction blisters can heal naturally without requiring treatment. However, relieving pressure and discomfort, as well as preventing fluid accumulation, can be achieved through the drainage of blister contents using a small "window" in the blister roof. Alternatively, hydrocolloid or other types of dressings can be applied [44]

– Know that interdisciplinary consultations play a pivotal role in assembling a team of specialists to enhance understanding and management of the disease.

Inherited Blistering Disorders

Epidermolysis bullosa is the main inherited condition to determine skin fragility and blistering. Other rare conditions are represented by superficial epidermolytic ichthyosis, acrodermatitis enteropathica, ectodermal dysplasia, bullous congenital ichthyosiform erythroderma, congenital porphyria, incontinentia pigmenti [43]. Wound care in epidermolysis bullosa is detailed in the text below.

Autoimmune blistering diseases are a group of rare conditions where the immune system mistakenly attacks proteins within the skin, leading to the formation of blisters and erosions on the skin and mucous membranes. These diseases result from the immune system targeting specific proteins that are essential for maintaining the structure and integrity of the skin. The goals of the management in these conditions are to alleviate pain, prevent infections, promote epithelialization and increase the quality of life. Treatment for autoimmune blistering diseases often involves immunosuppressive medications to suppress the immune response and reduce blister formation. Corticosteroids, immunosuppressants, and other medications that modulate the immune system's activity are commonly used.

Wound care in these patients can be challenging as they display increased skin and mucosal fragility, the areas affected may be large and immunosuppressants may slow wound healing. Additionally, the affected patients may have extreme ages, either elderly with decreased mobility and lesions difficult to dress [2, 51], or newborns up to toddlers.

Proper wound care is crucial to manage the blisters and prevent complications like infection. Steps for management:

- **Gentle wound cleaning** with a mild, non-irritating cleanser and lukewarm water to gently clean the affected areas. Saline can also be used. Three techniques are available for cleaning wounds: compresses (the gauze should be squeezed to avoid excess fluid), soaking (saturated gauze), and irrigation (not suitabe for deep wounds that may retain the cleanser) [52]. Scrubbing or rubbing the blisters or erosions vigorously should be avoided, as this can cause further damage and rupture of the blisters. Patients with large skin lesions may benefit from taking baths with antiseptics like chlorhexidine [35]. Potassium permanganate soaks may also be beneficial for moist, weepy erosions [53].
- **Drainage**: The optimal method for treating blistering skin has not yet been determined. Currently, there is debate over the best course of action for small blisters. While some authors recommend daily puncture of tense blisters to reduce lateral extension of the blister edges, others advocate for leaving blisters intact, to prevent secondary infection. Large blisters can be punctured with a sterile needle (as in inherited epidermolysis bullosa) and the roof of the blister can be left in place [2, 53].
- **Protective dressings**: non-adherent dressings can be used to cover the blisters or erosions. Silicone-based dressings or non-stick pads can be useful to protect the affected areas and promote healing without causing trauma upon

removal. A soft silicone mesh dressing functions well as a *primary dressing*. Before applying it to the skin, it can be covered with a topical antimicrobial or an adequate emollient. Usually, *the secondary dressing*—such as a soft silicone foam or other foam dressing—must be absorbent. Soft knit tube dressings can be used to fasten these dressings. In order to reduce discomfort and prevent additional harm, dressings that have dried on the skin should be soaked before being removed. Although there is no data to support the ideal number of dressing changes, one should take into account the stage of wound healing, the exudation through the secondary dressing, and the necessity to check for signs of infection. To evaluate the lesions, bandages in the acute stage should be changed every day. Later in the healing process, it would be appropriate to just change the secondary dressing and keep the original dressing in place, allowing the underlying erosion to continue undisturbed. In this case, additional topical applications might be applied on top of the silicon mesh primary dressing. It's important to remove crusts to promote healing [53]. *Etesami* et al. showed in a review article that the most commonly used topical care in pemphigus patients was silver-containing dressings [54].

- **Topical treatments**: topical medications like corticosteroids or calcineurin inhibitors to reduce inflammation and promote healing [36]. To maintain barrier function, a bland emollient can be applied directly to the skin or initially to primary dressings [53].
- **Oral care**: Adequate dental care and gel-containing local anesthetics are part of supportive treatment for oral lesions. Topical corticosteroid preparations, topical tacrolimus, intralesional corticosteroids, but also topical ciclosporin and topical prostaglandin E2 have been found helpful in some patients. Diluted mouthwashes with hydrogen peroxide or chlorhexidine mouthwash may be beneficial [53].
- **Avoid irritants**: avoid harsh soaps, perfumes, or other products that can irritate the skin. Opt for hypoallergenic, fragrance-free products when cleansing or moisturizing the affected areas [55].
- **Pain management**: to relieve discomfort or pain associated with the blisters or erosions. A multidisciplinary team including a pain specialist may be needed [53].
- **Avoiding trauma**: Minimize friction and trauma to the affected areas. Loose-fitting, soft clothing can help prevent rubbing against the blisters or erosions.
- **Monitoring for infection**: increased erythema, swelling, warmth, purulent exudate, or fever may be signs of infection. Mupirocin and retapamulin are effective against gram-positive organisms and topical metronidazole is an option in cases of infection with anaerobic organisms. In severe cases, systemic antibiotics may be required [54].
- **Nutrition and hydration**: A well-balanced diet rich in nutrients is essential for overall healing. Patients should be consuming adequate protein, vitamins, and minerals that support cutaneous healing. A multidisciplinary team including a nutritionist is recommended [35].

Stevens–Johnson syndrome (SJS) and toxic epidermal necrolysis (TEN) are rare, acute and life-threatening mucocutaneous diseases that are nearly always drug-related in adults. For TEN drug exposure is the cause in 80% of cases; infections and immunizations have also been incriminated. For SJS about 50% of cases are linked to drug consumption [56]. SJS and TEN are a consequence of extensive keratinocyte cell death that results in the separation of significant areas of skin at the dermal–epidermal junction, producing the appearance of scalded skin.

Fever, conjunctivitis, and pain when swallowing are among the initial signs of both TEN and SJS, and they can all appear one to three days before cutaneous manifestations. First appearing on the trunk, skin lesions typically migrate to the face, neck, and proximal upper extremities. Mucosal erosions cause excruciating discomfort, and skin lesions are typically sensitive [56].

These patients must therefore be handled with extreme care. Tense blisters are usually seen only on the palmoplantar surfaces, where the epidermis is thicker and, therefore, more resistant to mild trauma.

- If there is epidermal detachment affecting 10–20% (or more) of BSA, meticulous daily wound care, hydration, and nutritional support are necessary and should ideally be performed in an intensive care unit. It is advised to use an aluminum survival sheet, a thermoregulated bed with controlled pressure, instead of a standard bed and sheets.
- Venous catheters should, if possible, be inserted in an area of the patient's skin that is not affected. All patient procedures should be carried out aseptically.
- It is ideal to treat wounds once a day in the presence of a dermatologist or with their assistance.
- Minimal manipulation of the patient is recommended since any movement has the potential to trigger epidermal detachment.
- The face, eyes, nose, mouth, ears, anogenital region, axillary folds, and interdigital areas should all be the focus of cutaneous care.
- Vaseline® gauze should be applied to detached regions, especially the back and other pressure sites that come into contact with the bed, until re-epithelialization is complete. Biobrane®, a temporary semi synthetic skin substitute dressing is associated with reduced pain, decreased fluid loss and faster re-epithelialization. Biologic dressings like porcine xenografts or human skin allografts can also be used. Silver nitrate impregnated gauzes along with topical antibiotics can also be used. Chlorhexidine mouthwash helps in maintaining good oral hygiene and preventing secondary infection [10].
- Isotonic sterile sodium chloride solution can be used every day to clean the face of serous and/or bloody crusts.
- Around orifices, such as the mouth, nose, and ears, an antibiotic ointment (such as mupirocin) or petrolatum ointment (if the patient is on systemic antibiotics) should be applied.
- Skin that has been denuded can be covered with silicone dressings. The silicone dressing can be left in place until re-epithelialization occurs without the need

for replacement; however, it does require daily surface cleaning with an isotonic sterile sodium chloride solution [56].

Epidermolysis bullosa (EB) is the main inherited blistering condition. This is an umbrella term for a genetic group of diseases that are characterized by skin fragility and are caused by mutations in the genes encoding different proteins with a role in cell adhesion [57]. There are several types of EB, each with varying degrees of severity, but they generally involve issues with structural proteins that help bind the layers of skin together. The most recent consensus report in 2020 reclassified inherited epidermolysis bullosa and other disorders with skin fragility with an increased focus on the molecular origin of each subtype of EB when possible to investigate the gene involved and the type of mutation present. The four major types were retained: intraepidermal (EB simplex), junctional (junctional EB), dermolytic (dystrophic EB) and mixed (Kindler EB) [58].

Wound healing in individuals with EB can be a complex process due to the constant blistering and skin fragility. EB associates a vast spectrum of clinical manifestations, leading to different clinical forms.

The wound healing process in individuals with EB follows a similar pattern to normal wound healing but is often complicated due to the fragile nature of their skin. Some key aspects of wound healing in individuals with EB are:

- Formation of blisters: blister formation is a hallmark of EB. These blisters can occur spontaneously or due to minor trauma. They are fragile and prone to rupture, leading to open wounds or erosions on the skin.
- Delayed healing: the constant cycle of blistering and skin damage can affect the normal wound healing process. The fragile skin makes it challenging for wounds to heal properly, and they may take longer to heal than in individuals without EB.
- Risk of infection: open wounds in individuals with EB are susceptible to infection due to the compromised skin barrier. Infections can further delay healing and increase the risk of complications.
- Pain management: wound care in EB often involves pain management strategies, as these individuals may experience significant pain due to their skin condition.
- Specialized wound care: management of wounds in EB requires specialized approaches. This may include using non-adherent dressings, gentle wound cleansing techniques, and protecting the skin from further damage [59].
- Multidisciplinary approach: individuals with EB often benefit from a multidisciplinary team involving dermatologists, wound care specialists, nurses, nutritionists, and other healthcare professionals to manage their complex needs.

Research and emerging therapies: Research into potential treatments and therapies for EB, such as gene therapy and other innovative approaches, is ongoing to improve wound healing and overall management of the condition.

Management

Currently, day-to-day EB management focuses on wound care, preventing mechanical trauma and infection. It can be beneficial to use protective bandaging, cushioning around bony prominences, and loose-fitting, soft clothing. Reducing bacterial colonization can be achieved by various modalities described in the following text. It is best to take antibiotics sparingly and to avoid using oral antibiotics or topical mupirocin for prolonged periods of time [60, 61]. Topical antibiotics/antimicrobials should only be used for short periods of time to prevent resistance and sensitization and should be alternated every 2–6 weeks.

- **Gentle wound cleansing** should be done with a gentle, noncytotoxic cleanser. Saline solution, water, benzalkonium chloride 0.1% solution, or chlorhexidine hydrochloride 0.1% can be used [62]. In order to remove the dressings, most patients are bathing or soaking for 5–10 min in the bathtub. This can also reduce pain and trauma associated with dressing changes. A dilute acetic solution (5% white vinegar diluted to 0.25–1.0%) or bleach (5–10 mL in 5 L of water) may decrease the bacterial colonization [60–62]. Bathing frequency depends on the type of dressing and lesion characteristics: from daily or in alternate days in case of infected wounds or dressings which stick to the lesions, to 3–4 days up to a week when advanced dressings are available [63]. Salt baths have become popular among some patients, presumably because the osmotic impact is beneficial in pain relief. To make a 0.9% solution, add around 90 g of table salt to 10 L of water. Salt can be used in combination with antiseptics to minimize their tendency to sting [64].
- **Blister management and drainage:** the blisters can be punctured with a sterile needle; this is necessary to prevent blister extension. The needle should be passed through the blister roof, parallel to the skin, to create an entry and exit hole through which fluid can be drained. The roof of the blister can be left in place acting like a natural dressing [59, 60, 62–64]
- **Monitoring for infection**: increased erythema, swelling, warmth, purulent exudate, or fever may be signs of infection. Early diagnosis of critically colonized or infected wounds should consider:
  - *wound history*: several week duration, recent size extension and exudate increase;
  - *wound bed:* presence of debris, dead slough, friable tissue and foul smelling;
  - *wound margins and surrounding skin*: edema, erythema, increased temperature [63].
- **Protective dressings**: there are several dressings available. In general, only nonadhesive dressings should be applied on EB skin. Soft silicone dressings are widely used; silver-impregnated dressings may be helpful for wounds that are heavily colonized or infected, although long-term use should be avoided in order to minimize the systemic absorption of silver. Less expensive paraffin impregnated gauzes are another suitable dressing for uninfected wounds. The

choice of dressing should be individualized based on EB subtype, wound characteristics: site, exudate, critical colonization/infection, size and patient age, as well as patient/parent preference, frequency of dressing, cost, and availability [59, 62].

- *dry wounds or wounds with light exudate* can benefit from non-adhesive soft silicone or lipido-colloid contact dressings, and hydrogels. Hydrogel dressings need to be replaced every day or as soon as they start to dry out. The other types could be changed every 3–4 days.
- *wounds with heavy exudate* have a significant infection risk and call for particular dressings. It is preferable to use hydrofiber dressings or soft silicone foam with super-absorbers that can absorb heavy exudate. Polymeric membranes and soft silicone foams are also recommended. Secondary dressings to fixate or absorb excess exudate may be needed [62, 63].

Layering the bandages (Fig. 7.1) with primary contact layer dressings, secondary silicone foam dressings and retention bandages is the common approach also in EB, although some patients (EBS patients usually) may prefer to leave blisters undressed. To dry up the blistered areas and create a low friction surface, corn starch can be used by patients who find dressings uncomfortable or that they worsen the blister sites. Silk socks have the potential to lessen friction [64].

- **Topical Treatments:** Oleogel-S10 was the first topical treatment to be approved in the European Union in 2023 for patients suffering from DEB and JEB. Oleogel-S10 (birch triterpenes, also known as birch bark extract) is a topical sterile gel containing 10% birch triterpenes formulated with sunflower oil. EASE was a double-blind, randomized, vehicle-controlled, phase III study to

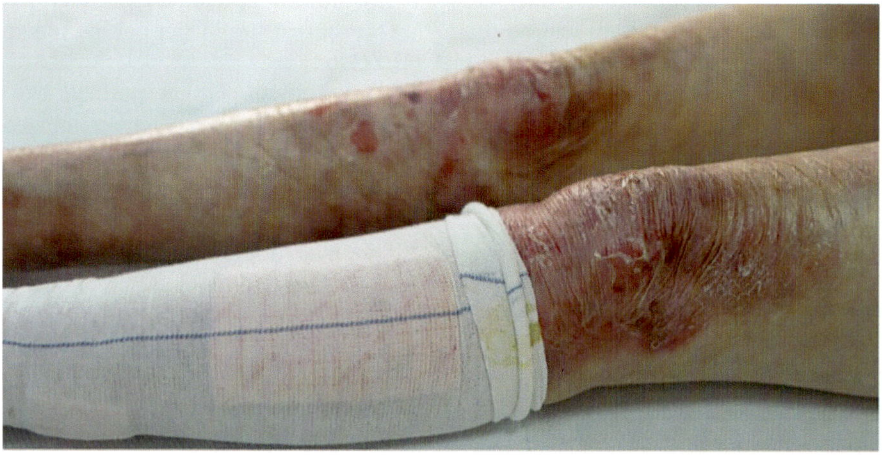

Fig. 7.1 Layers of dressings in RDEB patient

determine the efficacy and safety of the topical gel Oleogel-S10 (birch triterpenes) in EB. In EASE, the primary endpoint showed that Oleogel-S10 resulted in acceleration of wound healing with 41.3% of target wounds treated with Oleogel-S10 achieving first complete closure within 45 days compared with 28.9% for control gel [65].

- **Genetic therapies**: B-VEC (beremagene geperpavec) is a topical genetic therapy based on HSV-1 that restores the expression of collagen VII in keratinocytes and fibroblasts in patients with dystrophic EB [66]; it is limited by cost and availability.
- **Pain and pruritus management**: the aim is to relieve discomfort and pain associated with blisters or erosions. EB pain is caused by neuropathic and nociceptive mechanisms, which can be enhanced by central nervous system sensitization and psychological conditioning [59]. Pharmacological and nonpharmacological approaches are described in the management of pain in patients with [62, 64]. Pruritus is another prevalent and incapacitating symptom of all EB variants. Pharmacologic interventions employed for pruritus in EB include sedating and non-sedating antihistamines, antidepressants and CNS aiming drugs such as gabapentin and pregabalin [58].
- **Prevent complications**: non-healing wounds may be a clinical manifestation of squamous cell carcinoma in EB patients. Therefore, careful observation and, if necessary, biopsy is required [59, 67].
- **Nutrition**: dysphagia, oral blistering, and reduced appetite can all affect nutrition. Furthermore, much higher dietary needs are required to make up for losses and promote the healing of wounds [64]. The goal is to prevent anemia, hypoalbuminemia, mineral and vitamin deficiencies which result from decreased nutrient intake, inflammation and concomitant losses through severe and chronic wounds [59].
- **Special considerations**: neonates require special attention.
  - Preventive handling, emollient use, and cushioning are necessary for newborns with EB during most activities in order to lower the incidence of new blisters
  - Baby garments can be turned inside out to prevent the seams from rubbing the skin
  - The diapers can be lined with a soft material to reduce the rubbing from the elastic edges; the elastic edges can also be removed
  - Hands and feet require special technique dressings to prevent early digit fusion
  - Bathing should be delayed until prenatal and birth trauma have healed
  - Diluted vinegar or bleach for wound soaks are not recommended for neonates, nor are silver impregnated dressings [59, 62–64, 68]

Conclusions

Blistering conditions imply a complex management that require a multifaceted approach due to the diverse clinical manifestations and underlying causes. Treatment strategies encompass pain relief, infection prevention, wound care, and specialized interventions tailored to each condition's unique characteristics.

Proper wound care is crucial in all these conditions to prevent complications such as infection, promote healing, and alleviate discomfort. Techniques such as gentle cleansing, drainage of blisters, and the use of protective dressings are employed to maintain skin integrity and facilitate healing.

Blistering conditions may affect different age groups, from newborns to the elderly. Specialized care tailored to the unique needs of each age group is essential for optimal outcomes.

A multidisciplinary team involving dermatologists, wound care specialists, nurses, nutritionists, and other healthcare professionals is crucial for comprehensive management. Collaboration among experts ensures a holistic approach addressing various aspects of patient care, including wound management, pain control, and nutritional support.

Case 7.1. Epidermolysis Bullosa Simplex—Severe Form

Short Clinical Story of the Patient: A female neonate presented at birth multiple areas of aplasia cutis on the dorsal aspects of the hands, forearms, abdomen, knees and feet (Fig. 7.2A–C). Shortly after, she developed bullae and erosions on large areas of the skin, predominantly on the limbs. Her family medical history was unremarkable, as for her personal medical history, she was the second child of the family, her older brother having no medical history.

Considering the clinical manifestations at birth, the diagnosis of a bullous genetic disease was raised and the main differential diagnosis included the various

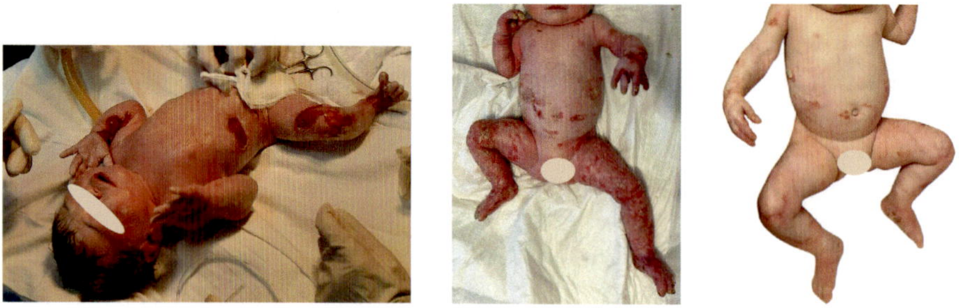

(a) (b) (c)

Fig. 7.2 A—Aspect at birth with birth multiple irregular areas of aplasia cutis; B, C—Improved skin fragility with reduced blistering and erosions (age 20 weeks compared to 11 weeks)

subtypes of epidermolysis bullosa with various life prognosis. Skin biopsy was obtained for transmission electron microscopy and genetic testing was performed (blood sample—Epidermolysis bullosa 26 genes Panel).

Laboratory Investigations

Skin biopsy for transmission electron microscopy concluded that the diagnosis was epidermolysis bullosa simplex (Dowling Meara type) (Fig. 7.3).

Genetic testing of the patient identified a pathogenic heterozygous mutation of KRT5 c.541 T > C, p.(Ser181Pro). This variant was previously reported in the literature [69–71] as appearing de novo; 3 others heterozygous mutations with uncertain significance were identified: LAMB3 c.1244C > T, p.(Pro415Leu), LAMB3 c.1516 T > A, p.(Phe506Ile) and PLEC c.7780C > T, p.(Arg2594Trp).

Genetic testing of the parents showed that the mutation of PLEC gene was inherited from the father and the mutations of LAMB3 gene were inherited from the mother. After the parents genetic testing, it was established that the mutation of KRT5 gene occurred de novo also in our patient.

Diagnosis: based on the above investigations results was of severe EBS.

Evolution: after birth the skin fragility increased, with large areas being affected by bullae and post bullous erosions, especially the limbs. She also developed marked acral hyperkeratosis of the fingers and toes around the age of 5 weeks up to the age of 12 weeks when it slowly started to improve. The skin fragility also improved with fewer new bullae appearing at the margins of the diapers and on trauma areas.

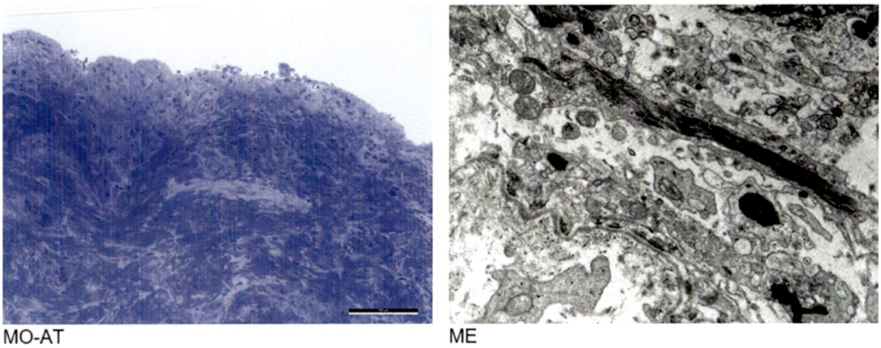

Fig. 7.3 HE staining (MO-AT) and TEM aspect (ME), courtesy of Prof. Dr. Mihaela Gherghiceanu, Ultrastructural Pathology and Bioimaging Laboratory National Institute of Pathology Victor Babeş—Bucharest

Management

The patient was admitted in a neonate intensive care unit (NICU) for almost 3 months. As for wound management, intact blisters were drained using a sterile needle. The fingers and toes were bandaged separately to prevent pseudo syndactyly. Non-adherent silicone dressing were used and retained with tubular and elastic dressings to prevent friction and formation of new bullae.

She developed some new lesions at the periphery of the dressings and after the age of 4 months the dressings were reduced to a minimum, according to data available in the literature [72].

Case 7.2. Bullous Pemphigoid in a 4-Month-Old Baby

Short Clinical Story of the Patient:

A 4-month-old female was admitted to the Pediatric Ward and referred to the Pediatric Dermatology Department for a vesiculobullous eruption affecting both palms and soles without mucosal involvement evolving for 9 days (Fig. 7.4A). The blisters were tense and other skin findings consisted of papules and annular, ring-shaped plaques with erythematous edges and a slightly hypopigmented center, distributed on trunk and limbs (Fig. 7.5A, B). The rash didn't affect the diaper area. From her family history we learned that her parents had multiple allergies.

Considering the tense bullae the suspicion of a bullous autoimmune disease was raised. The differential diagnosis included bullous pemphigoid, dermatitis herpetiformis or linear IgA disease (chronic bullous disease of childhood).

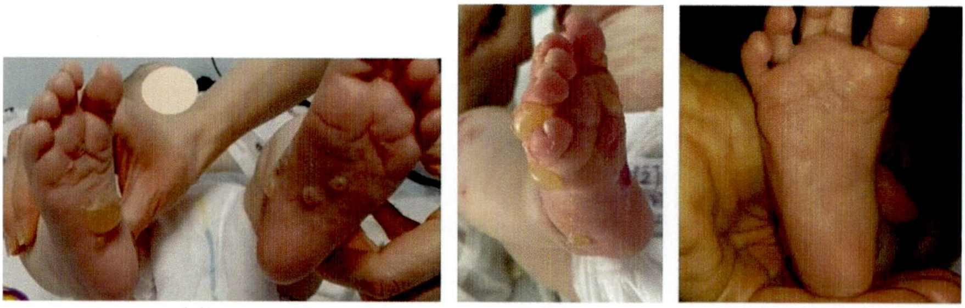

(a) (b) (c)

Fig. 7.4 Evolution of the plantar lesions; A, B—tense bullae on the soles; C—remission of the lesions on the soles

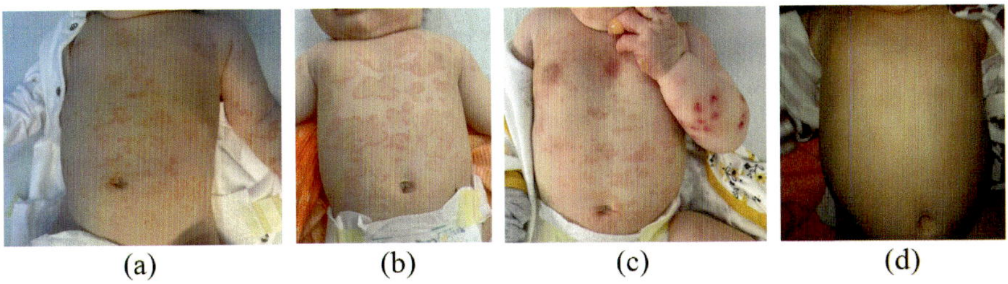

Fig. 7.5 Evolution of the trunk lesions; A, B—annular, ring-shaped plaques with erythematous edge and slight hyperpigmentation at center; C—erythematous papules and plaques; D—remission of trunk lesions

Laboratory Investigations:

The initial laboratory test showed eosinophilia with normal levels of IgE and negative IgM and IgG antibodies for Herpes Simplex Virus 1 and 2. Tzanck smear exhibited an acute nonspecific inflammatory process with leukocytes. The 3 mm punch biopsy for Hematoxylin–Eosin staining showed a subepidermal bulla consisting of eosinophils and lymphocytes which were also arranged around the perivascular space in the dermis and *DIF* was intensely positive with linear C3 staining along the basement membrane zone and less intense linear basement membrane zone for IgG and Fb. Also, anti-BP 180 and anti-BP 230 autoantibodies were recommended; only anti-BP 180 Ab were performed identifying high levels of anti-BP 180 autoantibodies (51 IU/ml, reference < 20 IU/ml).

Diagnosis: considering the clinical manifestations and the laboratory findings the diagnosis of bullous pemphigoid was established.

Management

The patient responded well to systemic corticosteroids to which systemic Erythromycin was added. After a week of treatment, no new bullae appeared, after a month the corticosteroid treatment was slowly tapered and stopped after five months. The evolution of the plantar and trunk lesions can be observed in Figs. 7.4A–C and 7.5A–D.

Local care: intact blisters were drained using a sterile needle inserted parallel to the skin. The blister roof was left in place. A local antiseptic was applied, as well as topical fusidic acid with hydrocortisone acetate cream and Copper-Zinc cream.

References

1. Cox NH, Coulson JH. Diagnosis of skin disease. In: Burns DA, Breathnach SM, CoxNH, Griffiths CEM, editors. Rook's textbook of dermatology. 1. 8th ed. Wiley; 2010.
2. Nadelmann E, Czernik A. Wound care in immunobullous disease. Autoimmune Bullous Diseases. 2018.
3. Welsh B. Blistering skin conditions. Aust Fam Physician. 2009;38(7):484–90.
4. Downing C, Mendoza N, Sra K, Tyring SK. Human herpesviruses. In: Bolognia JL, Schaffer JV, Cerroni L, editors. Dermatology. 4th ed. Philadelphia: Elsevier; 2018. p. 1400–15.
5. Trent JT, Kirsner RS. Herpesvirus infections and herpetic wounds. Adv Skin Wound Care. 2003;16(5):236–43.
6. Nardi NM, Schaefer TJ. Impetigo. In: StatPearls. StatPearls Publishing, Treasure Island (FL); 2017. PMID: 28613693.
7. Hay R, Adriaans B. Bacterial infections. In: Burns DA, Breathnach SM, CoxNH, Griffiths CEM, editors. Rook's textbook of dermatology, vol. 2. 8th ed. Wiley; 2010.
8. Xie F, Lehman JS, editors. Bullous Tinea Pedis. In: Mayo clinic proceedings. Elsevier; 2022.
9. Elewski BE, Hughey LC, Marchiony Hunt K, Hay RJ. Fungal diseases. In: Bolognia JL, Schaffer JV, Cerroni L, editors. Dermatology. 4th ed. Philadelphia: Elsevier; 2018. p. 1329–35.
10. Verma R, Vasudevan B, Pragasam V. Severe cutaneous adverse drug reactions. Med J Arm Forces India. 2013;69(4):375–83.
11. Micheletti RG. Treatment of cutaneous vasculitis. Front Med. 2022;9:1059612.
12. Sangolli PM, Lakshmi DV. Vasculitis: A checklist to approach and treatment update for dermatologists. Indian Dermatol Online J. 2019;10(6):617.
13. Carlson JA, Cavaliere LF, Grant-Kels JM. Cutaneous vasculitis: diagnosis and management. Clin Dermatol. 2006;24(5):414–29.
14. Sunderkötter C, Bonsmann G, Sindrilaru A, Luger T. Management of leukocytoclastic vasculitis. J Dermatol Treat. 2005;16(4):193–206.
15. Micheletti RG, Pagnoux C. Management of cutaneous vasculitis. La Presse Médicale. 2020;49(3):104033.
16. Bhat AG, Malleshappa SKS, Pasupula DK, Duke W, Shaaban R, Bhat AG. Bullous variant of Sweet's syndrome as a consequence of radioiodine contrast exposure. Cureus. 2018;10(10).
17. Joshi TP, Friske SK, Hsiou DA, Duvic M. New practical aspects of Sweet syndrome. Am J Clin Dermatol. 2022;23(3):301–18.
18. Verma SB. Recurrent bilaterally symmetrical bullous sweet's syndrome: A rare and confusing entity. Indian J Dermatol. 2012;57(6):483.
19. Leighton P, Amirfeyz R. Sweet syndrome: a lesson in the management of the cutaneous lesions of malignancy. J Surg Case Rep. 2015;2015(2):rjv003.
20. Rydz A, Lange M, Ługowska-Umer H, Sikorska M, Nowicki RJ, Morales-Cabeza C, et al. Diffuse cutaneous mastocytosis: a current understanding of a rare disease. Int J Mol Sci. 2024;25(3):1401.
21. Almheiri SK, Pakran J, AlFalasi AA, El Bahtimi R, Elbahtimi R. Bullous mastocytosis: a rare variant of diffuse cutaneous mastocytosis. Cureus. 2024;16(1).
22. Jin Q, Chen F, Zhou Y, Xu Z, Cheung JM, Chen R, et al. Hidden flaws behind expert-level accuracy of GPT-4 vision in medicine. arXiv preprint arXiv:240108396. 2024.
23. Norbert R, Peter O.F. Other eczematous eruptions. In: Bolognia JL, Schaffer JV, Cerroni L, editors. Dermatology, 4th ed. Philadelphia: Elsevier; 2018. p. 237.
24. Rallis E, Liakopoulou A, Christodoulopoulos C, Katoulis A. Successful treatment of bullous lichen planus with acitretin monotherapy. Review of treatment options for bullous lichen planus and case report. J Dermatol Case Rep. 2016;10(4):62.
25. Camisa C, Neff JC, Rossana C, Barrett JL. Bullous lichen planus: diagnosis by indirect immunofluorescence and treatment with dapsone. J Am Acad Dermatol. 1986;14(3):464–9.
26. Nousari HC, Goyal S, Anhalt GJ. Successful treatment of resistant hypertrophic and bullous lichen planus with mycophenolate mofetil. Arch Dermatol. 1999;135(11):1420–1.

27. Chyl-Surdacka K, Przepiórka-Kosińska J, Gerkowicz A, Krasowska D, Chodorowska G. Application of antimalarial medications in the treatment of skin diseases. Dermatol Rev/ Przegląd Dermatologiczny. 2016;103(4):316–22.
28. Liakopoulou A, Rallis E. Bullous lichen planus—a review. J dermatol Case Rep. 2017;11(1):1.
29. Van Tuyll van Serooskerken AM, Van Marion AM, De Zwart-Storm E, Frank J, Poblete-Gutiérrez P. Lichen planus with bullous manifestation on the lip. Int J Dermatol. 2007;46:25–6.
30. Khatib J, Wargo JJ, Krishnamurthy S, Travers JB. Hemorrhagic bullous lichen sclerosus: a case report. Am J Case Rep. 2020;21:e919353–61.
31. Vukicevic J. Extensive bullous lichen sclerosus et atrophicus. Bras Dermatol. 2016;91:81–3.
32. Lewis F, Tatnall F, Velangi S, Bunker C, Kumar A, Brackenbury F, et al. British Association of Dermatologists guidelines for the management of lichen sclerosus, 2018. Br J Dermatol. 2018;178(4):839–53.
33. Shah A, Bhatt H. Porphyria Cutanea Tarda.
34. Singal AK. Porphyria cutanea tarda: recent update. Mol Genet Metab. 2019;128(3):271–81.
35. Joly P, Horvath B, Patsatsi A, Uzun S, Bech R, Beissert S, et al. Updated S2K guidelines on the management of pemphigus vulgaris and foliaceus initiated by the European academy of dermatology and venereology (EADV). J Eur Acad Dermatol Venereol. 2020;34(9):1900–13.
36. Di Lernia V, Casanova DM, Goldust M, Ricci C. Pemphigus vulgaris and bullous pemphigoid: update on diagnosis and treatment. Dermatology practical & conceptual. 2020;10(3).
37. Santi CG, Gripp AC, Roselino AM, Mello DS, Gordilho JO, Marsillac PFd, et al. Consensus on the treatment of autoimmune bullous dermatoses: bullous pemphigoid, mucous membrane pemphigoid and epidermolysis bullosa acquisita-Brazilian Society of Dermatology. Anais brasileiros de dermatologia. 2019;94:33–47.
38. Zhang Y, Zhang J, Chen J, Xu Q, Zou Y, Chao J. Efficacy and safety of dupilumab in moderate-to-severe bullous pemphigoid. Front Immunol. 2021;12:738907.
39. Russo R, Capurro N, Cozzani E, Parodi A. Use of dupilumab in bullous pemphigoid: where are we now? J Clin Med. 2022;11(12):3367.
40. Zhao L, Wang Q, Liang G, Zhou Y, Yiu N, Yang B, et al. Evaluation of dupilumab in patients with bullous pemphigoid. JAMA Dermatol. 2023;159(9):953–60.
41. Odonwodo A, Vashisht P. Bullous systemic lupus erythematosus. StatPearls [Internet]: StatPearls Publishing; 2023.
42. Lipsker D. Bullous systemic lupus erythematosus. UpToDate [Internet] Waltham (MA): UpToDate Inc. 2020.
43. Zhao CY, Murrell DF. Blistering diseases in neonates. Curr Opin Pediatr. 2016;28(4):500–6.
44. José M. Mascaró Jr. Other Vesiculobullous Diseases. In: Bolognia JL, Schaffer JV, Cerroni L, editors. Dermatology, 4th ed. Philadelphia: Elsevier; 2018. p. 554–61.
45. Chatterjee D, Radotra A, Radotra BD, Handa S. Bullous diabeticorum: a rare blistering manifestation of diabetes. Indian Dermatol Online J. 2017;8(4):274.
46. Chouk C, Litaiem N. Bullosis Diabeticorum. StatPearls [Internet]: StatPearls Publishing; 2023.
47. Rocha J, Pereira T, Ventura F, Pardal F, Brito C. Coma blisters. Case Rep Dermatol. 2009;1(1):66–70.
48. Singh S, Mann BK. Insect bite reactions. Indian J Dermatol Venereol Leprol. 2013;79:151.
49. Ferguson NN. Edema Blisters. In: Inpatient dermatology. 2018. p. 399–401.
50. Uebbing CM, Walsh M, Miller JB, Abraham M, Arnold C. Fracture blisters. Western J Emerg Med. 2011;12(1):131.
51. Duipmans JC, Bolling MC. Wound care in autoimmune bullous diseases. Autoimmune bullous diseases: text and review. Springer; 2022. p. 193–8.
52. Alavi A, Kirsner R.S. Dressings. In: Bolognia J, Schaffer J, Cerroni L, editors. Dermatology, 4th ed. Philadelphia: Elsevier; 2018. p. 2462–76.
53. Harman K, Brown D, Exton L, Groves R, Hampton P, Mohd Mustapa M, et al. British Association of Dermatologists' guidelines for the management of pemphigus vulgaris 2017. Br J Dermatol. 2017;177(5):1170–201.
54. Etesami I, Dadkhahfar S, Kalantari Y. Topical care in pemphigus wounds: a systematic review of the literature. Dermatol Ther. 2022;35(11):e15808.

55. Mitoseriu-Bonteanu I, Butacu A, Grigore R-N, Cucu C, Zait M, Tiplica G-S, et al. Emollients–a cornerstone in the treatment of epidermolysis bullosa. Emolientele–elemente de bază în tratamentul epidermolizei buloase. Romanian J Clin Exp Dermatol. 2016;3(1).
56. Hötzenecker WPC, French LE. Erythema multiforme, Stevens–Johnson Syndrome, and toxic epidermal necrolysis. In: In: Bolognia JSJ, Cerroni L, editor. Dermatology, vol. 1. Philadelphia: Elsevier; 2018. p. 337–47.
57. Salavastru CM, Sprecher E, Panduru M, Bauer J, Solovan CS, Patrascu V, et al. Recommended strategies for epidermolysis bullosa management in Romania. Maedica. 2013;8(2):200.
58. Has C, Bauer JW, Bodemer C, Bolling MC, Bruckner-Tuderman L, Diem A, et al. Consensus reclassification of inherited epidermolysis bullosa and other disorders with skin fragility. Br J Dermatol. 2020;183(4):614–27.
59. Has C, El Hachem M, Bučková H, Fischer P, Friedová M, Greco C, et al. Practical management of epidermolysis bullosa: consensus clinical position statement from the European Reference Network for Rare Skin Diseases. J Eur Acad Dermatol Venereol. 2021;35(12):2349–60.
60. Pillay E, Clapham J. Development of best clinical practice guidelines for epidermolysis bullosa. Wounds Int. 2018;9(4):20–7.
61. Jo-David Fine JEM. Epidermolysis bullosa. In: Bolognia JSJ, Cerroni L, editor. Dermatology, vol. 2. Philadelphia: Elsevier; 2018. p. 538–53.
62. Pope E, Lara-Corrales I, Mellerio J, Martinez A, Schultz G, Burrell R, et al. A consensus approach to wound care in epidermolysis bullosa. J Am Acad Dermatol. 2012;67(5):904–17.
63. El Hachem M, Zambruno G, Bourdon-Lanoy E, Ciasulli A, Buisson C, Hadj-Rabia S, et al. Multicentre consensus recommendations for skin care in inherited epidermolysis bullosa. Orphanet J Rare Dis. 2014;9:1–20.
64. Denyer J, Pillay E. Best practice guidelines for skin and wound care in epidermolysis bullosa. An international consensus. Wounds International; 2017, p. 2023.
65. Kern JS, Sprecher E, Fernandez MF, Schauer F, Bodemer C, Cunningham T, et al. Efficacy and safety of Oleogel-S10 (birch triterpenes) for epidermolysis bullosa: results from the phase III randomized double-blind phase of the EASE study. Br J Dermatol. 2023;188(1):12–21.
66. Guide SV, Gonzalez ME, Bağcı IS, Agostini B, Chen H, Feeney G, et al. Trial of beremagene geperpavec (B-VEC) for dystrophic epidermolysis bullosa. N Engl J Med. 2022;387(24):2211–9.
67. Mellerio J, Robertson S, Bernardis C, Diem A, Fine J, George R, et al. Management of cutaneous squamous cell carcinoma in patients with epidermolysis bullosa: best clinical practice guidelines. Br J Dermatol. 2016;174(1):56–67.
68. Saad R, Duipmans J, Yerlett N, Plevey K, McCuaig C, Woolfe W, et al. Neonatal epidermolysis bullosa: a clinical practice guideline. Br J Dermatol. 2024:ljae006.
69. Has C, Küsel J, Reimer A, Hoffmann J, Schauer F, Zimmer A, et al. The position of targeted next-generation sequencing in epidermolysis bullosa diagnosis. Acta Derm Venereol. 2018;98(4):437–40.
70. Shemanko CS, Horn H, Keohane S, Hepburn N, Kerr A, Atherton D, et al. Laryngeal involvement in the Dowling-Meara variant of epidermolysis bullosa simplex with keratin mutations of severely disruptive potential. Br J Dermatol. 2000;142(2):315–20.
71. Chen F, Wei R, Deng D, Zhang X, Cao Y, Pan C, et al. Genotype and phenotype correlations in 441 patients with epidermolysis bullosa from China. J Eur Acad Dermatol Venereol. 2023;37(2):411–9.
72. Denyer J, Pillay E, Clapham J. Best practice guidelines for skin and wound care in epidermolysis bullosa. In: An international consensus wounds international; 2017.

Atypical Wounds

8

Kirsi Isoherranen, Ingel Soop, Justin Schlager, Jesse Karppinen, Anna Jylhä, Alexandra Irina Butacu, George-Sorin Tiplica, and Ionela Manole

Abstract

Atypical wounds can be suspected when the wound does not fall into the typical wound category, has an atypical location or appearance, pain out of proportion of the wound size, rapidly evolving necrosis, or shows poor healing on good treatment within 4–12 weeks. Dermatologists and dermatopathologists are key players in diagnosing atypical wounds. Treatment strategies are determined by the specific etiology and often require a multidisciplinary approach,

K. Isoherranen (✉)
Dermatology and Allergology, Wound Healing Centre, Helsinki University Hospital, Helsinki, Finland
e-mail: Kirsi.isoherranen@hus.fi

I. Soop
East-Tallinn Central Hospital, Tallinn, Estonia

J. Schlager
Dermatology and Allergology Clinic, München, Germany

J. Karppinen
Helsinki University Hospital, Skin and Allergy Hospital, University of Helsinki, Helsinki, Finland

A. Jylhä
Department of Dermatology, Kuopio University Hospital, Kuopio, Finland

Department of Dermatology, Institute of Clinical Medicine, University of Eastern Finland, Kuopio, Finland

A. I. Butacu · G.-S. Tiplica
2Nd Department of Dermatology, "Carol Davila" University of Medicine and Pharmacy, Colentina Clinical Hospital, Bucharest, Romania

I. Manole
2Nd Department of Dermatology, Colentina Clinical Hospital, Bucharest, Romania

G.-S.Tiplica and K. Isoherranen (eds.), *Wound Healing*,
https://doi.org/10.1007/978-3-031-84579-6_8

including immunosuppressive therapy, surgical intervention, antibiotic treatment, pain management, and compression therapy. Patient-centered approach is also needed to improve the reduced quality of life and treatment outcomes.

Keywords

Atypical wounds • Vasculitis • Pyoderma gangrenosum • Martorell hypertensive ulcers • Multidisciplinary approach • LUMBAR syndrome • Deficiency of adenosine deaminase 2 • Radiation therapy • Middle aortic syndrome • Leg ulcer

Introduction

Atypical wounds comprise about 10–20% of all chronic wounds treated at tertiary wound clinics [1–4]. The actual prevalence might be even higher due to under recognition and misdiagnosis. The recognition and diagnostics of an atypical wound is important, as diagnostic delay may lead in the worst case to limb amputation or patient's death [5–7].

The burden of atypical wounds for the health care system is enormous, as these wounds exhibit typically long healing times, and many patients are in their working life age [8]. Reduced quality of life and increased mortality are associated with atypical wounds. There is still a research gap in effective treatments, even if research especially in pyoderma gangrenosum is active [9].

Atypical wounds are wounds that do not fall into a typical wound category, i.e. venous, arterial, mixed venous arterial, pressure ulcer or diabetic foot ulcers. They are a heterogenous group of wounds caused by infection, inflammation, malignancy, genetic or congenital disorders [1]. Dermatologists and dermatopathologists are experts in diagnosing these wounds but several disciplines are needed in the treatment. Treatment is determined by the exact etiology and consists of i.e. immunosuppressive treatment, surgery, pain management, antibiotics, and compression therapy when wounds are located at lower limbs [10].

According to the ETR's of Wound Healing, a wound care professional must have the knowledge when to suspect an atypical wound and to refer the patient to a dermatologist specialist or other specialist experienced in atypical wounds. Typical signs include pain out of proportion of the wound size, atypical location or appearance, rapidly evolving necrosis, poor healing with traditional treatment within 4–12 weeks and if the wound cannot be classified as a typical one. Fast recognition and referral are key issues for a successful treatment outcome for the patient.

In addition to this chapter, atypical wound cases will be presented also in Chap. 6: Cutaneous wounds in systemic disorders.

Case 8.1. IgA Vasculitis

Introduction

Our case report presents a 13-year-old boy with a fast-appearing rash. His previous medical history was unremarkable except for obesity (with a BMI of 34) and attention deficit disorder well managed with methylphenidate. The rash consisted of purpura, vesicles, bullae and necrosis on his lower extremities and abdomen and the lesions were extremely painful to touch. Both legs were edematous. No auto-immune or skin diseases in the family were reported, nor were any allergies noted.

Differential Diagnosis

At the first visit, in a Pediatric emergency unit, laboratory tests showed low haemoglobin (89 g/L), hyponatremia (118 mg/L) and low albumin (16 mg/L), with raised CRP (139 mg/L) (but no fever), Anti-streptolysin O (608 mg/L) and amylase (699 mg/L). A urine sample showed protein- and hematuria consistent with mild nephrotic syndrome.

Coagulation markers, autoimmune antibodies and herpes cultures were negative. Bacterial cultures from the bullae on the lower legs showed both *Staphylococcus aureus* and Group B *Streptococcus*. Biopsies from skin showed leukocytoclastic vasculitis of postcapillary venules with IgA deposition and the immunofluorescence kidney biopsy presented with IgA deposition in the mesangium, thus the diagnosis of IgA vasculitis aka Henoch-Schönlein purpura was made (Fig. 8.1).

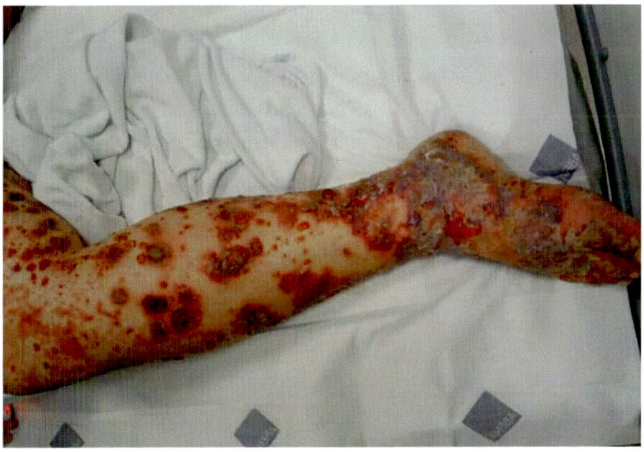

Fig. 8.1 IgA vasculitis (Henoch-Schönlein purpura)—case at admission

Treatment

The child was hospitalized in the Pediatrics department and high dose prednisolone (50 mg/day) plus topical wound care with silver products was started. Attempts to lower the dosage were met with exacerbations in condition. High dose prednisolone was continued over 2 months, with the child developing Cushingoid syndrome with classical upper body weight gain, striae and hypertension. Due to extreme pain of the lesions, wound dressing changes were done multiple times under general anesthesia by a plastic surgeon. Azathioprine (AZA) 100 mg $\times$ 2 was added after 2 months due to the necrotizing vasculitis continuing to being active.

A wound-care specialist was consulted about 3 months after hospitalization. Both legs were still edematous; large erosions with violaceous borders covered the lower extremities up to the groin area. Pressure ulcers on heels were also noted. Patient care was taken over by the wound-care department and carried out in an outpatient manner. Main intervention was the addition of compression therapy, wound-dressing changes being done under local anesthesia, and switching from silver dressings to honey-collagen products. With that, wound healing was markedly improved and notable re-epithelialization was seen at the two-week follow-up (Fig. 8.2). Wound-dressing changes were still very painful, but manageable with topical anesthetics and reduced with every visit to completely pain free in about 1 month. AZA was continued and prednisolone dose was gradually lowered with a goal of maintaining at 5 mg/day with no exacerbations in condition.

Discussion

IgA vasculitis (formerly known as Henoch-Schönlein purpura) is a leukocytoclastic vasculitis involving small vessels [11], where IgA1-containing immune complexes deposit within vessel walls, causing endothelial damage [12]. Upper respiratory tract infections often proceed IgAV, with *Streptococcus* strains being a frequent trigger [13–15]. Petechiae and palpable purpura can coalesce into bullous or necrotic lesions [16, 17]. Other organs often involved are the kidneys, gastrointestinal tract, and joints [13, 18]. Skin biopsy is the gold standard for diagnosing, but requires clinical correlation, as IgA vascular deposits can be found in other vasculitic syndromes [19].

There is no clear consensus on treating IgAV. Guidelines or reviews focus mainly on preventing kidney damage [20, 21], with latest case reports showing that with little or no kidney involvement, corticosteroids have no long-term benefit over placebo [22–24]. Extensive skin involvement has not been discussed much. Different immunosuppressive and immunomodulatory treatments have been used (mycophenolate mofetil, dapsone, cyclophosphamide, azathioprine) with little or no studies and few case reports. Compression is clinically believed to be important in atypical wound care, as it lessens edema and the deposition of immune complexes [1, 25]. Skin ulcerations can be difficult to manage due to pain and

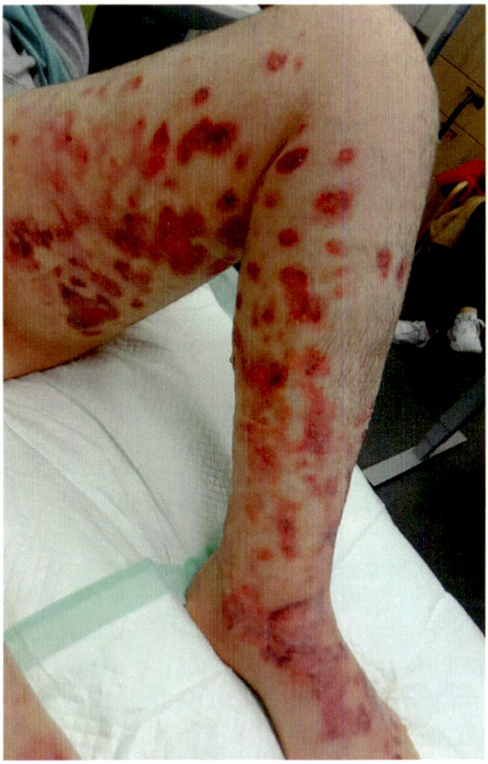

Fig. 8.2 IgA vasculitis after two weeks treatment showing markedly skin lesions

may require a multidisciplinary approach involving dermatology, plastic surgery, nephrology, pediatrics, and a specialized wound-care center.

Significant recovery in this case started only with the induction of regular compression therapy and proper wound therapy with local anesthesia and honey-collagen dressings. It is also arguable that some important side-effects (such as Cushingoid syndrome) would have been avoided with an early start of a steroid-spearing agent (such as AZA in this case). Proper therapy, both systemic and topical, has been shown to be cost-effective to the medical system [1], not to mention the monetary and emotional toll for the patient. This case report clearly illustrates the importance of consulting the appropriate departments early for optimal care as well as showing a wider need for educating specialists in different fields on proper atypical wound management.

Case 8.2. Deficiency of Adenosine Deaminase 2—A Rare Cause for Recurrent Painful Leg Ulceration

Introduction

A 35-year-old woman was hospitalized in our clinic with recurrent non-healing bilateral leg ulcers. Her past medical history was significant for multiple strokes of the brainstem region since early childhood, and recurrent livedo racemosa with painful ulcerations of the lower legs since the age of 18 years. The neurologic sequelae included dysarthria, tetra spasticity and cognitive impairment. She also suffered an episode of thrombotic occlusion of the right central retinal artery and peripheral facial nerve palsy of the right side. The recurrent painful ulcers led to multiple hospitalizations in external hospitals.

Diagnostics and Treatment

We performed a thorough diagnostic work-up. Differential blood count, liver enzymes, serum creatinine, serum protein electrophoresis and screening for thrombophilia were insignificant. Chronic venous insufficiency and peripheral arterial occlusion of the lower limbs were ruled out by ultrasound. There was no sign of ANCA-associated vasculitis or chronic infection including hepatitis B or C and syphilis. Wound biopsy did not show any specific changes. Given the neurologic and cutaneous manifestations, she was first diagnosed with Sneddon-Syndrome. However, oral anticoagulation with vitamin K antagonist phenprocoumon could not prevent new ischemic strokes and wounds only improved temporarily. Therefore, molecular testing was performed, which revealed mutation of the ADA2-gen with deficiency of adenosine deaminase 2 (DADA-2). Oral anticoagulation was discontinued and systemic treatment with adalimumab initiated. The wounds improved with standard care and no further ischemic event occurred.

After six months, however, the patient presented again due to a new painful ulceration on the left shin (Fig. 8.3). A deep skin biopsy yielded deposits of calcium, necrosis, and thrombotic occlusion of blood vessels at the ulcer border. The direct immunofluorescence showed IgM, C3 and fibrinogen positive vasculitis. Histology was thus consistent with ulceration due to DADA2. We then performed further laboratory testing, which yielded neutralizing antibodies against adalimumab. Hence, the ulceration was caused by insufficient disease control. We performed wound debridement with *Lucilia sericata* maggots followed by negative pressure therapy to support wound granulation. Finally, punch grafts from the left upper thigh were transplanted to the wound surface. Shortly thereafter, the patient experienced a significant relief of wound pain, thus, allowing rapid tapering of oral analgesia with oxycodone. She was discharged and the wound epithelialized within four weeks. After consultation with her neurologist, adalimumab was replaced with golimumab in combination with low-dose oral methotrexate (MTX). Up to date, no further stroke or leg ulceration occurred (Fig. 8.4).

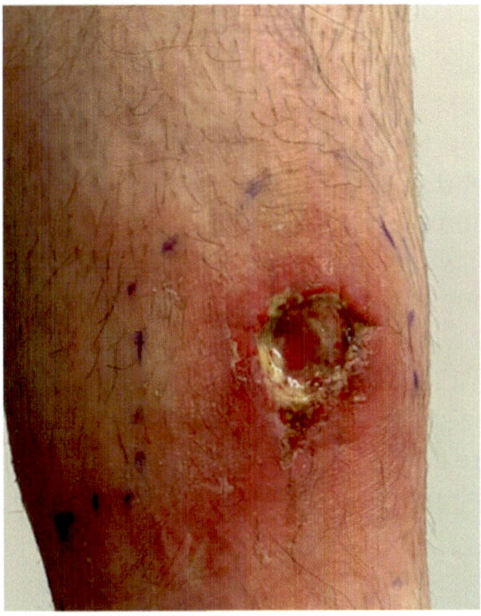

Fig. 8.3 Newly occurred leg ulceration in a patient with deficiency of adenosine deaminase 2

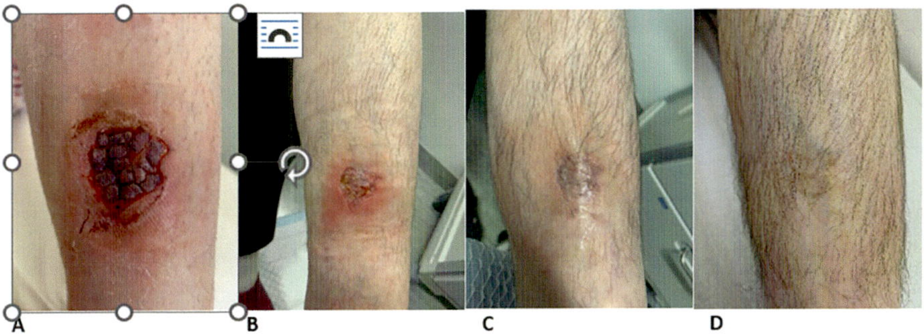

Fig. 8.4 Complete wound epithelialization within four weeks after wound debridement with *Lucilia sericata* maggots followed by negative pressure therapy to support wound granulation and, finally, punch grafts

Discussion

Deficiency in ADA-2 was first described in 2014. It is an extremely rare auto-inflammatory disorder caused by an autosomal-recessive loss-of-function mutation of the ADA-2 gen (former CECR-1 gen) [26, 27]. Adenosine deaminase-2 (ADA2) is produced by monocytes and myeloid cells. It plays an important role as growth factor and has immunoregulatory-properties. Reduction of ADA2 leads to impaired monocyte-differentiation with predominance of pro-inflammatory M1-monocytes and tumor necrosis factor (TNF) mediated perivascular inflammation [28]. Typical clinical manifestations include pan-arteritis nodosa-like vasculitis with fever, recurrent strokes of the brainstem region, livedo racemosa and skin ulceration, arthralgia and myalgia, impaired immune function (e.g. hypogammaglobulinemia) and hematologic abnormalities (e.g. lymphopenia, anemia) [29]. Diagnosis is based on clinical suspicion, which warrants testing for mutation of the ADA2-gene and low ADA2 activity [30]. However, the clinical picture may vary significantly. Fortunately, our patient did not show any hematologic abnormalities, nor signs of immunodeficiency. Although the evidence remains limited, anti-TNF-alpha agents, such as adalimumab, etanercept, infliximab or golimumab are considered as first-line treatment [31]. As in our patient, these biologicals may be combined with low-dose MTX to prevent the development of neutralizing antibodies [29].

This case demonstrates the importance of a systematic diagnostic work-up of atypical ulcers. However, it also highlights the importance of basic wound treatment and simple surgical techniques within treatment strategies of complex wounds.

Case 8.3. Martorell Hypertensive Ischemic Lower Leg Ulcer (HYTILU)

Introduction

A 75 years old male patient with chronic heart insufficiency, atrial fibrillation (with a history of warfarin usage, but cessation done four years ago), severe chronic obstructive pulmonary disease (cessation of smoking already 20 years ago), pulmonary *Pseudomonas* colonization, suspected polymyalgia rheumatica and a history of poorly healing lower leg ulcers was admitted to a Dermatological unit with a painful ulcer on the right Achilles tendon. During the initial visit, it was found out that the patient's blood pressure levels fulfilled the WHO criteria for arterial hypertension.

The ulcer itself had appeared three months prior due to minor trauma but had not healed with conservative care in primary care. The patient had peripheral pulses (arteria tibialis posterior and dorsalis pedis) ambidextrously palpable, and feet were warm. The leg presented with mild stasis dermatitis, some varicose veins and a mild level of lower leg oedema. The ulcer was 2×2 cm in size and it had a fibrinous ulcer bed with some necrosis at the proximal end. The ulcer had livid borders and also some red lining covering the central margin of the ulcer was seen (Fig. 8.5). The ulcer was tremendously painful.

Differential Diagnosis

Considering the patient's medical history and clinical characteristics of the ulcer, a mixed ulcer with venous and atypical components was suspected. A spindle shape biopsy from the proximal ulcer edge and blood samples were taken. Patient was referred to a vascular surgeon for arterial and venous examination where any arterial and venous insufficiencies requiring surgical intervention were ruled out.

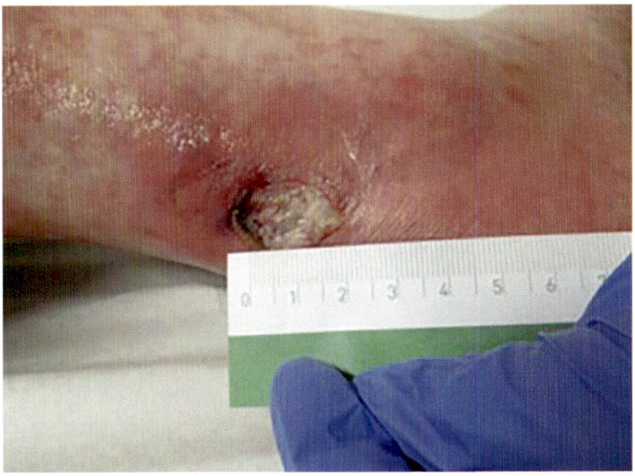

Fig. 8.5 Tremendously painful leg ulcer described as post-traumatic—at presentation

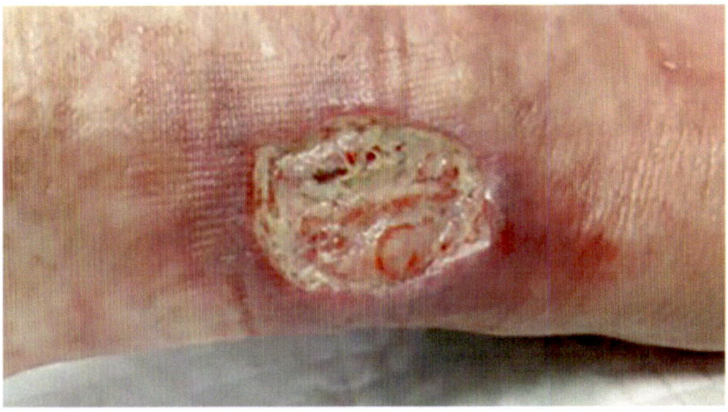

Fig. 8.6 Despite the usual treatment the ulcer grew in size and the pain did not diminish

Treatment

A calcium channel antagonist-medication was initiated for arterial hypertension and pain medication was optimized. In addition to an optimized local ulcer care, a moderate level of compression treatment was reinitiated. Nonetheless, the ulcer grew in size (Figs. 8.6 and 8.7), so the patient was hospitalized, maggot therapy was initiated, vitamin D supplementation was stopped, and the dosage of prednisolone (used for other diagnoses) was decreased. The ulcer still kept growing, so sodium-thiosulfate infusions (10 g/100 ml solution, 3x/week) were initiated. Subsequently, systemic antibiotic treatment was initiated for ulcer infection. Later, also surgical debridement and meshed skin transplant were performed and negative pressure wound therapy applied as well.

Discussion

HYTILU is a very painful lower leg ulcer that is typically found on the posterolateral ankle or on Achilles tendon [32, 33]. Patients are typically 70–80 years of

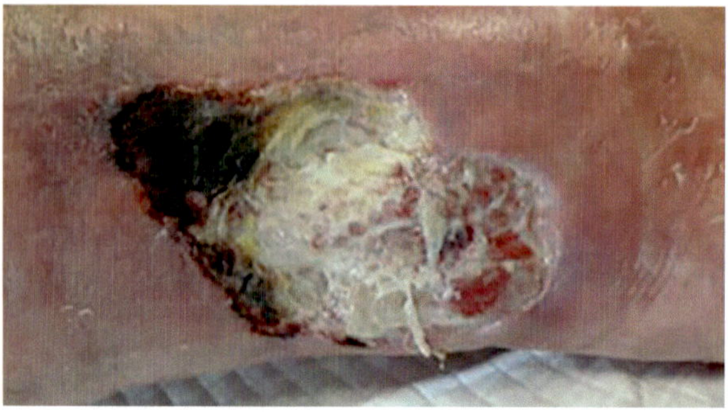

Fig. 8.7 Martorell Hypertensive Ischemic Lower Leg Ulcer (HYTILU)

age and present with arterial hypertension [35]. Approximately half of the patients also have diabetes mellitus (DM) [32–35]. The use of warfarin is also suggested as a significant risk factor [35]. Additionally, it has been suggested that HYTILU patients would have a heavy burden of other cardiovascular diseases as well [34, 35]. Concomitant peripheral arterial disease and venous insufficiency should be ruled out and if possible, treated.

The clinical picture of HYTILU consists of a fibrinotic/necrotic ulcer bed and livid, violaceous border with different features [32–37]. The immediate, central margin of the ulcer tends to have a bright red color resembling a red lipstick *(suggested as the red lipstick sign)* [34] and peripherally from this, also purple border and pathological livedo racemosa are usually seen. Histopathologically most common findings are arteriolosclerosis and Möckenberg medial calcinosis [32, 35].

The conservative treatment consists of optimizing the treatment of underlying diseases (*e.g.* hypertension, DM, arterial/venous insufficiency), an optimized local ulcer care (*i.e.* local dressing and compression therapy), cessation of warfarin as well as a prompt treatment of infections. Often, (repeated) surgical skin transplants are also needed and in extensively necrotic and large cases, also sodium-thiosulfate infusions may be recommended [1].

Case 8.4. Atypically Behaving Ulcer in a Young Patient with Congenital Combined LUMBAR Syndrome and Middle Aortic Syndrome

Introduction

A 16-year-old female with a congenital condition combining LUMBAR syndrome [38] and middle aortic syndrome [39] was referred to the University Hospital with an enlarging anterior leg ulcer on the right shin that had appeared 9 months earlier with no recordable trauma. She was born with bladder exstrophy, which was operated on as an infant and later also treated for bladder incontinence and hydronephrosis. Because of her condition she lacked one kidney, the infrarenal aorta and normal iliac veins. In her early childhood she also had pulsed dye laser

(PDL) treatments for multiple hemangiomas in her genital area and her right leg, which healed well, but were showing an unusually high inflammatory response.

Her condition has had little influence on her life: she had no claudication and was attending the sports class in school. Her prior health records showed that her blood pressure had been within a normal range. She had no regular medications and had been smoking since she was 13.

At clinical examination peripheral pulses were unpalpable. The duplex doppler sonography showed bilaterally monophasic curves, and the superficial femoral artery and the anterior tibial artery were detectable. Standard ABI was not performed due to ulceration, but toe pressure was 77/92 mmHg, showing a lower curve on the right. Transcutaneous oximetry (TcPO2) around the ulcer showed values between 55 and 62 mmHg. Both the superficial and the deep venous system were performing flawlessly.

The MRI angiography of the lower body and legs showed an anomaly of the lower abdominal aorta, where below the left kidney artery and superior mesenteric artery divides into several small branches leading to narrowed iliac arteries. The lower cava presented as duplicate that conjoined at the level of pancreas.

Differential Diagnosis

Considering the patient's history and physical examination and results of the specific studies described above, acute ischemic etiology, as well as venous insufficiency were excluded. A set of laboratory tests were performed in order to exclude underlying autoimmune conditions, such as rheumatoid arthritis or inflammatory bowel disease. Biopsies extending from the healthy skin to the wound bed were performed. The histopathology around the ulcerated skin showed changes in the capillary network, such as thickening of the capillary walls and coiling of the capillaries. Some features, such as panniculitis, increased number of granulocytes, micro abscesses and vasculitis-like reaction were seen in a single biopsy only and were considered secondary phenomena due to concurrent infection and edema, although pyoderma gangrenosum could not be excluded [40, 41]. The immunofluorescence staining of the biopsy was inconclusive.

Treatment

A multidisciplinary team of radiologists, plastic surgeons, vascular surgeons agreed that a conservative approach following a skin graft was recommended. Initially a clinical diagnosis of pyoderma gangrenosum was established by a dermatologist and prednisolone at a starting dose of 0.5 mg/kg had been initiated. The ulcer enlarged with prednisolone alone and later dapsone 50 mg/day in combination of prednisolone 0.3 mg/kg and compression therapy was initiated, which halted the ulcer progression and improved tissue granulation (Fig. 8.8). Smoking cessation was strongly supported.

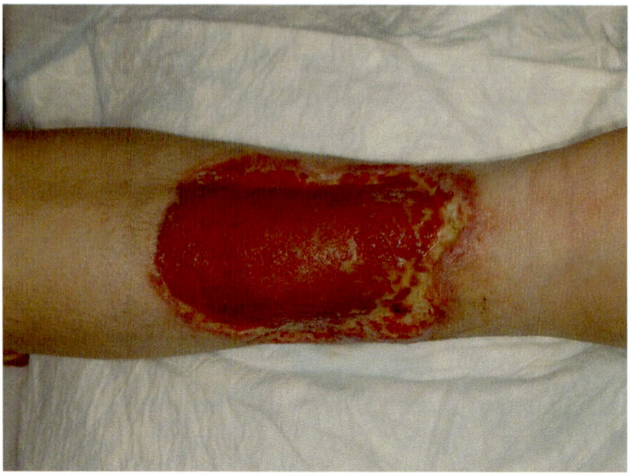

Fig. 8.8 Atypically behaving ulcer in a young patient with congenital combined LUMBAR syndrome and middle aortic syndrome

To improve the outcome, dapsone was switched to cyclosporine at 2 mg/kg along with prednisolone. During cyclosporine treatment an increase in blood pressure was noted and enalapril 5 mg × 1 was initiated and cyclosporine dosage was left at the lower end. During cyclosporine there was a wound infection that was treated with *po* clindamycine. Partial skin grafting was performed 10 weeks from the initiation of cyclosporine in co-operation with the plastic surgeons (Fig. 8.9).

After a successful skin graft cyclosporine was tapered down and switched to dapsone. Prednisolone was tapered down at a slow course during the next 3 months. At a control visit at 4 months only a small erosive area was still seen (Figs. 8.10 and 8.11).

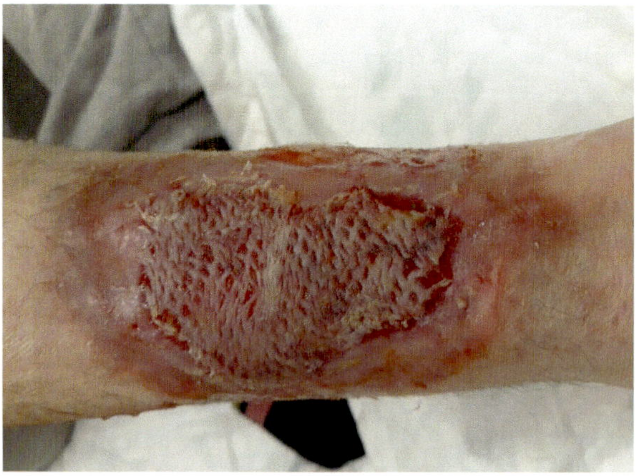

Fig. 8.9 Atypical leg ulcer after partial skin grafting (10 weeks from the initiation of cyclosporine)

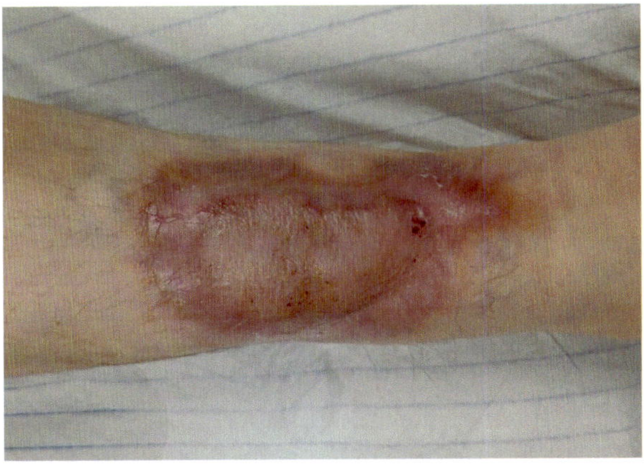

Fig. 8.10 Control visit at 4 months (general view)

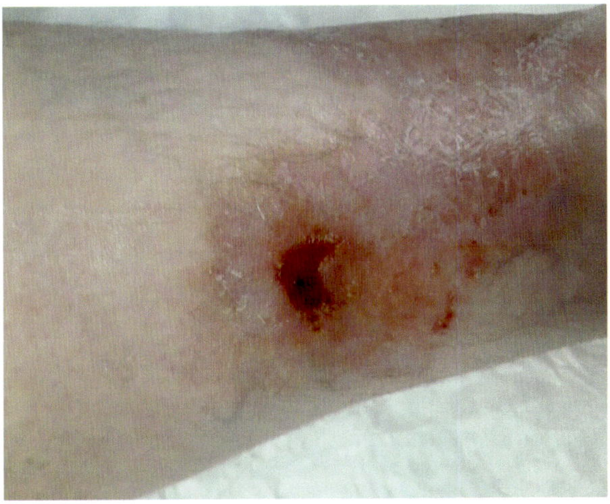

Fig. 8.11 Control visit at 4 months (detail view)—only a small erosive area still present

Discussions

Our case presents an example of a patient where the wound etiology is multifactorial with featuring both abnormalities in the capillary network as well as an increased inflammatory response. In the beginning of the treatment at lower doses of prednisolone there was substantial increase in inflammatory activity seen without bacterial infection. On the other hand, cyclosporine seemed to increase susceptibility to bacterial infection. Compression therapy was considered a golden standard for treatment and as a preventive measure.

Case 8.5. Impaired Wound Healing After Radiation Therapy

Introduction

Non-healing wounds have a multitude of pathogenic mechanisms, often acting in concert to exacerbate their detrimental effects. Effective diagnosis and treatment of these wounds require a multidisciplinary approach. A skilled team is essential to address all contributing factors, not just the most common or severe ones, in order to promote wound epithelialization. Chronic wounds, particularly in patients with adjacent skin neoplasms and a history of radiation therapy, have a poor prognosis as radiation disrupts the normal physiological processes of tissue repair. Moreover, superficial skin infections, which can become more aggressive in immunocompromised patients, must be managed effectively to facilitate healing.

Case Description and Medical History

A 57-year-old male patient presented to a Dermatology department in May 2022 with a non-healing wound on the left side of his neck in evolution for 3 months. The patient had a history of throat cancer and had received radiation therapy on the affected area 3 years ago. The wound appeared after a minor trauma in the previously radiated area, and the patient reported its presence for the last two months.

During his consultation, it was decided to have a swab for bacteriological examination and the patient was instructed to return for a follow-up visit in three days to initiate the proper treatment. However, the patient returned two months later, in July 2022, at which time the wound progressed in size and depth and the associated symptoms suggestive of local infection had worsened.

Clinical Findings

Upon first examination, the wound on the left side of the neck measured 2 cm in diameter and was covered by a purulent secretion (Fig. 8.12). The surrounding skin displayed late radiation injury with signs of fibrosis, tissue atrophy, telangiectasias and vascular damage. During the patient's second evaluation in July 2022, the wound had progressed in size to 3 cm in diameter with an increased depth. It was covered by a whitish, adherent purulent exudate (Fig. 8.13), suggestive for a bacterial infection. The peri-wound skin was erythematous and edematous, and the patient reported intense pain. Additionally, the patient reported a history of pruritus, a common symptom of radiation dermatitis he had in the past. The patient had no evidence of lymphadenopathy or other areas of infection. The presence of *Pseudomonas aeruginosa* identified through bacteriological examination in the wound bed required specific management strategies, including appropriate antibacterial therapy and wound care measures.

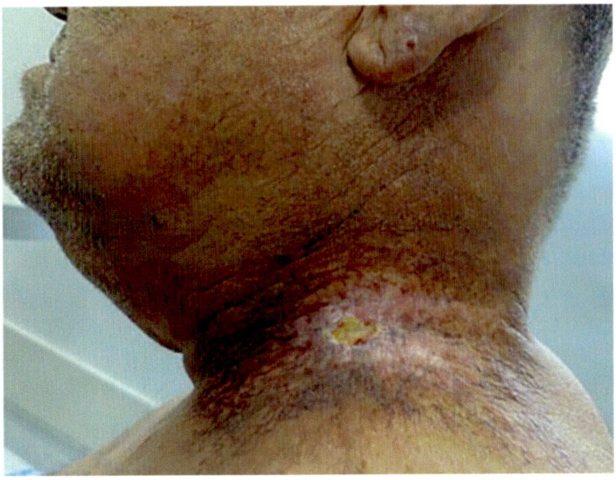

Fig. 8.12 Non-healing wound on the neck in a patient with history of throat cancer that received radiation therapy (general view)

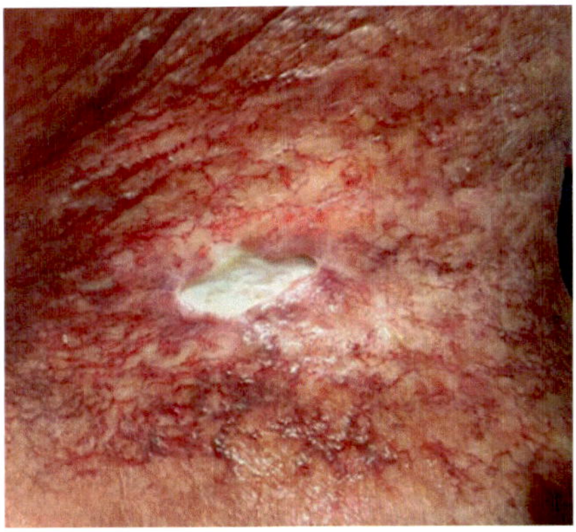

Fig. 8.13 Non-healing wound on the neck in a patient with history of throat cancer that received radiation therapy (detail)

Diagnostic Assessment

The diagnostic assessment for this patient included a combination of clinical examination, bacteriological examination, and laboratory tests to determine the extent of tissue damage and assess the patient's overall health status. The aim was to identify the underlying cause of the non-healing wound and to guide appropriate therapeutic interventions. The bacteriological examination revealed the presence of *Pseudomonas aeruginosa*, a common opportunistic bacterial pathogen that can cause severe infections in immunocompromised patients. Based on the antibiogram, *P. aeruginosa* showed complete resistance to ampicillin, erythromycin, and norfloxacin; intermediate resistance to gentamicin, amikacin, tobramycin, and cotrimoxazole and sensitivity to cefotaxime and ciprofloxacin. Considering the patient medical history, magnetic resonance imaging (MRI) of the neck region was performed, showing that there were no signs of metastasis, tumoral recurrences or deep tissue involvement.

Therapeutic Interventions

The therapeutic interventions for this patient included a combination of local wound care, debridement, and antimicrobial therapy. The aim was to control the infection, promote wound healing, and prevent recurrence. Antimicrobial therapy was initiated based on the bacteriological examination results, with topical antiseptics (chlorhexidine solution) and antibiotic therapy based on the antibiogram results (Ciprofloxacin, 1 g per day). The antimicrobial therapy was continued for 10 days, and the patient was monitored for any signs of adverse effects. Debridement was performed to remove the non-viable (sloughy, compromised) tissue from the wound bed to encourage wound healing. Hydroactive dressings (HydroClean Advance®, Hartmann) were applied to the wound bed to promote a moist wound healing environment; dressings were changed every three days, and the wound was monitored for any signs of infection. Hydroactive dressings were chosen for their properties of protecting the wound from external contaminants, promoting granulation tissue formation, and reducing pain associated with wound dressing changes. Silver dressings (Atrauman Ag®, Hartmann) were combined with hydroactive dressings as an adjunctive therapy, for their antimicrobial properties and support in infection control. Silver dressings are considered to be effective against a broad range of microorganisms. They are especially useful for managing wounds that are difficult to heal, such as burns, surgical wounds, and chronic wounds.

Follow-Up and Outcome

The patient was evaluated after four months when the wound was clean and almost closed (Fig. 8.14). The last consultation took place in March 2023, when the wound was completely healed for almost 3 months, with no recurrence (Fig. 8.15). The therapeutic interventions were successful in treating the wound, and the patient was satisfied with the outcome.

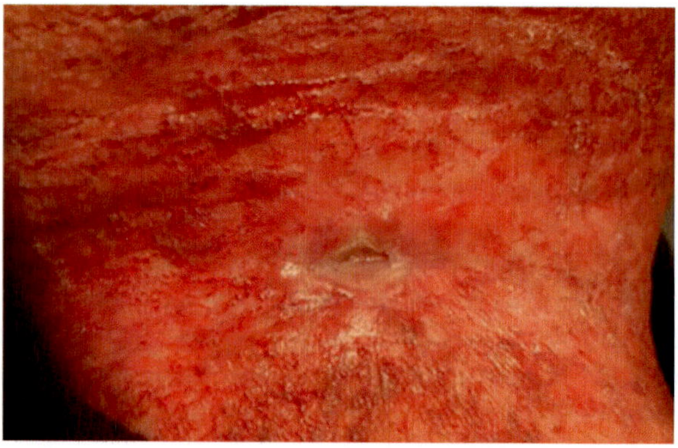

Fig. 8.14 Follow-up visit after the systemic antibiotic and local treatment (4 months after treatment)

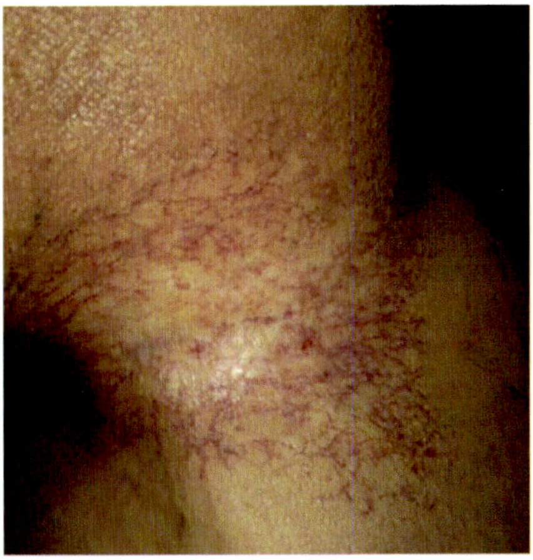

Fig. 8.15 Second follow-up visit with complete closure of the wound (7 months after treatment)

Discussion

The presented case highlights the challenges associated with wound healing in patients who have undergone radiation therapy. Radiation therapy is known to cause damage to the skin and underlying tissues, leading to fibrosis, atrophy, and vascular injury, which can impair the healing process and increase the risk of complications, such as infection and delayed wound closure [42, 43]. The patient's wound was initially superficial, but it progressed over time and became deeper, larger, and more painful, likely due to the impaired healing process.

The diagnostic assessment revealed the presence of *Pseudomonas aeruginosa* in the wound, which is a common pathogen associated with wound infections, especially in patients with compromised immune systems or impaired wound healing [44]. The therapeutic interventions included the use of topical antiseptics and antibiotics, as well as debridement and carefully chosen local dressings, to be effective in managing radiation therapy-related skin toxicity and promotion of wound healing. These interventions were effective in controlling the infection and favoring wound healing, as the wound was clean and almost closed after 4 months of treatment.

The presented case underscores the importance of a multidisciplinary approach to the management of non-healing wounds, especially in patients with a history of radiation therapy. Dermatologists, oncologists, and wound care specialists should work together to develop an individualized treatment plan that considers the patient's medical history, the location and severity of the wound, and the underlying pathophysiology of impaired wound healing. The use of advanced wound care modalities, such as negative pressure wound therapy, growth factors, topical fibronectin and tissue engineering, may also be considered in some more severe cases [45, 46].

In conclusion, impaired wound healing after radiation therapy is a challenging clinical problem that requires a comprehensive and multidisciplinary approach to diagnosis and management. The presented case highlights the importance of timely diagnosis, appropriate wound care interventions, and close follow-up to achieve optimal outcomes in patients with non-healing wounds.

References

1. Isoherranen K, Jordan O'Brien J, Barker J, et al. Atypical Wounds. Best clinical practices and challenges. J Wound Care. 2019;28(Sup6):S1–S92.
2. Shanmugan VK, Angra D, Rahimi H, McNish S. Vasculitic and autoimmune wounds. J Vasc Surg Venous Lymphat Disord. 2017;5(2):280–92.
3. Shanmugan VK, Schilling A, Germinario A, et al. Prevalence of immune disease in patients with wounds presenting to a tertiary wound healing centre. Int Wound J. 2012;9(4):403–11.
4. Körber A, Klode J, Al-Benna S, et al. Etiology of chronic leg ulcers in 31,619 patients in Germany analyzed by an expert survey. JDDG: J Dtsch Dermatol Ges. 2011;9(2):116–21.
5. Hradil E, Jeppsson C, Hamnerius M, Svensson Å. The diagnosis you wish you had never operated on: pyoderma gangrenosum misdiagnosed as necrotizing fasciitis—a case report. Acta Orthop. 2017;88(2):231–3.
6. Janowska A, Oranges T, Chiricozzi A, et al. Synergism of therapies after postoperative autograft failure in a patient with melanoma of the foot misdiagnosed as a pressure ulcer. Wounds. 2018;30(4):E41–3.
7. Santos PW, He J, Tuffaha A, Wetmore JB. Clinical characteristics, and risk factors associated with mortality in calcific uremic arteriolopathy. Int Urol Nephrol. 2017;49(12):2247–56.
8. Langan SM, Groves RW, Card TR, Gulliford MC. Incidence, mortality, and disease associations of pyoderma gangrenosum in the United Kingdom: a retrospective cohort study. J Invest Dermatol. 2012;132(9):599–608.
9. Tan MG, Tolkachjov SN. Treatment of pyoderma gangrenosum. Dermatol Clin. 2024;42:183–92.
10. Janowska A, Dini V, Oranges T, Iannone M, Loggini B, Romanelli M. Atypical ulcers: diagnosis and management. Clin Interv Aging. 2019;14:2137–43.
11. Yang YH, Tsai IJ, Chang CJ, Chuang YH, Hsu HY, Chiang BL. The interaction between circulating complement proteins and cutaneous microvascular endothelial cells in the development of childhood Henoch-Schonlein purpura. PLoS ONE. 2015;10:e0120411.
12. Palit A, Inamadar AC. Childhood cutaneous vasculitis: a comprehensive appraisal. Indian J Dermatol. 2009;54:110–7.
13. Trnka P. Henoch-Schonlein purpura in children. J Paediatr Child Health. 2013;49:995–1003.
14. Rigante D, Castellazzi L, Bosco A, Esposito S. Is there a crossroad between infections, genetics, and Henoch-Schonlein purpura? Autoimmun Rev. 2013;12:1016–21.
15. Dursun I, Dusunsel R, Poyrazoglu HM, Gunduz Z, Patiroglu T, Ulger H, et al. Circulating endothelial microparticles in children with Henoch-Schonlein purpura; preliminary results. Rheumatol Int. 2011;31:1595–600.
16. Chen JY, Mao JH. Henoch-Schönlein purpura nephritis in children: incidence, pathogenesis and management. World J Pediatr. 2015;11:29–34.
17. Landecho MF, Ros NF, Alegre F, Idoate MA, Lucena JF. Henoch-Schonlein purpura associated with celiac disease. J Am Acad Dermatol. 2011;64:e120-121.
18. Hong J, Yang HR. Laboratory markers indicating gastrointestinal involvement of Henoch-Schonlein purpura in children. Pediatr Gastroenterol Hepatol Nutr. 2015;18:39–47.
19. Carlson J. Cutaneous vasculitis update: small vessel neutrophilic vasculitis syndrome. Am J Dermatopathol. 2006;28:486.
20. Hahn D, Hodson EM, Willis NS, Craig JC. Interventions for preventing and treating kidney disease in Henoch-Schonlein purpura (HSP). Cochrane Database Syst Rev. 2015;Cd005128.

21. Mitsuaki I, et al. JCS 2017 guideline on management of vasculitis syndrome. Digest version. Circ J. 2020;84(2):299–359. https://doi.org/10.1253/circj.CJ-19-0773.
22. Dudley J, Smith G, Llewelyn-Edwards A, Bayliss K, Pike K, Tizard J. Randomised, double-blind, placebo-controlled trial to determine whether steroids reduce the incidence and severity of nephropathy in Henoch-Schonlein purpura (HSP). Arch Dis Child. 2013;98:756–63.
23. Jauhola O, Ronkainen J, Autio-Harmainen H, Koskimies O, Ala-Houhala M, Arikoski P, et al. Cyclosporine A vs. methylprednisolone for Henoch-Schonlein nephritis: a randomized trial. Pediatr Nephrol. 2011;26:2159–2166.
24. Ronkainen JJ. Early prednisone therapy in Henoch-Schönlein purpura: a randomized, double-blind, placebo-controlled trial. J Pediatr. 2006;149:241–7.
25. Sunderkötter C, Bonsmann G, Sindrilaru A, Luger T. Management of leukocytoclastic vasculitis. J Dermatolog Treat. 2005;16(4):193–206. https://doi.org/10.1080/09546630500277971.
26. Zhou Q, Yang D, Ombrello AK, Zavialov AV, Toro C, Zavialov AV, et al. Early-onset stroke and vasculopathy associated with mutations in ADA2. N Engl J Med. 2014;370(10):911–20. https://doi.org/10.1056/NEJMoa1307361.
27. Navon Elkan P, Pierce SB, Segel R, Walsh T, Barash J, Padeh S, et al. Mutant adenosine deaminase 2 in a polyarteritis nodosa vasculopathy. N Engl J Med. 2014;370(10):921–31. https://doi.org/10.1056/NEJMoa1307362.
28. Chasset F, Fayand A, Moguelet P, Kouby F, Bonhomme A, Franck N, et al. Clinical and pathological dermatological features of deficiency of adenosine deaminase 2: A multicenter, retrospective, observational study. J Am Acad Dermatol. 2020;83(6):1794–8. https://doi.org/10.1016/j.jaad.2020.03.110.
29. Barron KS, Aksentijevich I, Deuitch NT, Stone DL, Hoffmann P, Videgar-Laird R, et al. The spectrum of the deficiency of adenosine deaminase 2: an observational analysis of a 60 patient cohort. Front Immunol. 2022;12:811473. https://doi.org/10.3389/fimmu.2021.811473.
30. Aksentijevich I, Sampaio Moura N, Barron K. Adenosine deaminase 2 deficiency. In: Adam MP, Mirzaa GM, Pagon RA, et al., editors. GeneReviews®. Seattle: University of Washington, Seattle. p. 1993–2023.
31. Ombrello AK, Qin J, Hoffmann PM, Kumar P, Stone D, Jones A, et al. Treatment strategies for deficiency of adenosine deaminase 2. N Engl J Med. 2019;380(16):1582–4. https://doi.org/10.1056/NEJMc1801927.
32. Hines E, Farber E. Ulcer of the leg due to arteriolosclerosis and ischaemia, occurring in the presence of hypertensive disease (hypertensive-ischemic ulcers). Proc Staff Meet Mayo Clin. 1946;21(18):337–46.
33. Davison S, Lee E, Newton ED. Martorell's ulcer revisited. Wounds. 2003;15:208–12.
34. Karppinen JJ, Kallio M, Lappalainen K, Lagus H, Matikainen N, Isoherranen K. Clinical characteristics of Martorell hypertensive ischaemic leg ulcer. J Wound Care. 2023;32(12):797–804.
35. Hafner J, Nobbe S, Partsch H, et al. Martorell hypertensive ischemic leg ulcer: a model of ischemic subcutaneous arteriolosclerosis. Arch Dermatol. 2010;146(9):961–8.
36. Alavi A, Dieter M, Hafner J, Sibbald RG. Martorell hypertensive ischemic leg ulcer: an underdiagnosed entity. Adv Skin Wound Care. 2012;25(12):563–72.
37. Vuerstaek J, Reeder S, Henquet C, Neumann H. Arteriolosclerotic ulcer of Martorell. J Eur Acad Dermatol Venereol. 2010;24(8):867–74.
38. Iacobas I, Burrows PE, Frieden IJ, Liang MG, Mulliken JB, Mancini AJ. LUMBAR: association between cutaneous infantile hemangiomas of the lower body and regional congenital anomalies. J Pediatr. 2010;157:795–801.
39. Brunet-Garcia L, Prada Martínez FH, Lopez Sainz A, Sanchez-de-Toledo J, Carretero Bellon JM. Mid-aortic syndrome in a pediatric cohort. Pediatr Cardiol. 2023;44(1):168–78.
40. Maronese CA, Pimentel MA, Li MM, Genovese G, Ortega-Loayza AG, Marzano AV. Pyoderma Gangrenosum: an updated literature review on established and emerging pharmacological treatments. Am J Clin Dermatol. 2022;23(5):615–34.
41. Maverakis E, Marzano AV, Le ST, Callen JP, Brüggen MC, Guenova E, et al. Pyoderma gangrenosum. Nat Rev Dis Primers. 2020;6(1):81.

42. Jacobson LK, Johnson MB, Dedhia RD, Niknam-Bienia S, Wong AK. Impaired wound healing after radiation therapy: a systematic review of pathogenesis and treatment. JPRAS Open. 2017;13:92–105.
43. Dormand EL, Banwell PE, Goodacre TE. Radiotherapy and wound healing. Int Wound J. 2005;2(2):112–27.
44. Ruffin M, Brochiero E. Repair process impairment by Pseudomonas aeruginosa in epithelial tissues: major features and potential therapeutic avenues. Front Cell Infect Microbiol. 2019;9:182.
45. Haubner F, Ohmann E, Pohl F, Strutz J, Gassner HG. Wound healing after radiation therapy: review of the literature. Radiat Oncol. 2012;7:1–9.
46. Johnson MB, Pang B, Gardner DJ, Niknam-Benia S, Soundarajan V, Bramos A, et al. Topical fibronectin improves wound healing of irradiated skin. Sci Rep. 2017;7(1):1–10.

Wound Infections

9

Ewa Klara Stuermer and Mohnned Alghamdi

Abstract

Every chronic wound is colonised with microorganisms. *Pseudomonas aeruginosa*, *Staphylococcus aureus*, and *Enterobacteriae* are the dominant bacterial species in chronic wounds. They are derived from the environment and the surrounding skin but can also be spread oropharyngeal or anal from endogenous sources. However, detecting bacteria in a wound swab or biopsy does not necessarily imply a wound infection. Accordingly, a positive microbiological result cannot be the only indication for antibiotic therapy. The decision for the latter is based entirely on the clinical (systemic) findings. Wound infections can occur postoperatively (case 1), can be triggered by diabetes mellitus (cases 2 and 4), can be prologuised by insufficient perfusion (case 3) or can also occur in combination with immunological skin and vascular diseases (case 5). Therefore, treating the underlying disease is essential to wound healing and should not be ignored. Topical antiseptic therapy with or without accompanying systemic antibiotics is mandatory as an infection therapy. Its intensity depends on the amount and virulence of the microorganisms. The need to continue infection therapy should be reconsidered at least weekly, as topical antiseptic treatment is always associated with varying degrees of impairment of the human cells involved in wound healing. Involving the patient with accompanying information about the wound infection and its therapeutic options is mandatory and increases adherence.

Keywords

Wound infection • Biofilm • Slough • Debridement • Antiseptics • Antibiotics

E. K. Stuermer (✉) · M. Alghamdi
Comprehensive Wound Center, Department for Vascular Medicine, University Hospital Hamburg-Eppendorf, Hamburg, Germany
e-mail: e.stuermer@uke.de

G.-S.Tiplica and K. Isoherranen (eds.), *Wound Healing*,
https://doi.org/10.1007/978-3-031-84579-6_9

Introduction

Approximately 35% of all chronic wounds lead to recurrent (systemic) infections; and up to 40% of wound infections trigger prolonged healing [1]. Every wound, acute or chronic, is quickly colonised with microorganisms of the skin microbiome, which also contain pathogenic bacteria. In the case of good perfusion and health, the immune system counteracts the spreading of infection. Additionally, wound cleansing, usually performed on chronic and infected wounds, reduces microbial colonisation. Staphylococcus aureus, including its methicillin-resistant variant (MRSA), *Pseudomonas aeruginosa,* and *Enterobacteriae are the leading bacterial species colonising chronic wounds* [2, 3]. The Progress from wound colonisation to local or systemic infection is fluent [4] and often difficult to determine by clinical assessment only.

Most patients suffering from wound infection show typical signs of an acute infection like heat, redness, swelling of the wound area, worsening of pain, and sometimes even pus coming out of the wound. Systemic signs such as fever, chills, and general fatigue may accompany those symptoms. However, in chronic wounds, patients' comorbidities, particularly the metabolic syndrome associated with diabetes mellitus, should be considered because they can mask bacterial infections [5]. Other conditions that cover up the signs are malnutrition [6] and immune suppression. For these patients, secondary signs of wound infection had been defined as discoloration of granulation tissue, friable granulation tissue, delayed healing of wound breakdown, serous exudate with concurrent inflammation, pocketing at the base and malodor [7].

The following chapter is intended to raise awareness about the unique characteristics of infections in chronic wounds. It empowers to choose the right time and type of debridement, antiseptics, and systemic antibiotics. It helps to improve the ability to observe the wound and surrounding skin, making it easier to differentiate between a local infection and a potential systemic infection. Case 1 shows that AMS-compliant infection therapy concepts can only be successfully implemented in an interdisciplinary and interprofessional team. Case 2 illustrates the importance of involving patients in therapy, regardless of their age and cognitive limitations, taking their needs into account, and providing education. Case 3 illustrates that it is always worth the effort to avoid transtibial amputation in localized surgical site infection (SSI), as it is predictive of patient outcome and health-related quality of life (HRQoL). Case 4 highlights the importance of off-loading for DFU healing. However, it always requires individualized approaches (e.g., felting) that the patient (can) support. Case 5 encourages constant reflection on the cause of a chronic wound, even during the healing process. Prolonged inflammation can also trigger an autoimmunologic reaction. Regardless of the nature and cause of the wound infection, the choice of therapy should be re-assessed on a weekly basis.

For an adequate management, both diagnostic and therapeutic, of wound infections, it is important to be trained to:

- Know the (cutaneous) signs of local and systemic and understand their prognostic significance.
- Remember that wound infections, especially in the elderly, are not usually triggered by an isolated cause.
- Assess the bacterial burden (species, virulence, load, etc.) and the resulting treatment implications.
- Recognize when it is appropriate to involve other professionals of the interprofessional and interdisciplinary team.
- Perform debridement (preferably sharp) to reduce bacterial load and necrotic tissue.
- Control the wound environment and moisture to deprive bacteria of their nutrient source.
- Know the principles of AMS and decide which antimicrobial therapy is most effective for each patient.
- Identify the leading microbial species of the infection (swab, biopsy) to prescribe the right antibiotic at the right dose.

Case 9.1

Introduction

A 60-year-old male patient was admitted via the emergency department with a clinical presentation of perimandibular abscess. However, the clinical, radiologic and laboratory analysis revealed a necrotising fasciitis of the head-neck region. The diagnosis prompted an immediate surgical resection. The focus of the necrosis appeared to be dentogenic, secondary to a molar root resection. The dominant pathogen of the necrotising fasciitis was *Streptococcus anginosus*. Due to the resection-related, intraoperative palm-sized soft tissue defect of the neck region, a free transplantation of a fasciocutaneous flap (ALT flap) from the upper leg was performed. The tissue defect on the right upper leg ($12 \times 6 \times 2$ cm) was primarily covered with a split-thickness skin graft. On day eight postoperatively, surgical wound dehiscence (SWD) and local infection occurred in the upper leg. (Fig. 9.1a); the split skin graft was lost. The microbiological swabbing revealed a SSI secondary to *Pseudomonas aeruginosa* and *Enterobacter cloacae* complex colonisation. The patient had diabetes mellitus, coronary heart disease, atrial fibrillation, heart failure and hypertension as underlying comorbidities. It is known that systemic, severe infection may lead to significant metabolic variations amongst diabetic patients. that could be difficult to control [8, 9]. This may be a trigger factor of the infection but not the cause.

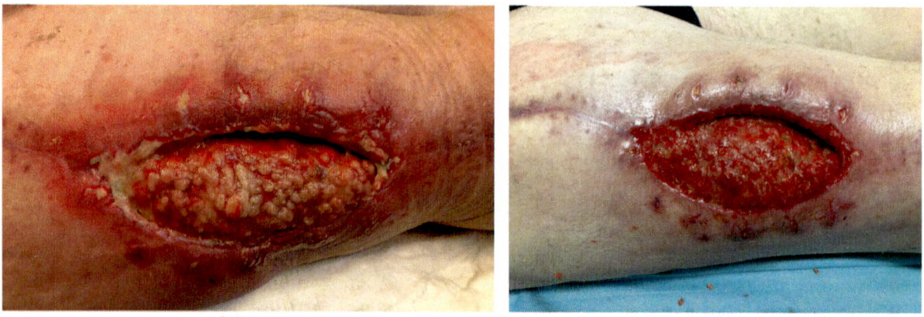

(a) (b)

Fig. 9.1 SSI and SWD at the right upper leg of a 60-year-old male patient after taking a fascio-cutaneous flap (ALT flap). **a** Hypergranulation and biofilm burden. Redness of the surrounding skin due to high exudation. **b** Decrease of local infection after antiseptic and anti-inflammatory therapy of the wound and wound edge

Treatment

The necrotising fasciitis of the head and neck region was surgically resected and treated with intravenous ampicillin-sulbactam for 21 days. Nevertheless, an SSI manifested on the upper leg on day eight postoperatively. The swab results showed a colonisation with ampicillin-sulbactam-resistant *P. aeruginosa*. However, the antibiotic treatment was not revised to cover the spectrum of the biogram as it was merely perceived as a localised infection of the wound. The infected SWD was treated topically and primarily with biofilm-dissolving antiseptic dressings (cardexomer-iodine) and superabsorbent. The bacterial burden led to high exudation, mandating a daily wound dressing change (Fig. 9.1a). The secondary moisture-associated dermatitis was managed with triamcinolone-zinc oxid paste and an advanced skin protectant (acrylate tetrapolymer+2-octyl cyanoacrylate); as a result the wound conditions improved significantly within a week (Fig. 9.1b). A split-thickness skin graft was planned four weeks after topical antimicrobials and an anticipated 100% granulation of the wound (Fig. 9.2a). However, the patient was deemed inoperable due to cardiac decompensation, which led to a protracted course of secondary wound healing. At the six-month follow-up, the wound had healed completely (Fig. 9.2b).

Discussion

The patient was primarily undergoing maxillofacial surgery, where the emergency of necrotising fasciitis of the neck region was recognised and treated. One of the pitfalls of this diagnosis is not to consider life-threatening necrotising fasciitis. The clinical presentation of fulminant pain with a comparatively modest clinical appearance was pathognomonic [10, 11]. Early surgical treatment with complete

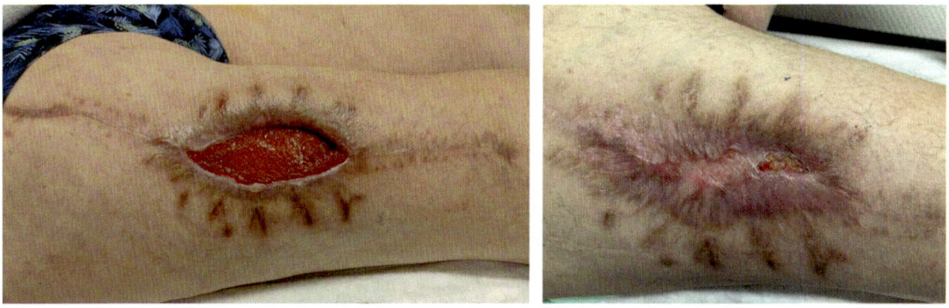

(a) (b)

Fig. 9.2 (**a**) Wound size reduction, healing of the undermining and 100% granulation of the wound surface just before the end of antiseptic local therapy. (**b**) Wound closure by secondary wound healing

resection of the infected area is indicated and was performed [12]. The multimorbidities of this case necessitated postoperative admission to the intensive care unit to manage metabolic and cardiac decompensation. The infected SWD at the flap site left the patient with a defect on the upper leg, which broadened the interdisciplinary care involving plastic surgery and wound care specialists. After careful interdisciplinary assessment of the SWD and in line with antimicrobial stewardship (AMS) [13], it was decided to only use local antiseptic therapy. This decision was taken after considering the following facts: first the patient showed no signs of systemic infection, second the *P. aeruginosa* evident in the wound swaps was merely sensitive to the reserve antibiotic meropenem. The possibility of the swift adaptation of the therapy concept granted in an in-patient care setting enabled the safe use of local antiseptics while maintaining the reserve antibiotics on a standby basis. Such a concept is applicable in an ambulatory setting if close monitoring every (24 h or 48 h) is assured. Finally, it can be concluded that thanks to cross-sectoral therapy (hospital, outpatient clinic, outpatient nursing service, GP) [14] and patient-centred care [15], acute cardiac decompensation was detected early and therefore treated efficiently at any time.

Case 9.2

Introduction

An 84-year-old female patient with a background of diabetes mellitus type II (HbA1c: 6.0%; reference 4.8–5.6%), peripheral polyneuropathy, hypertension and a history of colorectal adenocarcinoma, presented to the vascular outpatient clinic with high exudating chronic wounds on both lower legs. The gaiter-like, odorous wounds showed extensive necrotic and biofilm deposits as well as exudate-induced surrounding dermatitis (Fig. 9.3a, b). Microbiological swabbing revealed bacterial

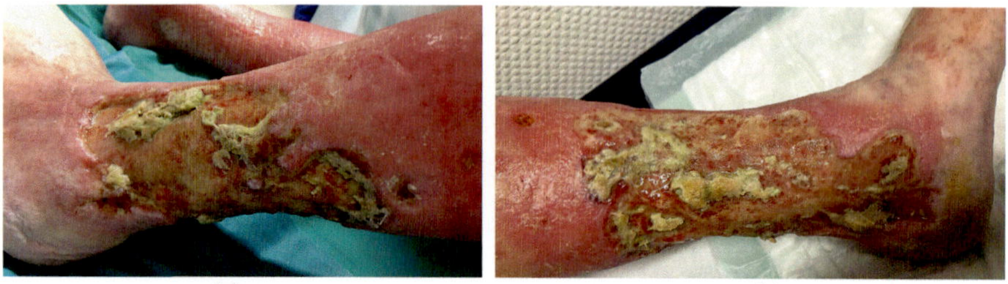

(a) (b)

Fig. 9.3 Left leg of 84-year-old female patient with big odorous, chronic wounds based on CVI and diabetes showing extensive necrotic and biofilm deposits as well as exudate-induced surrounding dermatitis. (**a**) Lateral view. (**b**) Medial view

colonization with *Enterobacter cloacae* complex, *Proteus mirabilis* and *Enterococcus avium.* The ankle-brachial index (ABI) was 1.1 on both sides but could not be rated due to diabetic-associated tonica media sclerosis. Duplex sonography of the leg arteries showed a triphasic A. femoralis communis (AFC), A. femoralis superficialis (AFS), A. femoralis profunda (AFP) and popliteal artery on both sides without high-grade stenosis and a biphasic flow profile of the A. tibialis anterior (ATA) and A. tibialis posterior (ATP) on both sides. Because of extensive ulceration and pain in both lower legs, no more distal arteries could be assessed sonographically, but oscillography of the feet and all toes revealed good arterial perfusion. Duplex sonography of the veins showed venous insufficiency (CVI) with complete varicosis of the V. saphena magna on the left (confluence of the great and small saphenous veins into the femal vein also insufficient) and incomplete varicosis of the right V. saphena magna with normal valve function on both sides. In this patient, CVI dominates the clinical picture of swollen, reddened lower legs with large, locally infected wounds.

Treatment

During the weekly visits over the first four weeks, extensive antimicrobial wound irrigation and sharp debridement under topical anesthesia were performed. The very severe, partly neuropathic wound pain of the patient was treated with metamizole and gabapentin, which was adapted to the current VAS scores during the healing process. For covering the infected, high-exuding wounds, antimicrobial dressings (containing cadexomer-iodine or silver) and superabsorbents for exudate management (daily dressing changes by the nursing service) were chosen. Initially, the patient received compression therapy -first as a compressive bandage, then as prefabricated compression wraps, which she could apply independently. Close intersectoral, interdisciplinary treatment and pointed patient education prevented hospitalization and usage of systemic antibiotics. After six weeks, the local antimicrobial therapy could be finished (Fig. 9.4a, b).

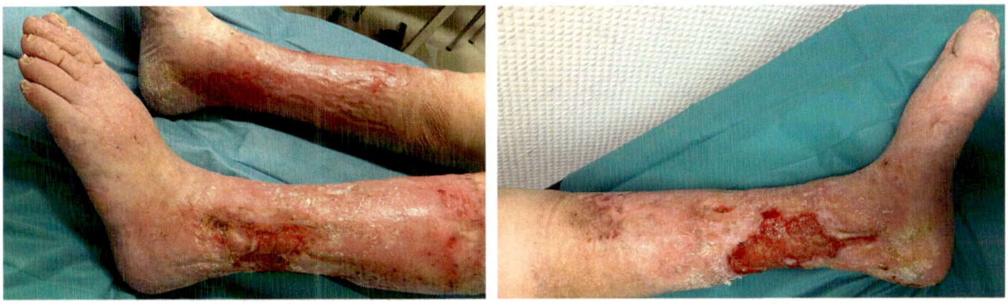

(a) (b)

Fig. 9.4 Six weeks after effective local antiseptic therapy (octenidine-dihydrochloride, cardexomer-iodine, hydrophobic meshes) of **a** the lateral and **b** the medial wound of the left lower leg

Discussion

The 84-year-old patient had treated the wounds herself for months, only consulting her GP intermittently. No specialist for vascular disease or wound care was involved, which is unfortunately not uncommon [15, 16]. Thus, the underlying disease of the chronic wound, CVI, was not diagnosed for months. Even in an international comparison, it is apparent that CVI is underdiagnosed, and a lot of patients needing compression therapy do not receive it [17]. This is difficult to understand because the only contraindications to compression therapy are advanced peripheral arterial disease (ABI < 0.5 or ankle artery pressure < 60 mmHg or toe pressure < 30 mmHg), decompensated heart failure (NYHA III + IV), septic phlebitis and phlegmasia coerulea dolens, but neither chronic nor exuding wounds [18]. The compression class (I-III) should be selected depending on the degree of venous insuffiency, the cardiovascular disease and the individual wound pain with and without compression. Inquiries about the current level of wound pain should be part of every outpatient visit, and drug and physical pain reduction should be initiated by an interdisciplinary and holistic approach [19]. Pain reduction means improving the HRQoL, autonomy and mobility of the elderly, usually multi-morbid patients. Patient's needs regarding their ADLs (e.g. performing activities of daily living), their body (e.g. pain or odor) and their psychological well-being (e.g. fear) can be easily assessed using a questionnaire, e.g. the Wound-QoL [20], both immediately and over time during consultations. It is a valuable tool for identifying patient needs in wound therapy and daily life, making it possible to address them in a time-saving and targeted manner. So, HCPs can thus tackle the most urgent problems directly, which helps the patient to overcome shame and fear.

Case 9.3

Introduction

A 70-year-old patient was admitted to the Vascular Wound Center for the treatment of critical ischemia of the right lower leg accompanied by wet gangrene of the right foot (Fig. 9.5a). His medical history revealed an obliterated right femoropopliteal bypass which was performed 18 months prior to his current presentation, PAD IV°, arterial hypertension, diabetic foot, obesity and a long history of nicotine abuse. Palpation elicited pulse at the right inguinal region with absence in the lower levels. Duplex sonography confirmed the femoropopliteal bypass occlusion, reduced femoral artery perfusion and occlusion of the popliteal and fibular arteries. A monophasic waveform with interrupted color filling corresponded to reduced perfusion of the anterior and posterior tibial artery. The progress of tissue destruction could not be halted despite the successful stenting of the right common iliac artery with frustrated recanalisation attempts at the lower levels. The polymicrobial deep soft tissue infection with *Pseudomonas aeruginosa, Enterococcus faecalis and Klebsiella pneumonia,* complicated by persistent ischemia and overall poor health conditions, prompted a transtibial amputation of the right lower extremity. Despite tension-free tissue approximation of the wound ends, a primary wound healing was not achieved and a surgical wound dehiscence (SWD) occured. Independent of the local antiseptic measures, the secondary healing was protracted due to a wound colonization of the presumed aforementioned pathogenic bacteria. The maximum extent of the surgical site infection (SSI) of the amputation stump was $2.7 \times 5 \times 2$ cm^3 lateral and $1.1 \times 1.7 \times 0.3$ mm^3 medial (Fig. 9.5b). The high bacterial load of the SSI could be visualized by UV-near light (e.g. MolecuLight®), which makes the autofluorescence of the bacteria at densities > 10^4 cells/mg tissue visible (Fig. 9.5c).

Treatment

The viable risk of deep soft tissue infection (SWD grade 3a) mandating a subsequent amputation at a higher level (e.g. above-knee amputation) and amplified by nosocomial pneumonia instigated i.v. administration of the antibiotics piperacillin/tazobactam for three weeks. The application of local antiseptics and wound tamponade at the cavity site facilitated the healing. Iodine-containing dressings, hydrophobic meshes and superabsorbent were initially used at the infected deep SWD. The heavy exudation secondary to the underlying infection led to moisture-dermatitis despite the daily wound dressing change. The erosive lesions were treated with triamcinolone-zinc oxide paste. The usage of local antiseptics was seized after seven weeks of ongoing intensive care. The application of tamponade at the cavity site proceeded for three months, whereby the skin cells were stimulated to subsequently close it (Fig. 9.6a, b). The stump was deemed ready for fitting of a lower leg prosthesis (Fig. 9.6c).

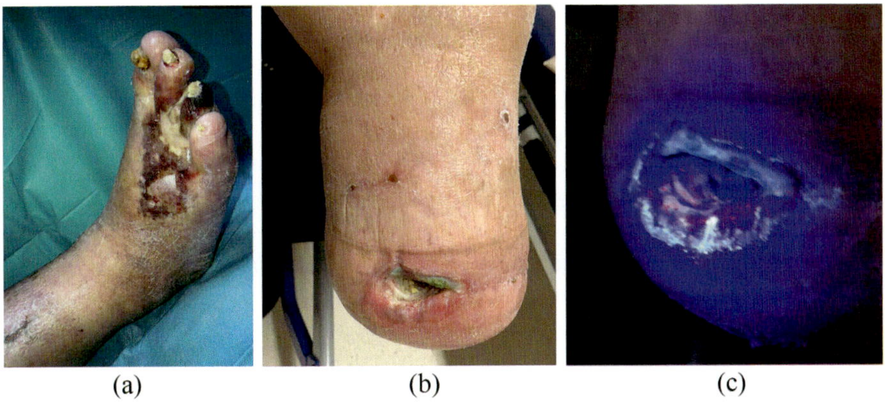

Fig. 9.5 Three images showing (a) the initial clinical situation with wet gangraene of the forefoot and (b) resulting right transtibial amputation. Dermatitis with small erosions on the distal stump pole due to heavy exudation induced by *P. aeruginosa* biofilm (c). Visualization of the bacterial burden in and on the wound by UV-near light. (*P. aeruginosa* = cyan blue; *E. faecalis* & *K. pneumonia* = red)

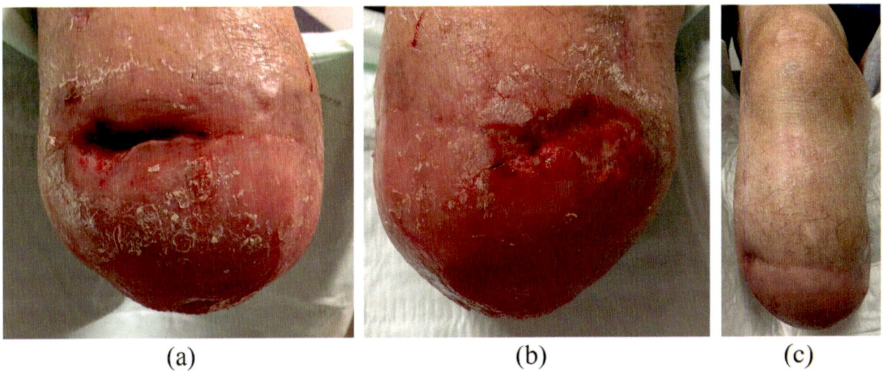

Fig. 9.6 Successful control of the infection on both SWD of the amputation wounds (**a**) lateral and (**b**) medial. Reduction of the wound cavities using antiseptic local therapy with frequent tamponade of both wound cavities with hydrophobic meshes. (**c**) healing result of the transtibial stump

Discussion

Chronic PAD wounds are a frequent cause for the transitioning from local bacterial and biofilm colonization [21] to systemic infection. The poor blood perfusion of affected extremities leads to a subtherapeutic concentration of systemic antibiotics regardless of their route of administration (i.v. or p.o.). If effective revascularization is deemed unlikely, amputation is often considered as a trivial logical consequence (life before limb). The dilemma lies in choosing the correct timing to warrant the indication, which is constantly under discussion [22–24]. Vascular centers are often confronted with high-risk cases where a transtibial amputation is complicated by reduced blood perfusion at the popliteal level which leads to protracted wound healing, increasing the likelihood of chronic bacterial wound colonization, wound dehiscence, or even revision surgeries. Targeted, systemic and local anti-infective therapy is required to avoid the latter [18]. Evidence-based recommendations advising on the specifics of antiseptic products are scarce; expert consensus provides direction here [25]. The goals have to be relevant and aligned with overall objectives. For example, regaining independent mobility via walking using a transtibial prosthesis has to be deferred in favor of soft tissue conditioning and wound healing. Early prosthesis adjustment often proves counterproductive and detrimental to residual limb tissue stability. This should be communicated on an interdisciplinary level (wound expert, surgeon, outpatient care, general practitioner, and physiotherapist) and, in particular, with the patient to achieve the therapeutic goal, albeit late. Such amputations burden the patients drastically and has a significant impact on the their quality of life, suppose there is a threat of prolonged healing, further surgeries or even subsequent amputation. In that case, a careful psychological evaluation is granted since most of those patients present with depressive symptoms and possible adjustment disorder [24, 26].

Case 9.4

Introduction

An 80-year-old male patient was clinically presenting with exacerbating pain secondary to a diabetic foot ulcer. The diabetic ulcer was clinically reported for over 14 weeks. It was located on the sole of the left foot over the metatarsal head V (Fig. 9.7a). In addition to the common polyneuropathy associated with type II diabetes, the patient suffered from chronic venous insufficiency, which was treated with compression stockings of class II, and arterial hypertension. The patient initially treated the wounds himself using local antiseptics and sterile compression bandage. Custom-made footwear enabled full mobility with no walking aids. Inspection of the wound area revealed slight swelling of the ankle and foot dorsum, with no redness. Fever, chills or malaise were denied. Areas of hyperkeratosis covered with hemorrhagic blood crusts were appreciated in the surrounding area. The foot exhibited no increase in warmth or tenderness upon palpation. However, pus was produced from the foot ulcer upon palpation (Fig. 9.7b). Swabs were taken for microbiology and yielded *P. aeruginosa*. The blood test revealed leukocytes and C-reactive protein (CRP) remained in the higher levels of normal values. In light of an unpredictable progression of a systemic infection ("foot attack") [27], a hospitalization was granted; however, it was rejected by the patient.

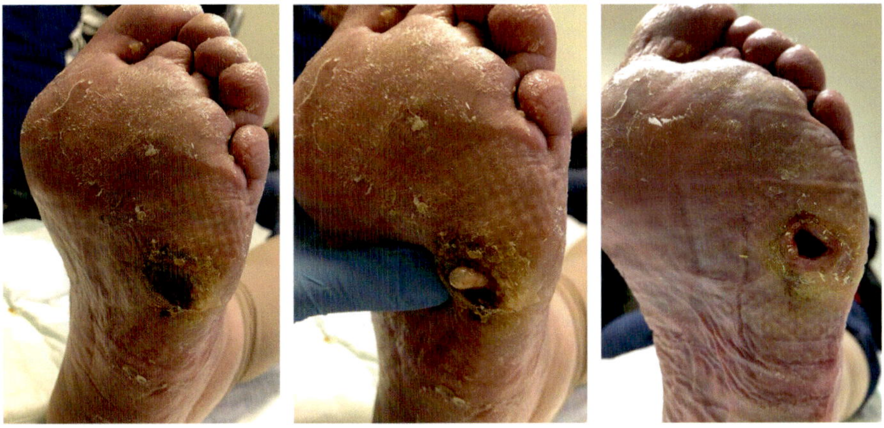

(a) (b) (c)

Fig. 9.7 Chronic, diabetic ulcer on the left foot of a 80-year-old male patient. (**a**) Crusty deposits on the ulcer without signs of infection (no surrounding redness, no swelling, no pain). (**b**) Drainage of pus under pressure. (**c**) ulcer approx. 10 mm in depth becomes visible after sharp debridement and removal of the hyperkeratosis

Treatment

The secondary evaluation of the wound revealed—after providing the necessary wound care by disinfection, pus drainage, sharp debridement of the wound and the hyperkeratosis—a perforating foot ulcer measuring $1.2 \times 2 \times 0.5$ cm^2 (Fig. 9.7c). The soft tissue of the perforating ulcer displayed no signs of significant necrosis. Sterile probing of the wound yielded no bone or joint involvement. The lesion was filled with a hydrophobic mesh and covered with a thin dressing. The pus draining, diabetic ulcer and the absence of swab results prompted a calculated course of oral antibiotics with clindamycin and ciprofloxacin. Preserving mobility while offloading the affected limb is a key factor for successful wound healing. However, the advanced age of the patient prevented him from offloading the affected limb using elbow or forearm crutches. Therefore, a plantar felting was custom-made with a cut-out in the ulcer region (Fig. 9.8a). The wound care, including sharp debridement to remove the rapidly growing hyperkeratosis and application of the plantar felting, was repeated every three days. Due to the underlying diseases combined with increasing pain despite reported polyneuropathy, oral antibiotics were applied immediately; for rapid remission only for seven days. Advanced healing of the diabetic foot ulcer was achieved within four weeks of diligent wound care (Fig. 9.8b). New compression stockings and diabetic footwear were prescribed. In addition, the patient was educated and advised to undergo regular podiatric treatment to prevent recurrence.

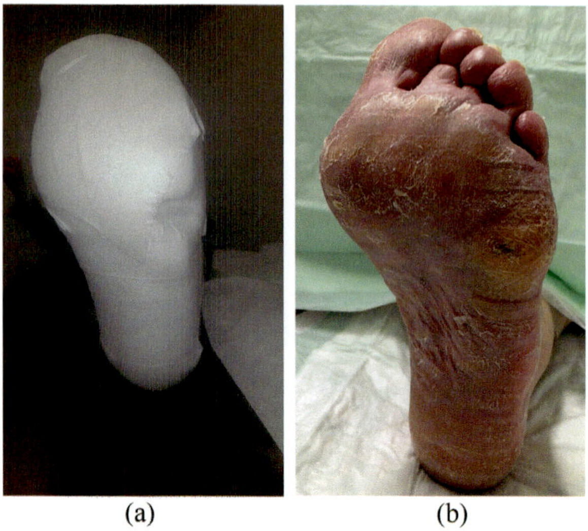

Fig. 9.8 (**a**) Padding of the entire sole of the foot to reduce the load on the ulcer region during continued antiseptic local therapy. (**b**) Diabetic foot ulcer with advanced healing after five weeks

Discussion

Diabetic polyneuropathy and presumed microangiopathy are associated with years of poorly controlled diabetes. Both pathologies constitute the underlying cause of diabetic foot syndrome. The recurrent foot ulcerations accompanied by increased susceptibility to develop subclinical infections unfold constant risk of developing fulminant diabetic foot infection with consequent minor and major amputations. [28]. An adequate and prompt therapy is therefore implicated in successfully managing such misleading trivial infections amongst diabetic patients [27]. In this case, the patient's refusal of hospitalization prompted the usage of broad-spectrum antibiotic therapy. Ongoing close monitoring of infection causes and signs predicts the outcome of diabetic foot management. Although the guidelines for managing diabetic foot provide clear recommendations when antibiotics should be used [29], there is a lack of evidence-based recommendations addressing the preference for certain antiseptics or antiseptic wound dressings. This lack is also apparent in the guidelines on local therapy of chronic wounds. The directives for using antiseptics and antiseptic wound dressing are governed by contextual international consensus and recommendations [25, 30]. High-concentrated hypochlorous solutions, chlorhexidine, iodophor-containing formulations, octenidine dihydrochloride-phenoxyethanol, PHMB and silver are recommended and assessed as equally effective. Although resting and offloading of the affected limb are pillars of the management of wound infections [29, 31], immobilizing diabetic patients, especially if they are older, is counterproductive and can carry some negative consequences for their overall health. Therefore, intelligent offloading solutions should be considered to promote the healing of chronic wounds—especially in pressure ulcers—without impairing the patient's well-being. Using custom-made sole felting as a bridge solution to alleviate the load bearing on diabetic foot ulcers is more effective and cost-efficient in comparison to orthopedic footwear [32]. Nursing staff and patients' relatives can easily familiarize with the felting technique. Patients should be made aware of the need for podiatric care and the need for skin care.

Case 9.5

Introduction

An 83-year-old male patient was sent to the outpatient clinic by the nursing service due to "wound aggravation". The chronic wound over the left achilles tendon ($3.5 \times 2.8 \times 0.2$ cm^2) existed for a year and now showed an exposed tendon, hardly any granulation, thick, fibrinous coatings and extensive surrounding dermatitis with excoriation due to heavy exudation (Fig. 9.9a). The patient had a history of a Stockmann bypass on the left leg for PAD IV° [33], coronary heart disease, post apoplexy with persistent aphasia, paroxysmal atrial fibrillation and hypertension. The ABI was 1.2 left and 1.0 right, so reduced perfusion could be ruled out as a trigger for the infection. The wound swab showed colonization with *Pseudomonas aeruginosa, Dolosigranulum pigrum* and *Staphylococcus caprae.* No leukocytosis was detectable in the serum with elevated C-reactive protein (CRP; 21 mg/l). After two weeks of antiseptic local therapy, there was an increased number of painful, point-like hemorrhages (petechiae) in the area around the wound (Fig. 9.9b), but also to a lesser extent on the entire right and left leg, which visually suspected the diagnosis of vasculitis. The histological examination of a skin biopsy revealed a necrotising, bullous non-Ig A small vessel vasculitis.

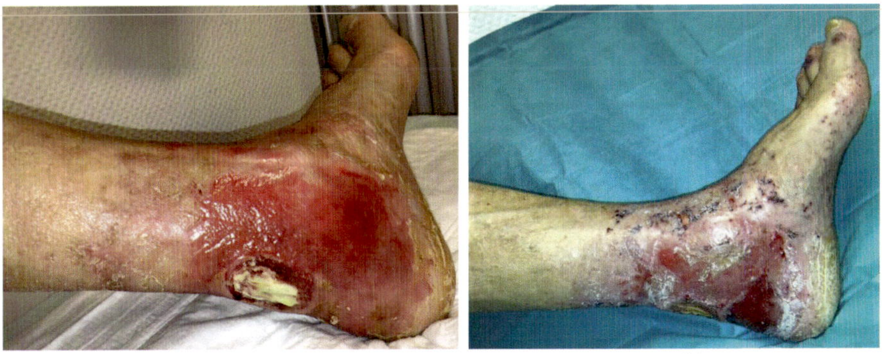

(a) (b)

Fig. 9.9 (**a**) Infected wound with exposed Achilles tendon on the left, fibrinous coating and heavy exudation of a 83-year-old male patient; (**b**) after 14 days development of painful, point-like hemorrhages (petechiae) in the area around the wound, feet and lower leg

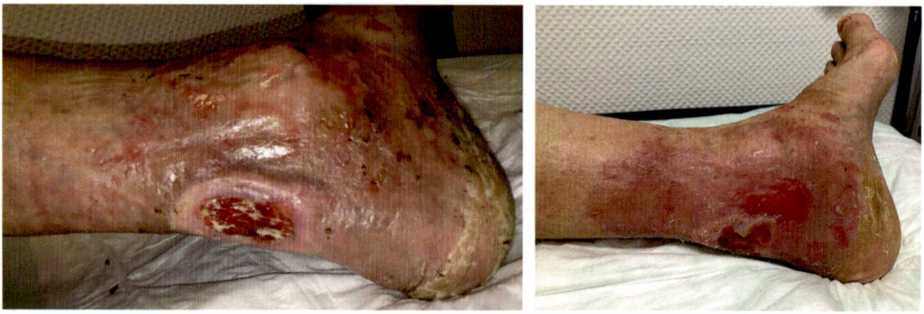

(a) (b)

Fig. 9.10 (**a**) After systemic and local immune-modulating (prednisolone, steroid-triclosan) combined with local antiseptics (iodine), quick, scabby healing of the petechial wounds and granulation of the wound over the Achilles tendon without (partial) resection of the latter. (**b**) Continuous, slow and infection-free wound healing—here after 6 weeks—with extremely fragile surrounding skin. Silicone dressings with/without border should be avoided

Treatment

Just a local infection was diagnosed when the patient was readmitted to the outpatient clinic, so systemic antibiotics could be avoided under close monitoring. The dominant *P. aeruginosa* in the wound had induced massive exudation as a tissue response, so the previous local therapy was now inadequate. The resulting exudate-induced dermatitis was treated with steroid-triclosan-containing cream, while the biofilm-infected wound was treated with a dressing containing cadexomer-iodine and a superabsorbent for exudate management. While the local conditions improved over the following 14 days, the patient developed small vessel vasculitis—the first episode of immunological disease in his long life. As it could not be ruled out that this will manifest systemically, the patient was admitted to the hospital and treated orally with prednisolone 2 mg/kg daily for three days, which was gradually reduced over the following seven days of in-hospital stay. The patient received paracetamol and metamizole for pain control. Therapy resulted in a fast regression of the vasculitic purpura with crusty healing as well as stabilization of the wound conditions over the achilles tendon (Fig. 9.10). Antiseptic wound therapy was carried out during the entire period of treatment and could only be discontinued after a total of six weeks.

Discussion

The infectious wound conditions, the age and the patient's pre-existing disease made it necessary to weigh up whether to use local antiseptic or systemic antibiotic therapy. Local antibiotics should be avoided in the treatment of chronic wounds to prevent allergic reactions and overall the development of antibiotic resistance

[30, 34]. With the availability of close clinical monitoring, application of systemic antibiotics could be avoided in this patient. Additionally, according to the resistogram obtained, only therapy with the reserve antibiotic meropenem would be effective. The use of reserve antibiotics should always be strictly weighed up in terms of antimicrobial stewardship [12]. Without any history of autoimmune disease and therefore unexpectedly, the patient developed small vessel vasculitis 14 days after starting treatment of infection with interestingly simultaneous improvement of the wounds. This vasculitis is induced by immune complexes deposited in the vessel walls [35]. It occurs, as in this patient, more frequently after infections—albeit rather infections caused by beta-hemolytic streptococci—which suggests an immune reaction as the cause. Clinically, multiple petechiae of the skin are impressive, preferably on dependent parts of the body. They cannot be pressed away with a glass spatula, i.e. there is no anemia. The petechiae can also be generalized (gastrointestinal tract, kidneys, joints), for which reason the patient was admitted to hospital under the presumed diagnosis of "immunological vasculitis". Due to the patient's existing multi-morbidity, glucocorticoid therapy was started, although the indication for steroid administration in this type of vasculitis should be rather strict. Wound healing was not impaired by the short-term immunosuppressive therapy.

References

1. Yao Z, Niu J, Cheng B. Prevalence of chronic skin wounds and their risk factors in an inpatient hospital setting in Northern China. Adv Skin Wound Care. 2020;33(9):1–10.
2. Gjodsbol K, Christensen JJ, Karlsmark T, Jorgensen B, Klein BM, Krogfelt KA. Multiple bacterial species reside in chronic wounds: a longitudinal study. Int Wound J. 2006;3(3):225–31.
3. Jockenhofer F, Gollnick H, Herberger K, Isbary G, Renner R, Stucker M, et al. Bacteriological pathogen spectrum of chronic leg ulcers: Results of a multicenter trial in dermatologic wound care centres differentiated by regions. J Dtsch Dermatol Ges. 2013;11(11):1057–63.
4. Swanson T, Ousey K, Haesler E, Bjarnsholt T, Carville K, Idensohn P, et al. IWII wound infection in clinical practice consensus document: 2022 update. J Wound Care. 2022;31(Sup12):S10–21.
5. Gardener SE, Frantz RA, Saltzman CL, et al. Diagnostic validity of three swab techniques for identifying chronic wound infection. Wound Repair Regen. 2006;14:548–57.
6. Ghaly P, Iliopoulos J Ahmad M. The role of nutrition in wound healing: an overview. Br J Nurs 2021; 30:38–42
7. Gardener SE, Frantz RA, Doebbeling BN. The validity of the clinical signs and symptoms used to identify localized chronic wound infection. Wound Repair Regen. 2001;9(3):178–86.
8. Martin ET, Kaye KS, Knott C, Nguyen H, Santarossa M, Evans R, Bertran E, Jaber L. Diabetes and risk of surgical site infection: a systematic review and meta-analysis. Infect Control Hosp Epidemiol. 2016;37(1):88–99. https://doi.org/10.1017/ice.2015.249.
9. Berbudi A, Rahmadika N, Tjahjadi AI, Ruslami R. Type 2 diabetes and its impact on the immune system. Curr Diabetes Rev. 2020;16(5):442–9. https://doi.org/10.2174/1573399815666191024085838.
10. Acharya PP, Cohn JE, Shokri T, Bundrick P, Ducic Y. Surgical management of necrotizing fasciitis of the head and neck. J Craniofac Surg. 2022;33(8):e858–61. https://doi.org/10.1097/SCS.0000000000008787.

11. Chen LL, Fasolka B, Treacy C. Necrotizing fasciitis: a comprehensive review. Nursing. 2020;50(9):34–40. https://doi.org/10.1097/01.NURSE.0000694752.85118.62.
12. Probst S, Apelqvist J, Bjarnsholt T, Lipsky BA, Ousey K, Peters EJG. Antimicrobials and non-healing wounds: an update. J Wound Manage. 2022;23(3 Sup1):S1–33. https://doi.org/10.35279/jowm2022.23.03.sup01
13. Klein AA, Petermann J, Brosse F, Piller S, Kramer M, Hanf M, Dinh TS, Schulz-Rothe S, Engler J, Mergenthal K, Seidling HM, Klasing S, Timmesfeld N, van den Akker M, Voigt K. Implementation and evaluation of a complex intervention to improve information availability at the interface between inpatient and outpatient care in older patients with multimorbidity and polypharmacy (HYPERION-TransCare)—study protocol for a pilot and feasibility cluster-randomized controlled trial in general practice in Germany. Pilot Feasibility Stud. 2023;9(1):146. https://doi.org/10.1186/s40814-023-01375-2.
14. Gethin G, Probst S, Stryja J, Christiansen N, Price P. Evidence for person-centred care in chronic wound care: a systematic review and recommendations for practice. J Wound Care. 2020;29(Sup9b):S1–22. https://doi.org/10.12968/jowc.2020.29.Sup9b.S1.
15. Heyer K, Herberger K, Protz K, Glaeske G, Augustin M. Epidemiology of chronic wounds in Germany: analysis of statutory health insurance data. Wound Repair Regen. 2016;24:434–42.
16. Ahmajärvi K, Isoherranen K, Venermo M. Cohort study of diagnostic delay in the clinical pathway of patients with chronic wounds in the primary care setting. BMJ Open. 2022;12(11):e062673. https://doi.org/10.1136/bmjopen-2022-062673.
17. O'Meara S, Cullum N, Nelson EA, Dumville JC. Compression for venous leg ulcers. Cochrane Database Syst Rev. 2012; 11:CD000265.
18. Isoherranen K, Montero EC, Atkin L, Collier M, Høgh A, Ivory JD, Kirketerp-Møller K, Meaume S, Ryan H, Stuermer EK, Tiplica GS, Probst S. Lower leg ulcer diagnosis & principles of treatment. Including recommendations for comprehensive assessment and referral pathways. J Wound Manage. 2023;24(2 Sup1):s1–76
19. Holloway S, Ahmajärvi K, Frescos N, Jenkins S, Oropallo A, Slezáková S, Pokorná A. Holistic management of wound-related pain. J Wound Manage. 2024;25(1 Sup1).
20. Augustin M, Conde Montero E, Zander N, Baade K, Herberger K, Debus ES, Diener H, Neubert T, Blome C. Validity and feasibility of the wound-QoL questionnaire on health-related quality of life in chronic wounds. Wound Repair Regen. 2017;25(5):852–7. https://doi.org/10.1111/wrr.12583.
21. Stuermer EK, Besser M, Debus ES, Smeets R, Dietrich M. Bacterial infiltration in biofilm-colonized wounds: analyses in the hpBIOM ex vivo wound model and possible impact on swabbing and debridement. J Wound Care. 2023;23:446–55.
22. Martinez OP, Storo K, Provenzano Z, Murphy E, Tomita TM, Cox S. A systematic review and meta-analysis on the influence of sociodemographic factors on amputation in patients with peripheral arterial disease. J Vasc Surg. 2024;79(1):169-178.e1. https://doi.org/10.1016/j.jvs.2023.08.130.
23. McGinigle KL, Minc SD. Disparities in amputation in patients with peripheral arterial disease. Surgery. 2021;169(6):1290–4. https://doi.org/10.1016/j.surg.2021.01.025.
24. Spoorendonk JA, Krol M, Alleman C. The burden of amputation in patients with peripheral arterial disease in the Netherlands. J Cardiovasc Surg (Torino). 2020;61(4):435–44. https://doi.org/10.23736/S0021-9509.19.1.
25. Nair HKR, Mrozikiewicz-Rakowska B, Sanches Pinto D, Stuermer EK, Matiasek J, Sander J, Lázaro-Martínez JL, Ousey K, Assadian O, Kim P, Percival SL. International consensus document: use of wound antiseptics in practice. Online at www.woundsinternational.com
26. Peters CML, de Vries J, Steunenberg SL, Ho GH, Lodder P, van der Laan L. Is there an important role for anxiety and depression in the elderly patients with critical limb ischemia, especially after major amputation? Ann Vasc Surg. 2019;58:142–50. https://doi.org/10.1016/j.avsg.2018.10.045.
27. Vas PRJ, Edmonds M, Kavarthapu V, Rashid H, Ahluwalia R, Pankhurst C, Papanas N. The diabetic foot attack: "'Tis Too Late to Retreat!" Int J Low Extrem Wounds. 2018;17(1):7–13. https://doi.org/10.1177/1534734618755582.

28. Lin C, Liu J, Sun H. Risk factors for lower extremity amputation in patients with diabetic foot ulcers: a meta-analysis. PLoS One. 2020;15(9):e0239236. https://doi.org/10.1371/journal.pone.0239236.
29. Schaper NC, van Netten JJ, Apelqvist J, Bus SA, Hinchliffe RJ, Lipsky BA.on behalf of the International Working Group on the Diabetic Foot (IWGDF). IWGDF Guidelines on the prevention and management of diabetic foot disease. 2019; www.iwgdfguidelines.org.
30. AWMF guideline S3-Leitlinie 091-001 [Lokaltherapie chronischer Wunden bei den Risiken CVI, PAVK und Diabetes mellitus]. https://register.awmf.org/de/leitlinien/detail/091-001.
31. Armstrong DG, Tan TW, Boulton AJM, Bus SA. Diabetic foot ulcers: a review. JAMA. 2023;330(1):62–75. https://doi.org/10.1001/jama.2023.10578.
32. Gefen A. Alternatives and preferences for materials in use for pressure ulcer prevention: an experiment-reinforced literature review. Int Wound J. 2022;19(7):1797–809. https://doi.org/10.1111/iwj.13784.
33. Stockmann U, Albiker C. Peripheral prosthesis bypass for saving the extremity. Langenbecks Arch Chir Suppl. 1998;115:544–6.
34. Falcone M, De Angelis B, Pea F, Scalise A, Stefani S, Tasinato R, Zanetti O, Dalla PL. Challenges in the management of chronic wound infections. J Glob Antimicrob Resist. 2021;26:140–7. https://doi.org/10.1016/j.jgar.2021.05.010.
35. DeHoratius DM. Cutaneous small vessel vasculitis. Postgrad Med. 2023;135(sup1):44–51. https://doi.org/10.1080/00325481.2022.2159207.

Active Wound Phase Adapted Dressings

10

Sebastian Probst and Damien Pastor

Abstract

Managing chronic wounds presents a big challenge due to the increasing prevalence of this pathology within society. In Europe alone, an estimated 4 million patients suffer with chronic wounds annually. Additionally, the management of chronic wounds imposes significant financial burdens on healthcare systems and often leads to diminished quality of life for patients and their families. Consequently, a multitude of wound dressings have been developed over time with the goal of improving the treatment of chronic ulcers, utilizing Active Wound Phase Adapted Dressings, inspired by Winter's "moist wound healing theory" introduced in 1962.

Keywords

Chronic wounds • Adapted dressings • Hydrogels • Hydrocolloids • Gauzes • Foams • Transparent films • Alginate dressings • Hydrofiber dressing • Superabsorbent dressings • Medicated wound dressings • Bioactive wound dressings

S. Probst (✉)
Geneva School of Health Sciences, HES-SO University of Applied Sciences and Arts Western Switzerland Geneva, Geneva, Switzerland
e-mail: sebastian.probst@hesge.ch

Medical Faculty, University of Geneva, Geneva, Switzerland

Care Directory, Geneva University Hospitals, Geneva, Switzerland

College of Medicine Nursing and Health Sciences, University of Galway, Galway, Ireland

Faculty of Medicine Nursing and Health Sciences, Monash University, Melbourne, Australia

D. Pastor
Department of Dermatology, Geneva University Hospitals, Geneva, Switzerland

G.-S.Tiplica and K. Isoherranen (eds.), *Wound Healing*,
https://doi.org/10.1007/978-3-031-84579-6_10

Introduction

Chronic wounds are a result of stalled wound healing mechanisms influenced by multifaceted factors such as advanced age, impaired vascularization, and concurrent medical conditions, compounded by microbial colonization [1]. Conventional therapeutic modalities often prove inadequate, impairing the considerable socioeconomic and healthcare burdens associated with chronic wounds [2]. Despite the available possibilities of wound care interventions, persistent hurdles persist, notably the absence of universally efficacious dressings and a disjunction between scientific inquiry and product availability [3]. The moist wound healing paradigm, pioneered by Winter [4], emphasizes the necessity of a moist milieu to expedite tissue repair processes. Recent developments in wound management are focused on meeting the complex needs of chronic wound care [5]. Successfully bridging the gap between scientific research and real-world application is crucial for improving the effectiveness of wound care and reducing the burden on healthcare systems and society as a whole [6].

Traditional Wound Dressings

Gauzes

Gauzes, made of woven or synthetic fibers, are the oldest, most widely available and economical wound dressing. They are absorbent and adaptable to various wound shapes including cavity ones and easy to use. However, they are non-moisture-retentive and can dry easily. Its removal can cause discomfort and pain, and in particular woven gauzes can leave residues behind that activate the immune system and potentially contribute to granuloma formation [3]. As they are non-occlusive, they are susceptible to bacterial contamination [7] and might require frequent changing for exudative or infected wounds. Nowadays, they are most useful as secondary dressings in most wounds, especially low exudative ones.

Low Adherent Dressings

Low adherent dressings consist of tulles or porous silicone. They are quite cheap and widely available. Porous dressings allow exudate to pass through into a secondary dressing while maintaining a moist wound bed. The use of low-adherent fabrics such as silicone and /or fatty acid coats limits pain and trauma to newly formed tissues at dressing removal and thus improves wound healing [8]. These dressing are suitable for delicate tissue (e.g. burns, skin grafts and donor sites) and for patients with fragile skin (e.g. dermatoporosis), They are used as a primary dressing for lightly exudating, granulating or epithelializing wounds and can stay in place up to seven days for silicone dressings.

Transparent Films

Transparent film dressings are thin flexible transparent sheets with adhesive backing, composed of polyurethane or co-polyester. They are semipermeable meaning they retain moisture and create a moist wound environment, allow gas exchange and prevent external bacterial contamination. However, they lack swelling capability and are not suitable for wounds with high exudate or infections [3]. Evidence has emphasized the importance of mechanical properties in wound dressings, with new poly-(dimethylsiloxane)-based bi-layer films showing promising results in diabetic chronic wound treatment due to their flexibility and adaptability [9]. Since they are transparent, they allow monitoring of the wound. They are suitable for shallow wounds, split-thickness skin graft donor sites and secondary dressings. The frequency of dressing changes varies from every few days a week to up to 10–14 days for skin graft donor site.

Foams

Foam dressings are made of semipermeable polyurethane or silicone foam. They are proficient in absorbing low to medium quantities of fluid while concurrently offering thermal insulation and facilitating gas exchange. The outer layer is often hydrophobic or waterproof to keep out bacteria and other contaminants. Some include extra features such as a semipermeable backing that can prevent outside fluid leakage and bacterial contamination and adhesive borders to maintain the dressing in place. They can remain in position for up to 7 days in wounds [3, 10]. Comparative clinical analyses have evaluated diverse foam dressings, emphasizing discrepancies in their absorbency capacities and their consequential influence on the frequency of dressing changes and related expenses [11–15]. The contact area of a foam dressing is non-adherent and non-linting, so the dressing is easy to remove. They are used for exudative wounds. They can also be used when there is an infection and under compression therapy. Because of their thickness, they allow extra protection from external trauma.

Hydrogels

Hydrogel-based wound dressings are commonly used due their hydrophilic nature (containing up to 90% of water) maintaining a moist wound environment [16]. They primarily utilize alginate, known for its ability to absorb fluids and promote tissue regeneration. While natural polymers like collagen offer similar benefits, they face limitations such as pathogen transmission and enzymatic degradation. Synthetic hydrogels, although devoid of these issues, lack active participation in the healing process. Combining natural and synthetic materials in bioartificial hydrogel dressings shows promise in addressing these limitations [17]. They can facilitate autolytic debridement by softening and liquefying necrotic tissue and can soothe pain and discomfort via their cooling effect. Some hydrogels are infused with antimicrobial agents, aiding in infection prevention. They are an effective option for low exudative, necrotic or fibrinous wounds and burns. Hydrogels can conform with any type of wounds, including cavity ones, are applied directly to the wound bed and can be combined with a secondary dressing for additional protection. They can be left in place for several days (up to three or four days) depending on exudate level.

Hydrocolloids

Hydrocolloid dressings, composed of gel forming agents such as carboxymethylcellulose combined with other materials like pectin or gelatin, efficiently absorb fluids, maintain a moist environment, and accelerate wound healing by promoting autolysis [18]. They are typically backed with a film or foam layer to provide a semi-permeable and waterproof barrier. They also prevent any mechanical injury by cushioning the wound. After fluids interaction, hydrocolloids tend to have a purulent-like appearance and produce a characteristic and foul odor that is often mistaken as a wound infection. While they are effective in many cases, hydrocolloids may not be suitable for infected wounds due to their occlusive nature and potential for trauma upon removal. Research comparing hydrocolloid dressings with other types reveals varied outcomes, with some studies suggesting enhanced healing capabilities compared to traditional dressings like gauzes [19]. They are applied directly over the wound and beyond the margins and can last several days depending on the saturation of the dressing.

Alginate Dressing

Alginate dressings are made from nonwoven fibers extracted from brown seaweed and consist of alginic acid and are coated with calcium or sodium salts. These dressings are capable of absorbing 20 times their weight, do not stick to the wound since they jellify after fluid contact and degrade naturally over time. They are suitable for wounds with moderate to heavy drainage, maintain a moist wound environment and support autolytic debridement. Alginates possess hemostatic properties, rendering them beneficial for managing bleeding wounds. They can conform well to the wound bed, ensuring complete coverage and effective absorption even for cavity wounds. However, these dressings are not recommended for use on dry wounds as they readily absorb moisture and lack hydrating properties. Additionally, some alginate dressings may incorporate controlled-release ionic silver [20]. These dressings may be changed every one to three days, depending on the level of exudate and the condition of the wound.

Gelling Fiber Dressing

Gelling Fiber dressings are composed of sodium carboxymethylcellulose (CMC). These fibers are highly absorbent (up to 30 times their weight) and turn into a gel after wound exudate contact. Their great absorbent qualities have been demonstrated to effectively decrease levels of matrix metalloproteinases (MMPs) and microbial contamination [21]. They provide and maintain a moist wound environment, reduce maceration risk by locking moisture into a gel and support autolytic debridement. Additionally, some dressings incorporate controlled-release ionic silver. They are used as a primary dressing for managing wounds with moderate to heavy exudate and or infected. These dressings may be left in place for up to 3–7 days or until saturated.

Superabsorbent Dressings

Superabsorbent dressings, composed of superabsorbent polymers (SAPs) that can absorb and trap fluids inside by forming a gel, are engineered with a superior capacity to manage exudate compared to standard dressings, thereby mitigating the risk of leakage and maintaining fluid retention even under compression. Furthermore, they effectively sequester exudate components such as bacteria and MMPs within the dressing core, consequently reducing the likelihood of infection and maceration. They can be used as a primary or secondary dressing. Dressing change will depend on the amount of exudate from a few days to longer wear times compared to standard dressings. A recent systematic review and meta-analysis, encompassing studies on eight different superabsorbent dressings, revealed heterogeneity in patient populations and outcome measures [22]. Despite this variability, superabsorbent dressings show promise in yielding favorable outcomes, potentially resulting in reduced frequency of dressing changes and improved pain score [22].

Medicated and Bioactive Wound Dressings

Medicated Wound Dressings

Medicated wound dressings represent an advancement in wound care by incorporating functional components that actively participate in the wound healing process. These dressings, categorized as bioactive wound dressings and drug-loaded wound dressings, release therapeutic agents or biological factors such as antimicrobial, anti-inflammatory, and analgesic substances.

Bioactive Wound Dressings

Bioactive wound dressings consist of precursors with inherent activity that actively enhance tissue regeneration. They are often composed of naturally-derived polymers like alginate, chitosan, collagen, or synthetic materials engineered to exert specific functions [23]. Strategies to enhance bioactivity include incorporating metal ions like zinc, exploiting the antimicrobial properties of polymers, or blending materials to improve healing rates and reduce inflammation. Hyaluronic acid-based dressings have gained traction for their ability to promote collagen deposition and wound vascularization. Collagen dressings, derived from natural or synthetic collagens, are highly effective for hard to heal wounds by supporting the deposition and organization of newly formed collagen fibers, promoting tissue regeneration and modulating matrix metalloproteinases (MMPs) that can impede healing [24]. Additionally, the use of antimicrobial peptides (AMPs) shows promise in combating a wide range of pathogens without inducing resistance, although challenges in stability and delivery hinder their clinical application. Medicated wound dressings may also incorporate natural or synthetic antiseptics such as Manuka honey or polyhexamethylene biguanide (PHMB), which have demonstrated antimicrobial efficacy and wound healing acceleration in clinical studies [25]. They can also incorporate dialkylcarbomoyl chloride (DACC), a fatty acid derivative that is highly hydrophobic and irreversibly binds to bacteria and fungi and diminishes bacterial load after subsequent dressing removals. They have demonstrated efficacy for surgical site infection prophylaxis [26].

Drug-Loaded Wound Dressings; Wound Dressings Releasing Antimicrobial Agents

One common strategy involves incorporating antimicrobial agents into wound dressings. Silver ions, renowned for their antimicrobial properties against bacteria, viruses, and fungi, have been utilized for centuries. Silver ions disrupt bacterial cell walls, enzymes, and DNA synthesis, though they may struggle to penetrate thick wounds [27]. Numerous commercially available dressings release silver ions at varying concentrations to combat infections. However, challenges include balancing high silver concentrations with cytotoxic effects and prolonging release kinetics. Researchers are exploring innovative approaches such as embedding silver nanoparticles into materials like alginate fibers or chitosan hydrogels to improve wound healing outcomes [28]. Despite promising in vitro results, clinical studies have yielded mixed findings regarding the superiority of silver-containing dressings in reducing infections, although they may enhance ulcer healing rates [27]. Iodine, another commonly used antiseptic agent, is often bound into carrier molecules like povidone-iodine [29] or cadexomer iodine [30] to mitigate side effects.

Wound Dressings Releasing Anti-inflammatory Drugs

Pain management is a crucial aspect of the management of chronic wounds different etiologies, as it not only affects patients' quality of life but also impacts the immune system's response and wound healing [31]. Anti-inflammatory and analgesic drugs such as ibuprofen, lidocaine, and opioids have been extensively studied by researchers to address this issue. Various studies have investigated the sustained release of ibuprofen from different wound dressing materials, including chitosan-based hydrogels, conductive polymeric films, and electrospun nanofibers [32–34].

Activated Charcoal

Activated charcoal is a form of carbon that has undergone activation to enhance its adsorption capabilities, achieved through steaming or heating in a vacuum environment. When applied to a wound, activated charcoal dressings bind odor-causing molecules and bacteria, locally released toxins, and wound degradation products, thereby facilitating wound healing. These dressings have been designed to manage wound odors, exudate and reduce infection risk. They are often combined with an absorbent layer to absorb wound exudate and a non-adherent wound contact to minimize pain and trauma upon dressing changes. Some dressings also incorporate antimicrobial agents such as silver or copper for a direct bactericidal activity [35]. They are suitable for moderate exudative wounds with strong odors such as malignant fungating wounds, wounds with necrosis and/or infected. They can be used as a primary or a secondary dressing over a primary wound contact layer. They are typically changed every one to three days, or when the dressing becomes saturated with exudate.

Wound Dressings Embedding Biological Factors

Recent research has focused on developing wound dressings capable of actively participating in the wound healing process by releasing biological factors. Growth factors (GFs) play a significant role in wound closure, with granulocyte–macrophage colony-stimulating factor (GM-CSF), basic fibroblast growth factor (bFGF), platelet-derived growth factor (PDGF), and vascular endothelial growth factor (VEGF) showing the greatest potential [36, 37]. Various delivery systems have been engineered to locally release GFs, including free form or encapsulated within nanoparticles, electrospun membranes, or nanofibers [38, 39]. Despite promising results in research studies, the clinical translation of GF-loaded wound dressings has been limited due to factors such as high costs, loss of GF activity, and potential safety concerns.

Advanced Wound Dressings

Advanced wound dressings are smart systems designed to release their payload in response to external stimuli, such as temperature, pH, oxygen, and moisture composition, to enhance therapeutic efficacy while minimizing side effects [40]. These dressings can be self-responsive, externally triggered, or automated based on their mode of operation. Self-responsive systems autonomously change their structure in response to environmental stimuli, leading to payload release [41]. Such dressings offer promising avenues for improving wound care by providing precise drug delivery, automating treatment processes, and tailoring dressings to individual patient needs, ultimately enhancing healing outcomes and patient quality of life.

References

1. Frykberg RG, Banks J. Challenges in the treatment of chronic wounds. Adv Wound Care (New Rochelle). 2015;4(9):560–82. https://doi.org/10.1089/wound.2015.0635.
2. Falanga V, Isseroff RR, Soulika AM, Romanelli M, Margolis D, Kapp S. Chronic wounds. Nat Rev Dis Primers. 2022;8(1):50. https://doi.org/10.1038/s41572-022-00377-3
3. Sood A, Granick MS, Tomaselli NL. Wound dressings and comparative effectiveness data. Adv Wound Care (New Rochelle). 2014;3(8):511–29. https://doi.org/10.1089/wound.2012.0401.
4. Winter GD. Formation of the scab and the rate of epithelization of superficial wounds in the skin of the young domestic pig. Nature. 1962;193(4812):293–4.
5. Liang Z, Lai P, Zhang J, Lai Q, He L. Impact of moist wound dressing on wound healing time: a meta-analysis. Int Wound J. 2023;20(10):4410–21. https://doi.org/10.1111/iwj.14319.
6. Ongarora BG. Recent technological advances in the management of chronic wounds: a literature review. Health Sci Rep. 2022;5(3): e641. https://doi.org/10.1002/hsr2.641.
7. Lawrence JC. Dressings and wound infection. Am J Surg. 1994;167(1a):21s–4s. https://doi.org/10.1016/0002-9610(94)90006-x.
8. Wiegand C, Abel M, Hipler U-C, Elsner P. Effect of non-adhering dressings on promotion of fibroblast proliferation and wound healing in vitro. Sci Rep. 2019;9(1):4320. https://doi.org/10.1038/s41598-019-40921-y.
9. Wei S, You Y, Ma Y, Huang W, Liang X, Zhang A, Lin Y. Bi-layer supramolecular polydimethylsiloxane elastomer film: synthesis, characterization, and application in wound dressing on normal and diabetic rat. React Funct Polym. 2019;141:21–32.
10. Seaman S. Dressing selection in chronic wound management. J Am Podiatr Med Assoc. 2002;92(1):24–33.
11. Alvarez OM, Granick MS, Reyzelman A, Serena T. A prospective, randomized, controlled, crossover study comparing three multilayered foam dressings for the management of chronic wounds. J Comp Eff Res. 2021;10(6):481–93. https://doi.org/10.2217/cer-2020-0268.
12. Bianchi J, Gray D, Timmons J, Meaume S. Do all foam dressings have the same efficacy in the treatment of chronic wounds? Wounds UK. 2011;7.
13. Call E, Oberg C, Streit I, Rappl LM. Comparing fluid handling and microclimate conditions under superabsorbent polymer and superabsorbent foam dressings over an artificial wound. World Council Enterostomal Therapists J. 2019;39(4):11–23.
14. Namviriyachote N, Lipipun V, Akkhawattanangkul Y, Charoonrut P, Ritthidej GC. Development of polyurethane foam dressing containing silver and asiaticoside for healing of dermal wound. Asian J Pharm Sci. 2019;14(1):63–77.
15. Oh G-W, Nam SY, Heo S-J, Kang D-H, Jung W-K. Characterization of ionic cross-linked composite foams with different blend ratios of alginate/pectin on the synergistic effects for wound dressing application. Int J Biol Macromol. 2020;156:1565–73.

16. Su J, Li J, Liang J, Zhang K, Li J. Hydrogel preparation methods and biomaterials for wound dressing. Life (Basel). 2021;11(10). https://doi.org/10.3390/life11101016.
17. Zhang L, Yin H, Lei X, Lau JNY, Yuan M, Wang X, et al. A systematic review and meta-analysis of clinical effectiveness and safety of hydrogel dressings in the management of skin wounds. Front Bioeng Biotechnol. 2019;7:342. https://doi.org/10.3389/fbioe.2019.00342
18. Heyneman A, Beele H, Vanderwee K, Defloor T. A systematic review of the use of hydrocolloids in the treatment of pressure ulcers. J Clin Nurs. 2008;17(9):1164–73. https://doi.org/10.1111/j.1365-2702.2007.02218.x.
19. Kamińska MS, Cybulska AM, Skonieczna-Żydecka K, Augustyniuk K, Grochans E, Karakiewicz B. Effectiveness of hydrocolloid dressings for treating pressure ulcers in adult patients: a systematic review and meta-analysis. Int J Environ Res Public Health. 2020;17(21). https://doi.org/10.3390/ijerph17217881.
20. Aderibigbe BA, Buyana B. Alginate in wound dressings. Pharmaceutics. 2018;10(2). https://doi.org/10.3390/pharmaceutics10020042.
21. Krejner A, Grzela T. Modulation of matrix metalloproteinases MMP-2 and MMP-9 activity by hydrofiber-foam hybrid dressing—relevant support in the treatment of chronic wounds. Cent Eur J Immunol. 2015;40(3):391–4. https://doi.org/10.5114/ceji.2015.54605.
22. Veličković VM, Macmillan T, Lones E, Arlouskaya Y, Prieto PA, Webb N et al. Systematic review and quality assessment of clinical and economic evidence for superabsorbent wound dressings in a population with chronic ulcers. Int Wound J. 2024;21(3):e14750. https://doi.org/10.1111/iwj.14750.
23. Oliveira C, Sousa D, Teixeira JA, Ferreira-Santos P, Botelho CM. Polymeric biomaterials for wound healing. Front Bioeng Biotechnol. 2023;11:1136077. https://doi.org/10.3389/fbioe.2023.1136077.
24. Shu H, Xia Z, Qin X, Wang X, Lu W, Luo Q et al. The clinical efficacy of collagen dressing on chronic wounds: a meta-analysis of 11 randomized controlled trials. Front Surg. 2022;9:978407. https://doi.org/10.3389/fsurg.2022.978407.
25. Saghazadeh S, Rinoldi C, Schot M, Kashaf SS, Sharifi F, Jalilian E. Drug delivery systems and materials for wound healing applications. Adv Drug Deliv Rev. 2018;127:138–166. https://doi.org/10.1016/j.addr.2018.04.008.
26. Totty JP, Bua N, Smith GE, Harwood AE, Carradice D, Wallace T, Chetter IC. Dialkylcarbamoyl chloride (DACC)-coated dressings in the management and prevention of wound infection: a systematic review. J Wound Care. 2017;26(3):107–14. https://doi.org/10.12968/jowc.2017.26.3.107.
27. Yousefian F, Hesari R, Jensen T, Obagi S, Rgeai A, Damiani G. Antimicrobial wound dressings: a concise review for clinicians. Antibiotics(Basel). 2023;12(9). https://doi.org/10.3390/antibiotics12091434.
28. Krishnan PD, Banas D, Durai RD, Kabanov D, Hosnedlova B, Kepinska M et al. Silver nanomaterials for wound dressing applications. Pharmaceutics. 2020;12(9). https://doi.org/10.3390/pharmaceutics12090821.
29. Bigliardi PL, Alsagoff SAL, El-Kafrawi HY, Pyon JK, Wa CTC, Villa MA. Povidone iodine in wound healing: a review of current concepts and practices. Int J Surg. 2017;44:260–8. https://doi.org/10.1016/j.ijsu.2017.06.073.
30. Woo K, Dowsett C, Costa B, Ebohon S, Woodmansey EJ, Malone M. Efficacy of topical cadexomer iodine treatment in chronic wounds: Systematic review and meta-analysis of comparative clinical trials. Int Wound J. 2021;18(5):586–97. https://doi.org/10.1111/iwj.13560.
31. Bechert K, Abraham SE. Pain management and wound care. J Am Col Certif Wound Spec. 2009;1(2):65–71. https://doi.org/10.1016/j.jcws.2008.12.001.
32. Aycan D, Selmi B, Kelel E, Yildirim T, Alemdar N. Conductive polymeric film loaded with ibuprofen as a wound dressing material. Eur Polymer J. 2019;121: 109308.
33. Boffito M, Pontremoli C, Fiorilli S, Laurano R, Ciardelli G, Vitale-Brovarone C. Injectable thermosensitive formulation based on polyurethane hydrogel/mesoporous glasses for sustained co-delivery of functional ions and drugs. Pharmaceutics. 2019;11(10):501.

34. Djekic L, Martinović M, Ćirić A, Fraj J. Composite chitosan hydrogels as advanced wound dressings with sustained ibuprofen release and suitable application characteristics. Pharm Dev Technol. 2020;25(3):332–9.
35. Balasubramanian P, Mari Selvam S. Valorization of biomass to activated carbon for wound dressing applications: recent trends and future challenges. Bioresour Technol Rep. 2023;23: 101562. https://doi.org/10.1016/j.biteb.2023.101562.
36. Chen F-M, Zhang M, Wu Z-F. Toward delivery of multiple growth factors in tissue engineering. Biomaterials. 2010;31(24):6279–308.
37. Ulubayram K, Cakar AN, Korkusuz P, Ertan C, Hasirci N. EGF containing gelatin-based wound dressings. Biomaterials. 2001;22(11):1345–56.
38. Choi JS, Leong KW, Yoo HS. In vivo wound healing of diabetic ulcers using electrospun nanofibers immobilized with human epidermal growth factor (EGF). Biomaterials. 2008;29(5):587–96.
39. Yang Y, Xia T, Zhi W, Wei L, Weng J, Zhang C, Li X. Promotion of skin regeneration in diabetic rats by electrospun core-sheath fibers loaded with basic fibroblast growth factor. Biomaterials. 2011;32(18):4243–54.
40. Derakhshandeh H, Kashaf SS, Aghabaglou F, Ghanavati IO, Tamayol A. Smart bandages: the future of wound care. Trends Biotechnol. 2018;36(12):1259–74. https://doi.org/10.1016/j.tibtech.2018.07.007.
41. Rani Raju N, SilinaE, Stupin V, Manturova N, Chidambaram SB, Achar RR. Multifunctional and smart wound dressings—a review on recent research advancements in skin regenerative medicine. Pharmaceutics. 2022;14(8). https://doi.org/10.3390/pharmaceutics14081574.

Negative Pressure Wound Therapy in Leg Ulcers

11

Mihaela Leventer, Elena Soare, Johan Löfgren, Lotta Purola, Valentin Popescu, Mirela-Elena Vasile, Bogdan-Stelian Mastalier-Manolescu, and Outi Kaarela

Abstract

Negative Pressure Wound Therapy (NPWT), also known as vacuum-assisted closure (VAC), has revolutionized wound care by applying controlled negative pressure to wound sites using specialized vacuum systems. NPWT accelerates wound healing by reducing oedema, promoting angiogenesis and blood flow, and encouraging granulation tissue formation. It also minimizes bacterial growth, reduces infection risks, and supports wound closure by promoting wound edge contraction. NPWT is widely used across medical specialties for chronic wounds, acute injuries, surgical incisions, and complex wounds. However, careful patient assessment is essential due to specific contraindications, including untreated osteomyelitis and certain anatomical considerations. In surgical dermatology, NPWT enhances post-operative recovery by maintaining a controlled environment, improving graft adherence, and expediting wound closure. The future of NPWT holds promise with advancements in portable

M. Leventer (✉) · E. Soare
Dr. Leventer Centre, Bucharest, Romania
e-mail: mihaelaleventer@drleventercentre.com

M. Leventer
"Carol Davila" University of Medicine and Pharmacy, Bucharest, Romania

J. Löfgren
Department of Surgery, Oulu University Hospital, Oulu, Finland

L. Purola · O. Kaarela
Department of Plastic Surgery, Oulu University Hospital, Oulu, Finland

V. Popescu · B.-S. Mastalier-Manolescu
General Surgery Clinic, Colentina Clinical Hospital, Carol Davila University of Medicine and Pharmacy, Bucharest, Romania

M.-E. Vasile
Pediatric Surgery Clinic, Grigore Alexandrescu Clinical Hospital, Carol Davila University of Medicine and Pharmacy, Bucharest, Romania

G.-S.Tiplica and K. Isoherranen (eds.), *Wound Healing*,
https://doi.org/10.1007/978-3-031-84579-6_11

devices and personalized wound management strategies, offering continued improvements in patient care and outcomes.

Keywords

Negative pressure wound therapy (NPWT) • Wound reconstruction • Granulation tissue • Skin grafting • Adjuvant therapy

Abbreviations

NPWT	Negative pressure wound therapy
WLE	Wide local excision
DFSP	Dermatofibrosarcoma protuberans

Introduction

In the ever-evolving landscape of medical technology, innovative approaches to wound care continue to revolutionize patient outcomes. One such advancement that has significantly transformed wound management is Negative Pressure Wound Therapy (NPWT). This therapy has emerged as a powerful tool in the hands of healthcare professionals, offering new avenues for treating complex wounds.

Negative Pressure Wound Therapy, often referred to as vacuum-assisted closure (VAC), involves the application of controlled negative pressure to a wound site using a specialized vacuum pump and dressing system. The basic principle is straightforward, yet effective: a sealed dressing is applied over the wound, and air and excess fluid are drawn out from the wound area through a connected vacuum pump [1]. This controlled suction helps in several ways. NPWT promotes wound healing by reducing oedema and excess fluid, which can impede the body's natural healing processes. The controlled negative pressure also stimulates blood flow to the wound bed, encouraging granulation tissue formation and ultimately promoting tissue regeneration. NPWT creates an environment less susceptible to bacterial growth by removing excess exudate and debris. This reduction in bacterial load minimizes the risk of infection and supports the body's immune response. It also can assist in wound closure by promoting the contraction of wound edges, which is particularly beneficial for large or irregularly shaped wounds [2].

The versatility of NPWT has led to its widespread adoption across various medical specialties [3]. From chronic wounds like diabetic ulcers and pressure injuries to acute traumatic wounds and surgical incisions, NPWT has demonstrated efficacy in a spectrum of clinical scenarios [4, 5].

Some notable benefits of NPWT include accelerated healing, improved patient comfort and management of complex wounds. Studies have shown that NPWT can significantly shorten healing times compared to traditional wound care methods, reducing hospital stays and healthcare costs. Despite applying negative pressure, patients often report reduced pain and discomfort, which is attributed to the stabilization and protection of the wound bed provided by the NPWT dressing. NPWT has proven particularly effective in managing complex wounds with significant tissue loss or compromised vascularity, where conventional treatments may be insufficient. While NPWT has undoubtedly transformed wound care, challenges persist. The cost of NPWT devices and dressings, coupled with the need for specialized training in their application, can pose barriers to widespread adoption. Furthermore, optimizing NPWT protocols for different wound types and patient populations remains an ongoing area of research [6].

NPWT is indicated for a variety of wound types and clinical scenarios. This innovative therapy is commonly used for chronic wounds such as diabetic ulcers, venous ulcers, and pressure injuries, where conventional wound care methods have proven inadequate. NPWT is also valuable in the management of acute traumatic wounds, surgical incisions, and burns, facilitating faster healing and reducing the risk of complications. Additionally, NPWT is employed in complex wounds with large tissue defects or exposed bone, providing a controlled environment that supports tissue regeneration and wound closure. The versatility of NPWT extends across medical specialties, making it a cornerstone in modern wound care protocols for improving patient outcomes. Contraindications to NPWT include wounds with untreated osteomyelitis, untreated malignancy in the wound bed, exposed blood vessels or organs, and necrotic tissue with eschar that has not been adequately debrided. NPWT should also be used cautiously in patients with active bleeding, fistulas, or with certain anatomical locations such as the bowel, bladder, or exposed nerves. Additionally, NPWT may be unsuitable for patients with inadequate perfusion or in whom negative pressure could cause harm or discomfort. It's crucial for healthcare professionals to assess each patient's condition carefully and weigh the benefits against potential risks before initiating NPWT [6, 7].

NPWT has become an invaluable adjunct in surgical dermatology, offering unique benefits in the management of complex wounds and enhancing post-operative recovery [8].

In this field, NPWT is frequently employed following extensive dermatologic procedures such as Mohs surgery (as presented in case report 11.2), skin grafts, and flap reconstructions [9].

One of the primary advantages of NPWT in surgical dermatology is its ability to promote wound healing and minimize complications [10].

By maintaining a controlled environment with negative pressure, NPWT facilitates the removal of excess fluid and reduces o edema, which can improve graft adherence and reduce the risk of seroma or hematoma formation [11]. Moreover, NPWT helps to promote the formation of healthy granulation tissue, thereby expediting wound closure and enhancing aesthetic outcomes. In cases where primary closure is challenging, NPWT can assist in wound contraction and prepare the wound bed for subsequent surgical interventions (case report 11.1) [2]. The use of NPWT in surgical dermatology underscores its versatility and efficacy in optimizing outcomes for patients undergoing complex dermatologic procedures, such as reconstruction after wide local excision of acral melanoma (case report 11.2) [1].

NPWT can be effectively utilized in the treatment of burns following wound bed preparation (case report 11.3). Additionally, NPWT has shown positive outcomes in chronic conditions such as arteriosclerosis (case report 11.4). It is possible to potentiate the efficiency of different methods used in wound healing by including NPWT as it is demonstrated by using NPWT in combination with a collagen matrix impregnated with platelet-rich plasma (PRP) (case report 11.5).

In conclusion, NPWT stands as a testimony to the power of innovation in modern healthcare. By harnessing the principles of negative pressure, this therapeutic approach has reshaped the approach to wound management, offering new hope and healing to patients facing complex wounds. As research continues and technology evolves, the future of NPWT holds immense potential in shaping the landscape of wound care for years to come. Advancements such as portable NPWT devices, novel dressing materials, and intelligent algorithms for personalized wound management hold promise in further improving patient outcomes and accessibility.

The wound healing training curricula should include NPWT. The trainees will be able to understand that NPWT treatment must be based on a diagnosis, evidence-based and patient-centered. They will be able to create and follow a treatment plan according to the aetiology and characteristics of the wound, taking into account other factors that have contributed to the wound and that are relevant in the care. The trainee will be able to apply the NPWT and will identify the situations in which surgical revision is appropriate. The treatment plan, including NPWT will be assessed realistically, and the trainee will determine the appropriate treatment limitations and will be able to identify and solve problems related to care and support of the patient (e.g. adherence to treatment and organizing the treatment). The evolution of the patient under NPWT should be accurately recorded by the trainees.

Case 11.1. NPWT—An Adjuvant Therapy in the Reconstruction of a Large Defect After Wide Local Excision of Acral Melanoma

Introduction

A 63-year-old male patient came to our clinic complaining of a recent bleeding nodule grown on the surface of a preexisting dark-brown, slowly growing lesion on his left heel (Fig. 11.1A). A 6 mm punch biopsy was performed from the nodular lesion, and the pathology report revealed an ulcerated acral melanoma with a Breslow thickness of 4.2 mm. The patient underwent melanoma management, and after wide local excision (WLE), the resulting defect was large and deep, with loss of the subcutaneous fat pad.

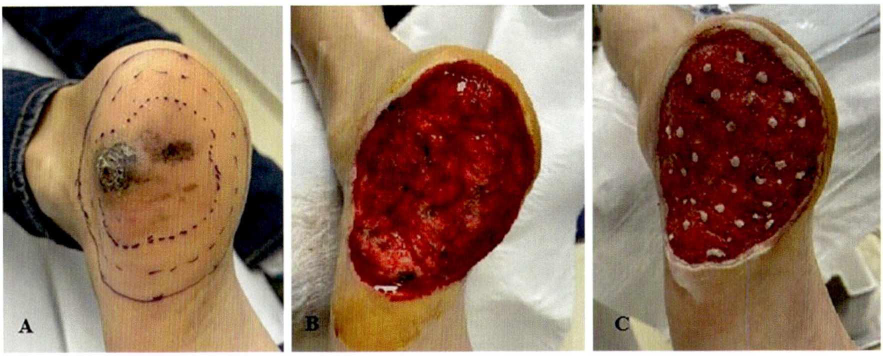

Fig. 11.1 (**A**) Clinical aspect and 2 cm margin drawing before WLE; (**B**) the resulting surgical defect with formed granulation tissue after applying NPWT for one week; (**C**) aspect of the granulated wound bed and applied punch grafts

Treatment

The acute wound resulting after surgical treatment was difficult to reconstruct because of the dimensions and anatomical region. The treatment plan was to promote healthy granulation tissue before autologous punch grafting by applying intermittent negative pressure wound therapy (NPWT) immediately after the WLE. After cleaning the wound with saline irrigation and surgical soap, silicone gauze covered the wound bed. The underlying tegument was protected by applying zinc paste. We followed the protocol for NPWT: the specialized porous foam dressing was cut to the dimensions of the wound and placed on top of the silicone gauze; the foam was sealed with transparent adhesive tape. The suction device was connected to the canister of the NPWT machine. At one week's check-up, the canister had minimal fluid accumulation, and granulation tissue was formed. The NPWT on an intermittent regimen was maintained for another two weeks before the reconstruction to ensure a thick, granulated bed for the grafts (Fig. 11.1B). Under local anesthesia, skin grafts were harvested from the right inguinal fossa using 2-mm and 4-mm punch biopsies and placed on the defect (Fig. 11.1C). We applied intermittent NPWT again, as dressing, to facilitate the integration of the grafts. In case of intense pain, we discussed with the patient the option of changing the device to a continuous regimen. Also, the patient was instructed to seal any perforation with a transparent film dressing to prevent vacuum loss.

Discussions

In this case, the NPWT had a dual role as adjuvant therapy to create a granulated wound bed before reconstruction and as dressing to help integrate the punch grafts. The heel is a weight-bearing site, so the reconstruction with split-thickness skin grafting was inappropriate because the plantar location impairs the vascularization

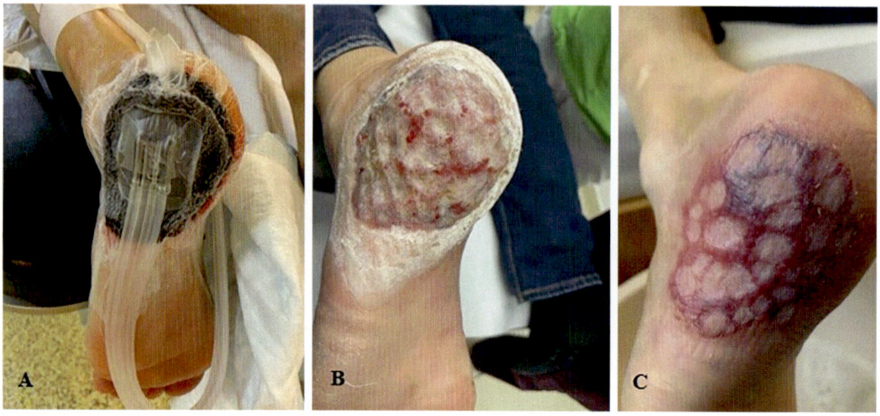

Fig. 11.2 (**A**) NPWT device applied after reconstruction with punch grafts; (**B**) clinical improvement at two weeks; note the zinc paste applied on the margins of the wound; (**C**) final outcome after one month

of the graft, resulting in partial or full-thickness necrosis [12]. Also, the absence of the subcutaneous fat pad after surgical excision was another argument against direct skin grafting [13]. Punch grafting is a straightforward and commonly utilized method in the treatment of persistent non-healing ulcers. These grafts, composed of epidermal and superficial dermal layers, cover the wound's defect and facilitate the migration of keratinocytes. Moreover, post-grafting, cytokine response, and expression of growth factors can be anticipated [14]. NPWT emerges as an efficacious adjunctive therapy for managing complex wounds. Applying subatmospheric pressure to the skin defect makes the healing faster through various mechanisms, including reducing local tissue edema, preventing infection, and enhancing microperfusion and angiogenesis in wounds [15]. In our case, NPWT was first used for wound bed preparation for the delayed closure and as a dressing, preventing infection and ensuring a better immobilization of the grafts (Fig. 11.2).

Case 11.2. NPWT as Adjuvant Therapy Before Reconstruction of a Large and Deep Defect After Surgical Treatment of DFSP

Introduction

A 33-year-old male patient presented to our clinic complaining of a painless bump on his right dorsal foot, which had slowly grown in the last seven years. Two years ago, he had removed a tumor from his right dorsal forefoot in another hospital, and the histopathologic diagnosis on Hematoxylin–Eosin was of dense cell dermatofibroma with deep resection margins in contact with the tumor. No immunohistochemical stains were performed. He noted three other tumors growing near the old scar one year after the first excision. Two were excised, and the pathology report was positive for dermatofibrosarcoma protuberans. The magnetic resonance showed that the tumor is in contact with the extensor digitorum longus on the right dorsal forefoot.

Differential Diagnosis

In the differential diagnosis of dermatofibrosarcoma protuberans, we include hypertrophic/keloid scars, dermatofibroma, lipoma, Kaposi sarcoma, fibrosarcoma, peripheral nerve sheath tumor, and spindle cell melanoma.

Treatment

In this case of recurrent dermatofibrosarcoma, the treatment of choice was the Slow Mohs micrographic procedure. We drew the clinical margins of the tumor, a margin of 1 cm (Fig. 11.3A), oriented the specimen, and excised deep until the fascia. The histopathology report showed invaded resection margins, so we excised the tumor-positive region, including the second toe's extensor digitorum longus and brevis. The final defect measured 9×8 cm, exposing tendons and the second and third metatarsophalangeal joints (Fig. 11.3B). The reconstruction with local flaps was not an option because of the large size and depth of the resulting defect. The surgical team opted for a two-step reconstruction approach. Intermittent negative pressure therapy (125 mmHg) was applied for two weeks before the closure of the defect with a split-thickness skin graft. The NPWT reduced the size of the defect from 9×8 cm to 7.5×7 cm, allowing epithelization of the margins and forming granulation tissue on the bed of the resulting cutaneous defect (Fig. 11.3C). After the two-week delayed period, the defect was covered with a dermal substitute after superficial debridement of the newly formed tissue to create a bleeding recipient wound bed. The dermal matrix was covered with a split-thickness skin graft from the anterolateral right thigh (Fig. 11.4A). We re-applied continuous NPWT (70–80 mmHg) for five more days to fix the graft, enhance the survival rate, and reduce the infection risk. At the three-month checkup, the skin graft was fully integrated. (Fig. 11.4B).

Discussions

DFSP is a rare, intermediate-grade soft tissue sarcoma with low metastatic potential, usually presenting as a violaceous, red, brown, or skin color plaque-like skin thickening. The main characteristics are slow infiltrative growth and local recurrence when excision is incomplete [16, 17].

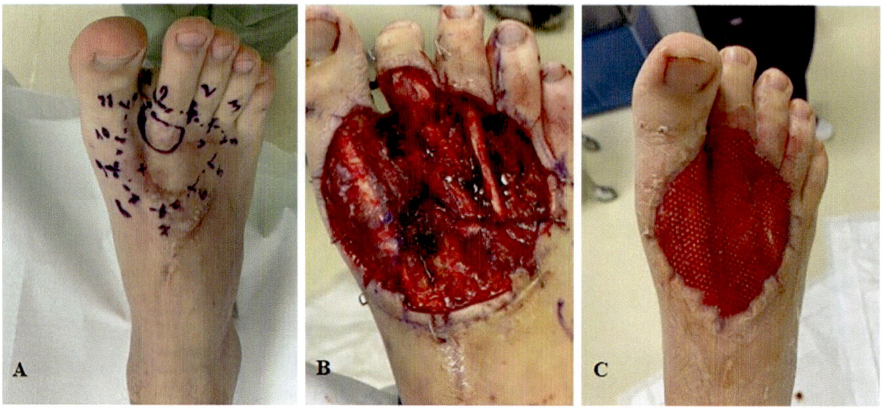

Fig. 11.3 (**A**) Mapping of the tumor for Slow Mohs micrographic procedure. (**B**) Final defect with extensive soft tissue loss, exposed tendons, and metatarsophalangeal joints. (**C**) Granulation of the wound bed after applying intermittent NPWT

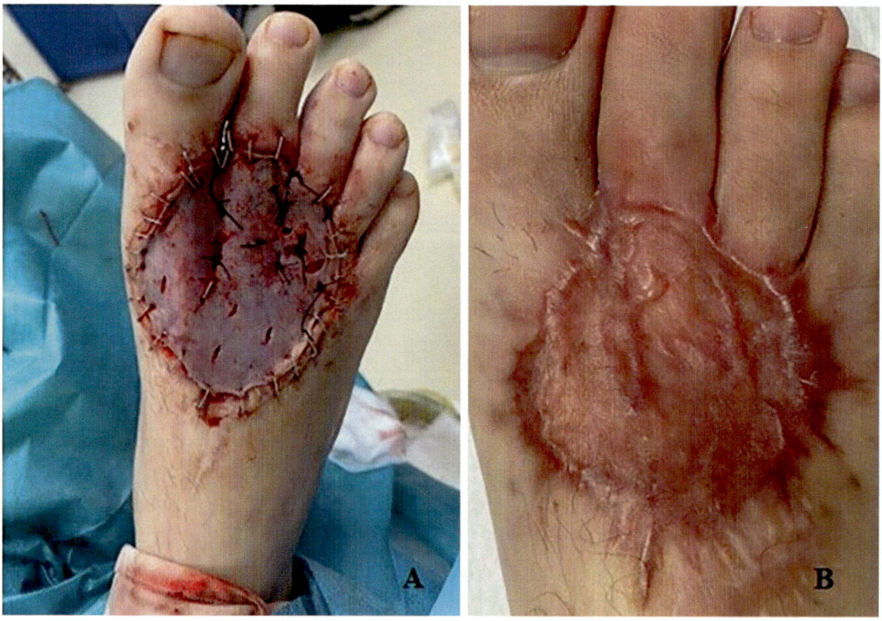

Fig. 11.4 (**A**) Aspect immediately after reconstruction with a partially split skin graft, (**B**) at three-month check-up

NPWT facilitates surgical reconstructions for large, deep skin and soft tissue defects without extensive flap surgery or skin graft loss. Applying controlled subatmospheric pressure creates mechanical stress on tissues, resulting in wound contraction. NPWT reduces local edema, increases microperfusion of the wound, reduces bacterial colonies, and stimulates granulation tissue growth in the wound bed. NPWT is useful when the wound is unsuitable for immediate reconstruction, as in our case [15]. In contrast to conventional wound care techniques, NPWT presents clear benefits. It accelerates the healing process and minimizes the necessity for frequent dressing changes.

Case 11.3. Burn Wounds Treated with Negative Wound Pressure, Dermal Substitute and Skin Grafts

Introduction

Our patient is a 77-year-old male, with hypercholesterolemia, hip arthrosis, and a suspected memory disorder. The patient had fallen against the sauna stove and received 3rd degree burns to the back of his head, the upper back, and shoulders. The left upper limb had 2nd degree burns in the upper half of the limb. Total burn surface area was assessed as 8%. The patient could not recall what had happened or if he had been unconscious. GCS score was 15 in the emergency department. The burns were first treated with Burn Relief wound products by emergency medical services on location. The patient was admitted to the hospital after initial assessment in the emergency department.

Differential Diagnosis

The cause of the burn wounds was clear, contact with a hot object. The depth of the burns changed with time and clinical deepening of the burns was observed during surgical operations. The exact events leading to the contact with the sauna stove remain unclear, due to the patient's memory problems.

Treatment

The patient was treated at a normal surgical ward; there was no need for ICU care. Initially the burn wounds were treated with Mepilex AgR silver dressings. The dressings were changed every 3 days. 5 days after the trauma (Fig. 11.5a), the burns in the upper back and left shoulder were excised to the fascial layer. The right shoulder and left upper limb burns were excised to a vital dermal layer. The burn behind the head was excised to the galea layer. All areas were covered with split skin grafts. The upper back, shoulders and back of head areas were covered

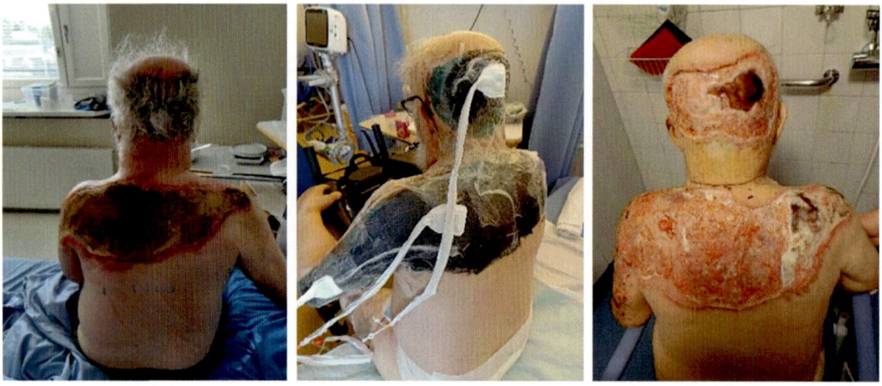

(a) (b) (c)

Fig. 11.5 (**a**) Deep 3rd degree burn 4 days after trauma just before operation. (**b**) Negative wound pressure dressing after burn wound excision and skin grafting. (**c**) After removing the dressing skin graft infected in shoulder site and skull partially exposed

with negative pressure wound (NPW) dressings using a Y connector and a single machine (Fig. 11.5b).

The skin grafts of the right shoulder and the back of the head were lost due to infection, *Staphylococcus aureus* and *Pseudomonas* bacteria was found in culture tests (Fig. 11.5c). 12 days after the initial surgery, the right shoulder was debrided to fascial layer and the back of the head all the way to bone. 8 days later, the right shoulder was covered with skin grafts. The exposed non-vascular dry surface of cranial bone in the back of the head was bled with a rose drill before covered with an Integra® dermal substitute (Fig. 11.6a and b). The patient was transferred to a primary care unit one week after the application of the Integra® substitute. At an outpatient wound clinic follow up 2 weeks later, the Integra® was seen starting to begin vascularized. Three weeks after application, the Integra's® silicone sheet was removed, and the area was covered with thin skin grafts and a NPW dressing was applied with 125 mmHg pressure. A week later the NPW dressing was removed, and the skin grafts were healing well (Fig. 11.7a). 4 weeks later most areas had healed appropriately (Fig. 11.7b). The right shoulder still had some small areas which had not healed, these areas had hyper granulation, which were treated with silver nitrate. The patient started wearing a pressure garment, covering the upper body and upper arms (T-shirt model). A half year since the burn occurred, the patient came for an outpatient checkup, and all areas had healed normally, and he had good mobility in both upper extremities and no restrictions in head movements. No major scar hypertrophy could be seen, and the pressure garment was advised to be used at least until 1 year of the accident.

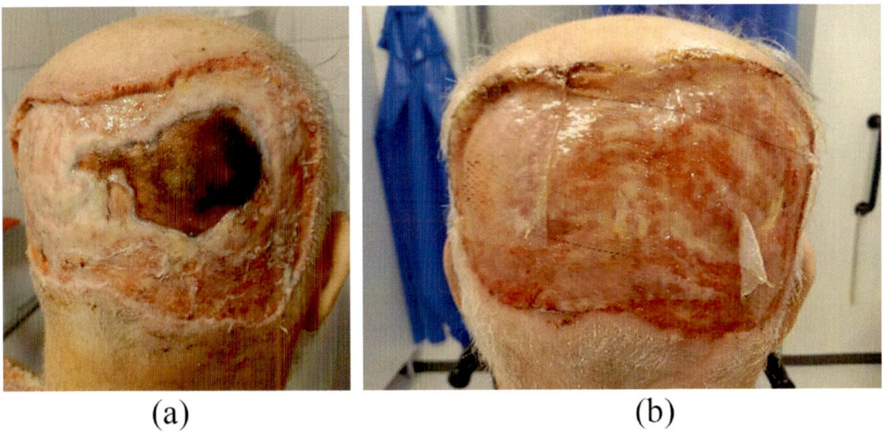

Fig. 11.6 (**a**) Exposed skull was dry and the surrounding area had some inflammatory tissue on the raw surface. A debridement was carried out. Exposed dead bone was removed tangentially with a rose drill. (**b**) Integra® was applied on the whole wound bed and it vascularized gradually in 3 weeks, part of the silicone layer peeling off on the right side

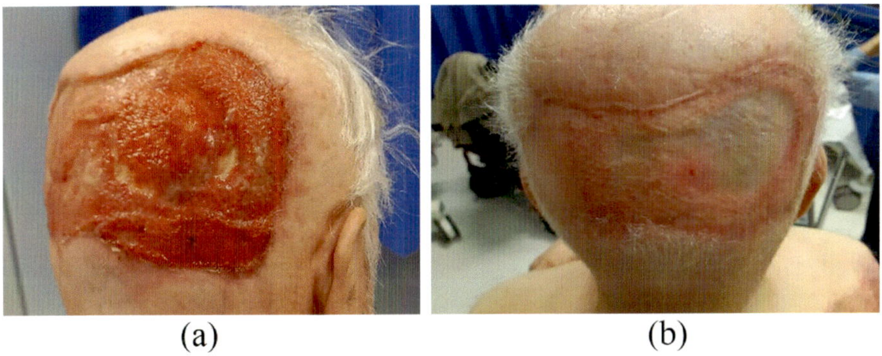

Fig. 11.7 (**a**) Skin grafts took well on Integra 3 weeks after coverage. (**b**) Skin grafts on skull 6 weeks after coverage operation

Discussions

Burns were excised when the burn depth and affected areas were defined. Some burn areas were later observed deeper than what was initially assessed, these areas required additional and deeper excisions. Negative pressure wound therapy was used on top of skin grafts to enable immediate mobilization and to promote healing of the skin grafts during both grafting operations. We also often use NPWT on the Integra® dermal substitute, but this time we decided not to use it because of the infection. The dermal substitute was used to ensure good adhesion and healing of skin grafts in the head area, where the wound bed was a bony surface, without galea or periosteum [18–22].

Case 11.4. Negative Pressure Therapy Helping the Wound Closure

Our patient is a 72-year-old man with very few healthcare visits before. He contacted the primary health care unit due to lower limb swelling and was diagnosed with heart failure and coronary artery disease. He had total right coronary artery (RCA) blockage and had percutaneous coronary intervention (PCI) on 10/2024. He had non-healing chronic wounds in both lower extremities. The first long-term swelling was thought to be the aetiology of chronic wounds. He was sent to the ER due to critical left leg ischemia. He had wide atherosclerotic changes in emergency CT angiography. He had stopped smoking but had a smoking history of decades.

The patient had general arteriosclerosis, affecting also the coronary arteries and a heart failure, which caused him swelling in lower extremities. No other etiological reasons for wounds.

Treatment

He had an urgent femoral-popliteal bypass with contralateral VSM due to critical left leg ischemia. Postoperative ABI 0.77/0.6, toe pressure 73/58 mmHg, TBI 0.82/0.55 being acceptable. Vascular surgeons noted numerous chronic, dry wounds with no sign of acute infection. One of these wounds was over the Achilles tendon. Two weeks later the patient's Achilles tendon ruptured while walking normally with a walking aid. The edges of the tendon were visible through the necrotic wound (Fig. 11.8a). When the patient came to his routine graft and wound control vascular surgeons consulted plastic surgeons and the wound debridement was carried out the next day. The entire tendon had to be removed, and the wound was left open (Fig. 11.8b). Bacterial cultures had polymicrobial growth.

The local traditional wound care provided good granulation tissue on the surface of the entire wound. The patient had an outpatient consultation appointment three weeks later (1/2024). The wound was improving but another smaller wound with visible tendon structures was noticed on the medial side of the ankle. The second operation was two weeks later and both wounds were covered with partial-thickness skin grafts. The grafts were covered with Sorbact Gel Side® dressing. NPWT with 85 mmHg and black foam was utilized (Fig. 11.9a and b). The patient was allowed to stand for a short while and move in a wheelchair. Prophylactic antibiotic therapy was utilized till the negative bacterial culture results were obtained.

The skin graft was controlled for five days and then seven days post-op (Fig. 11.10a). At control, in 4 weeks, some of the skin graft was lost (Fig. 11.10b), but the patient wished to be treated conservatively.

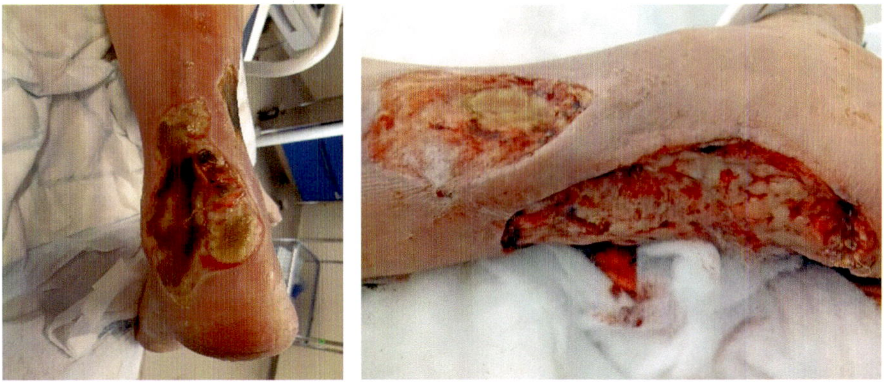

(a) (b)

Fig. 11.8 (**a**) Ankle wound Achilles tendon exposed. (**b**) Ankle wounds after the debridement

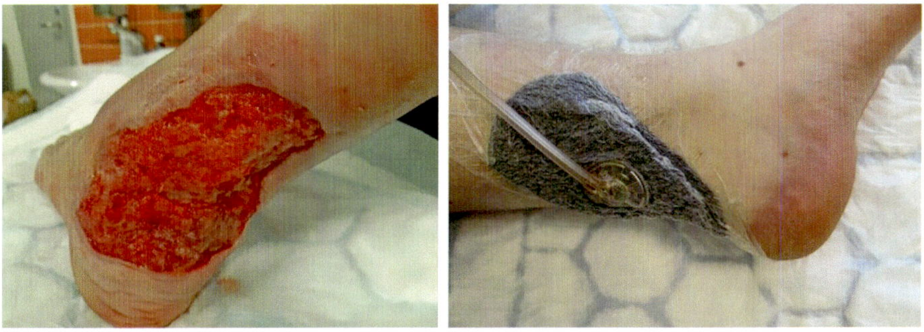

(a) (b)

Fig. 11.9 (**a**) Outpatient control in two months after conservative treatment. The area is well granulated after conservative treatment and ready for skin grafting. (**b**) Negative pressure wound treatment dressings on skin graft

Discussion

The original wound etiology was chronic swelling due to heart failure and accompanied by peripheral arterial disease-causing impaired circulation and healing capacity. Achilles tendon rupture was an unexpected event. After the bypass operation and active wound care the general situation improved. The Non-viable Achilles tendon had to be removed. The ankle did not have well vascularized tissue covering the defect after debridement, therefore the wound was covered with a split thickness skin graft.

NPWT has been popularized during the last few decades [23]. There are numerous studies and systematic reviews and meta-analyses focusing on them with

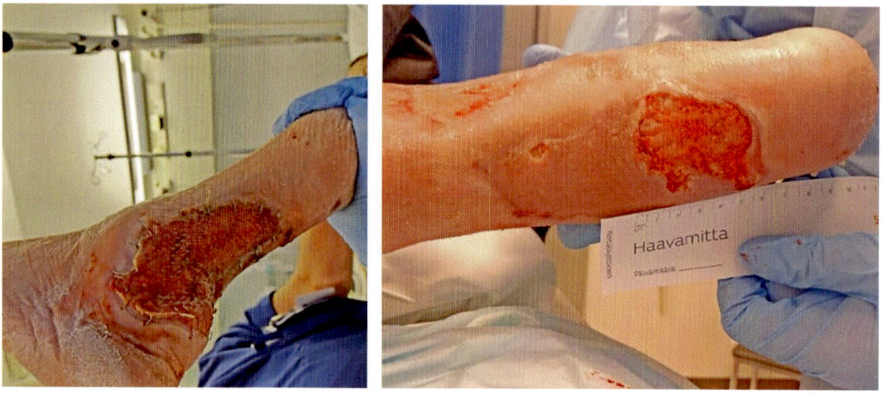

(a) (b)

Fig. 11.10 (**a**) Skin graft one week postoperatively after NPWT period. (**b**) Skin graft partially lost, about one third, and the patient was not immediately ready for another operation, therefore conservative treatment continued

somewhat controversial results [24–26]. However, it is currently a part of routine wound care [27]. Jian et al. [11] performed a systematic review showing that NPWT improves the healing of skin grafts.

In wound care the etiology of the wound is the most important thing and in this particular case heart failure and impaired vascularity had to be treated first. Focused and organized wound care is beneficial both from financial and individual points of view [28, 29]. NPWT is considered to be safe in patients with ischemia [25]. The wound must be properly debrided before NPWT therapy. Our patient had a two-stage operation: First, he had thorough debridement, and in second operation, skin grafting. Due to the challenging location, we chose negative pressure therapy after skin grafting post-operatively to allow active rehabilitation. This was the major advantage of the NPWT in this case.

The majority of the skin graft succeeded, and the patient was able to return home. During the last inpatient period, he actively practiced walking with a light splint.

Case 11.5. The Effectiveness of Collagen Matrix Impregnated with PRP Under NPWT (PRP Cupcake Technique) in a Patient with a Complex Wound

A 71-year-old female patient with multiple comorbidities including stage III obesity, mild cardiac dysfunction, diabetes mellitus type II, stage III hypertension, congestive heart failure, chronic venous insufficiency (CVI), asthma, and documented sepsis was seeking for surgical consultation for a highly exudative wound located on the lower third of the right calf. The tendons of the tibialis anterior and extensor digitorum longus muscles were exposed (Fig. 11.11). The wound was associated with *Morganella morganii* and *Pseudomonas aeruginosa* infections, as evidenced by laboratory findings.

This case presentation follows the Strengthening the Reporting of Observational Studies in Epidemiology (STROBE) guidelines. The patient was selected based on specific inclusion criteria, including the presence of a complex wound with exposed tendons, a history of diabetes mellitus type II, and signs of sepsis. The control in this case was defined by the standard wound care practice, which includes surgical debridement followed by dressings without the use of PRP or NPWT.

After surgical debridement to remove necrotic tissue, a 1 cm layer of a hemostatic collagen matrix impregnated with PRP was applied directly to the wound bed. This matrix serves as a scaffold for cellular infiltration and tissue regeneration [30, 31]. NPWT was applied over the collagen matrix for 4 days (Fig. 11.12). Following the removal of NPWT, the wound was covered with a silver-containing impregnated dressing and an absorbent dressing for an additional 3 days. The primary outcome measured was the percentage of wound volume reduction, assessed at the end of the treatment period.

At the time of admission, the patient's wound was presented with significant necrotic tissue and a high bacterial load, as indicated by laboratory cultures. The initial treatment with surgical debridement reduced the burden of necrotic tissue and exposed viable tissue. The application of the collagen matrix impregnated with PRP under NPWT was associated with a marked reduction in wound exudate and improved wound bed appearance.

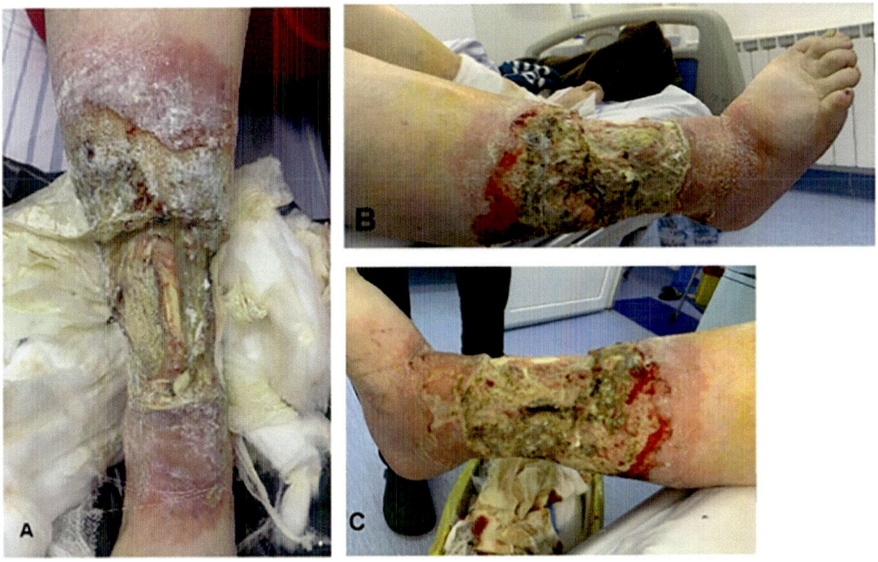

Fig. 11.11 Initial wound site after primary debridement (**A**) frontal view, (**B**) lateral view, (**C**) medial view

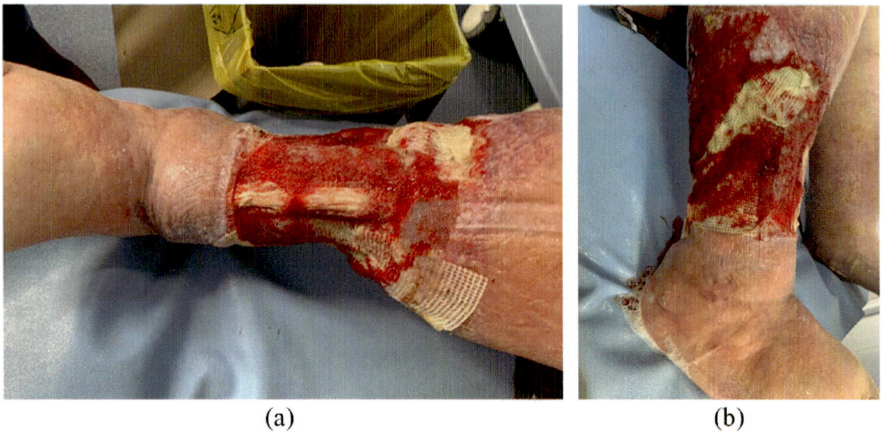

Fig. 11.12 Images of the wound after 4 days of NWPT PRP (**a**) anterior view, (**b**) lateral view

After 4 days of NPWT, a significant volume of granulation tissue had formed. Upon removal of the NPWT and the application of silver-containing dressings, further improvement was noted. By the end of the 7-day observation period, the wound had filled 72% of its volume with new tissue, a remarkable healing rate given the initial wound characteristics and the patient's comorbidities.

Discussion

The results suggest that the combined use of a collagen matrix impregnated with PRP and NPWT can significantly enhance wound healing, even in a patient with multiple systemic challenges, resulting in a significant reduction in wound size and a rapid formation of granulation tissue. The PRP provides a rich source of growth factors [32, 33], which are essential for tissue regeneration, while the collagen matrix offers a scaffold for cellular growth [34, 35]. The NPWT helps to maintain a moist wound environment [36], reduce edema [36], and remove infectious materials [37], thus creating optimal conditions for wound healing [38].

This case highlights the potential benefits of integrating advanced wound care technologies in managing complex wounds, particularly in patients with comorbidities that may otherwise impede healing. The use of silver-containing dressings post-NPWT helped in maintaining an antimicrobial environment [39, 40], further contributing to the positive outcome (Fig. 11.13).

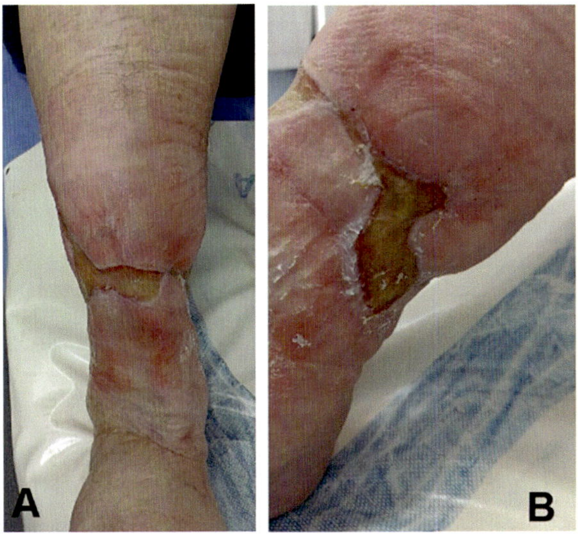

Fig. 11.13 Results after 6 months (**A**) anterior view, (**B**) medial view

References

1. Huang C, Leavitt T, Bayer LR, Orgill DP. Effect of negative pressure wound therapy on wound healing. Curr Probl Surg. 2014;51(7):301–31. https://doi.org/10.1067/J.CPSURG.2014.04.001.
2. Lalezari S, et al. Deconstructing negative pressure wound therapy. Int Wound J. 2017;14(4):649–57. https://doi.org/10.1111/iwj.12658.
3. El-Sabbagh AH. Negative pressure wound therapy: an update. Chin J Traumatol. 2017;20(2):103–7. https://doi.org/10.1016/j.cjtee.2016.09.004.
4. Webster J, Scuffham P, Stankiewicz M, Chaboyer WP. Negative pressure wound therapy for skin grafts and surgical wounds healing by primary intention. Cochrane Database Syst Rev. 2014. https://doi.org/10.1002/14651858.CD009261.pub3.
5. Zaver V, Kankanalu P. Negative pressure wound therapy; 2024.
6. Apelqvist J et al. EWMA document: negative pressure wound therapy. J Wound Care. 2017;26(Sup3):S1–154. https://doi.org/10.12968/JOWC.2017.26.SUP3.S1.
7. Cai SS, Gowda AU, Alexander RH, Silverman RP, Goldberg NH, Rasko YM. Use of negative pressure wound therapy on malignant wounds—a case report and review of literature. Int Wound J. 2017;14(4):661–5. https://doi.org/10.1111/iwj.12665.
8. Scalise A, et al. Improving wound healing and preventing surgical site complications of closed surgical incisions: a possible role of Incisional Negative Pressure Wound Therapy. A systematic review of the literature. Int Wound J. 2016;13(6):1260–81. https://doi.org/10.1111/IWJ.12492.
9. Putri IL, Adzalika LB, Pramanasari R, Wungu CDK. Negative pressure wound therapy versus conventional wound care in cancer surgical wounds: a meta-analysis of observational studies and randomised controlled trials. Int Wound J. 2022;19(6):1578–93. https://doi.org/10.1111/iwj.13756.
10. Norman G et al. Negative pressure wound therapy for surgical wounds healing by primary closure. Cochrane Database Syst Rev. 2020;5(5):CD009261. https://doi.org/10.1002/14651858.CD009261.PUB5.

11. Jiang ZY, et al. Negative-pressure wound therapy in skin grafts: a systematic review and meta-analysis of randomized controlled trials. Burns. 2021;47(4):747–55. https://doi.org/10.1016/J.BURNS.2021.02.012.
12. Zyman LM, da Cunha JAJ, Gimenez AO, Maia M. Acral melanoma: considerations about the surgical management of this tumor. An Bras Dermatol. 2019;94(5):632–3. https://doi.org/10.1016/j.abd.2019.09.019.
13. Nakamura Y, Teramoto Y, Sato S, Yamamoto A. Current surgical management of acral lentiginous melanoma. In: Melanoma—current clinical management and future therapeutics. Intech; 2015. https://doi.org/10.5772/59133.
14. Seo J, Kim J, Nam KA, Zheng Z, Oh BH, Chung KY. Reconstruction of large wounds using a combination of negative pressure wound therapy and punch grafting after excision of acral lentiginous melanoma on the foot. J Dermatol. 2016;43(1):79–84. https://doi.org/10.1111/1346-8138.13017.
15. Lee DL, Ryu AY, Rhee SC. Negative pressure wound therapy: an adjuvant to surgical reconstruction of large or difficult skin and soft tissue defects. Int Wound J. 2011;8(4):406–11. https://doi.org/10.1111/j.1742-481X.2011.00813.x.
16. St. Clair B, Clark A, Rollins B, Jennings TA. Mohs micrographic surgery for dermatofibrosarcoma protuberans in 15 patients: the University of Arkansas for Medical Sciences Experience. Cureus. 2022. https://doi.org/10.7759/cureus.24147.
17. Lowe GC, et al. A comparison of mohs micrographic surgery and wide local excision for treatment of dermatofibrosarcoma protuberans with long-term follow-up: the Mayo Clinic experience. Dermatol Surg. 2017;43(1):98–106. https://doi.org/10.1097/DSS.0000000000000910.
18. Molnar JA, DeFranzo AJ, Hadaegh A, Morykwas MJ, Shen P, Argenta LC. Acceleration of Integra incorporation in complex tissue defects with subatmospheric pressure. Plast Reconstr Surg. 2004;113(5):1339–46. https://doi.org/10.1097/01.PRS.0000112746.67050.68.
19. Kantak NA, Mistry R, Varon DE, Halvorson EG. Negative pressure wound therapy for burns. Clin Plast Surg. 2017;44(3):671–7. https://doi.org/10.1016/J.CPS.2017.02.023.
20. Alkhonizy SW, et al. Effectiveness of dermal regeneration templates in managing acute full-thickness and deep dermal burn injuries: a comparison with split-thickness skin grafts. Plast Reconstr Surg Glob Open. 2024;12(2):e5572. https://doi.org/10.1097/GOX.0000000000005572.
21. Asif M, Ebrahim S, Major M, Caffrey J. The use of IntegraTM as a novel technique in deep burn foot management. JPRAS Open. 2018;17:15–20. https://doi.org/10.1016/J.JPRA.2018.04.003.
22. González Alaña I, Torrero López JV, Martín Playá P, Gabilondo Zubizarreta FJ. Combined use of negative pressure wound therapy and Integra® to treat complex defects in lower extremities after burns. Ann Burns Fire Disast. 2013;26(2):90. https://pmc.ncbi.nlm.nih.gov/articles/PMC3793885/. Accessed 16 Dec 2024
23. Lambert KV, Hayes P, McCarthy M. Vacuum assisted closure: a review of development and current applications. Eur J Vasc Endovasc Surg. 2005;29(3):219–26. https://doi.org/10.1016/J.EJVS.2004.12.017.
24. Vikatmaa P, Juutilainen V, Kuukasjärvi P, Malmivaara A. Negative pressure wound therapy: a systematic review on effectiveness and safety. Eur J Vasc Endovasc Surg. 2008;36(4):438–48. https://doi.org/10.1016/J.EJVS.2008.06.010.
25. Cheng HT, Hsu YC, Wu CI. Efficacy and safety of negative pressure wound therapy for Szilagyi grade III peripheral vascular graft infection. Interact Cardiovasc Thorac Surg. 2014;19(6):1048–52. https://doi.org/10.1093/ICVTS/IVU289.
26. Sandy-Hodgetts K, Watts R. Effectiveness of negative pressure wound therapy/closed incision management in the prevention of post-surgical wound complications: a systematic review and meta-analysis. JBI Database Syst Rev Implem Rep. 2015;13(1):253–303. https://doi.org/10.11124/JBISRIR-2015-1687.
27. Negative pressure wound therapy an update for clinicians and outpatient care givers. J Wound Manage. 2024;(1). https://doi.org/10.35279/JOWM2024.25.02.SUP01.

28. Lindholm C, Searle R. Wound management for the 21st century: combining effectiveness and efficiency. Int Wound J. 2016;13(Suppl 2):5–15. https://doi.org/10.1111/IWJ.12623.
29. Morton LM, Phillips TJ. Wound healing and treating wounds: differential diagnosis and evaluation of chronic wounds. J Am Acad Dermatol. 2016;74(4):589–605. https://doi.org/10.1016/J.JAAD.2015.08.068.
30. Borzini P, Mazzucco L. Tissue regeneration and in loco administration of platelet derivatives: clinical outcome, heterogeneous products, and heterogeneity of the effector mechanisms. Transfusion. 2005;45(11):1759–67. https://doi.org/10.1111/J.1537-2995.2005.00600.X.
31. Powers JG, Higham C, Broussard K, Phillips TJ. Wound healing and treating wounds. J Am Acad Dermatol. 2016;74(4):607–25. https://doi.org/10.1016/j.jaad.2015.08.070.
32. Miron RJ, Fujioka-Kobayashi M, Bishara M, Zhang Y, Hernandez M, Choukroun J. Platelet-rich fibrin and soft tissue wound healing: a systematic review. Tissue Eng Part B Rev. 2017;23(1):83–99. https://doi.org/10.1089/TEN.TEB.2016.0233.
33. Badade P, Mahale S, Panjwani A, Vaidya P, Warang A. Antimicrobial effect of platelet-rich plasma and platelet-rich fibrin. Indian J Dent Res. 2016;27(3):300. https://doi.org/10.4103/0970-9290.186231.
34. Masuki H, et al. Growth factor and pro-inflammatory cytokine contents in platelet-rich plasma (PRP), plasma rich in growth factors (PRGF), advanced platelet-rich fibrin (A-PRF), and concentrated growth factors (CGF). Int J Implant Dent. 2016;2(1):19. https://doi.org/10.1186/s40729-016-0052-4.
35. Naik B, Karunakar P, Jayadev M, Marshal VR. Role of Platelet rich fibrin in wound healing: a critical review. J Conserv Dent. 2013;16(4):284–93. https://doi.org/10.4103/0972-0707.114344.
36. Deng W et al. Platelet-rich plasma, bilayered acellular matrix grafting and negative pressure wound therapy in diabetic foot infection 2016;25(7):393–397. https://doi.org/10.12968/JOWC.2016.25.7.393.
37. Zheng Z, et al. Polydopamine-modified collagen sponge scaffold as a novel dermal regeneration template with sustained release of platelet-rich plasma to accelerate skin repair: a one-step strategy. Bioact Mater. 2021;6(8):2613–28. https://doi.org/10.1016/J.BIOACTMAT.2021.01.037.
38. Eming SA, Martin P, Tomic-Canic M. Wound repair and regeneration: mechanisms, signaling, and translation. Sci Transl Med. 2014;6(265). https://doi.org/10.1126/SCITRANSLMED.3009337.
39. Dhivya S, Padma VV, Santhini E. Wound dressings—a review. Biomedicine. 2015;5(4):24–8. https://doi.org/10.7603/S40681-015-0022-9.
40. Vowden K, Vowden P. Wound dressings: principles and practice. Surg Infect. 2017;35(9):489–94. https://doi.org/10.1016/J.MPSUR.2017.06.005.

Adjuvant Therapies in Cutaneous Ulcers

12

Alexandra Irina Butacu, Ioana Simona Popa, Isabela Iancu, Ionela Manole, George-Sorin Tiplica, Mihaela Leventer, and Laura Banciu

Abstract

Cutaneous ulcers include a wide spectrum of disorders, from leg ulcers due to chronic venous insufficiency to neoplastic processes. There are numerous options available regarding adjuvant therapies in cutaneous ulcers depending on the underlying pathology and may include a) pharmaceutical interventions, (b) surgical interventions, (c) topical agents, (d) the use of devices, and (e) other, such as physiotherapy and psychological treatments. Examples of pharmacological treatments used for treatment of cutaneous ulcers include pentoxifylline, iloprost, calcium antagonists, systemic corticosteroids, analgesics and other medications less often used such as NSAIDs, colchicine and antiplatelets. Surgical interventions are mainly used for the management of advanced cases of peripheral arterial disease, including open bypass and endovascular procedures, and closing with skin grafts or flaps hard-to-heal ulcers. Topical products in wound healing may be directed against the associated infections, such as use of antimicrobials. Other topical agents may be glyceryl trinitrate, zinc, phenytoin and retinoids. The use of specific devices in wound healing represents an ascending trend and include various procedures such as negative-pressure wound therapy, platelet-rich plasma (PRP) infiltrations of the cutaneous ulcer, hyperbaric oxygen therapy, radiant heat dressings, ultrasound therapy, laser therapy, hydrotherapy, electromagnetic therapy. Nonetheless, physiotherapy procedures may be required in cases of prolonged immobilization or after complex surgical interventions and impaired mobility and psychological treatments are

A. I. Butacu (✉) · I. S. Popa · I. Iancu · I. Manole · G.-S. Tiplica
Department of Dermatology, Colentina Clinic Hospital, Carol Davila University of Medicine and Pharmacy, Bucharest, Romania
e-mail: alexandra.butacu@umfcd.ro

M. Leventer · L. Banciu
Dr. Leventer Center, Carol Davila University of Medicine and Pharmacy, Bucharest, Romania

G.-S.Tiplica and K. Isoherranen (eds.), *Wound Healing*,
https://doi.org/10.1007/978-3-031-84579-6_12

used to alleviate stress to achieve a rapid and complete rehabilitation of the patient.

Keywords

Adjuvant therapies • Pharmaceutical options • Surgical interventions • Topical agents • Psychological treatments • Systemic corticosteroids • Pyoderma gangrenosum • Breast neoplasm • Cribriform atrophic scars • Inflammatory bowel disease • Venous leg ulcer • Chronic venous insufficiency • Negative pressure wound therapy • Platelet-rich plasma • Arterial ulcer • Multidisciplinary approach • Doppler examination • Arteriography • Revascularization

Abbreviations

COPD	Chronic obstructive pulmonary disease
CVI	Chronic venous insufficiency
LVEF	Left ventricular ejection fraction
NPWT	Negative-pressure wound therapy
NRS	Numeric rating scale
NSAIDs	Nonsteroidal anti-inflammatory drugs
PRP	Platelet-rich plasma
PDGF	Platelet-derived growth factor

Introduction

Cutaneous ulcers include a wide spectrum of disorders, from leg ulcers due to chronic venous insufficiency or peripheral arterial disease to metabolic disorders including diabetes, to inflammatory or autoimmune diseases such as cutaneous vasculitis or neoplastic processes. Therefore, there are numerous options available regarding adjuvant therapies in cutaneous ulcers depending on the underlying pathology.

The classification of adjuvant therapies in cutaneous ulcers includes (a) pharmaceutical options, (b) surgical interventions, (c) topical agents, (d) the use of specific devices, and (e) other, such as physiotherapy and psychological treatments [1].

Pharmaceutical options in wound healing are represented by various agents used depending on the underlying condition. Pharmacological treatments used for treatment of cutaneous ulcers are several, with different mechanisms to promote healing. Pentoxifylline is a methylxanthine used mainly for patients with peripheral arterial disease, and it improves capillary microcirculation, and inhibits tumor necrosis factor-α [2]. It can also be used in cases of vasculitis or necrobiosis lipoidica [3] Iloprost is a prostacyclin analogue, that is used for severe limb ischemia, vasculitis and connective tissue disorders such as Raynaud phenomenon (reference needed). Calcium antagonists, such as diltiazem and nifedipine dilate small vessels and are used for vasculitis and connective tissue disorders (reference). Systemic corticosteroids promote healing by diminishing the inflammatory response, but they should not be used long term, as it may have a detrimental effect on wound healing. Systemic corticosteroids are mainly used in cutaneous ulcers associated with vasculitis, pyoderma gangrenosum, scleroderma and rheumatoid arthritis [2]. Analgesics are required in cases with associated pain and may vary from tricyclic antidepressants (amitriptyline) to antiepileptics (gabapentin) in cases of diabetic neuropathy; other medications less often used include NSAIDs (ibuprofen), colchicine, antiplatelets (aspirin), anticoagulants (heparin), warfarin, vasoconstrictors (nicotine, adrenaline); natural products are also used in some parts of the world in wound healing, such as manuka honey, yogurt or tea tree oil [4].

Surgical interventions are mainly used for the management of advanced cases of peripheral arterial disease, revascularization being the standard of choice, by different procedures such as open bypass or endovascular procedures such as balloon angioplasty (plain balloon, specialized balloon, or drug-coated); bare-metal, drug-eluting or covered stent placement; and plaque removal (atherectomy). Open surgical variants include endarterectomy and bypass grafting (autogenous or prosthetic). Hybrid procedures are also available [5]. Another surgical procedure used for leg ulcers, especially due to vascular disorders is represented by punch grafting, in which small size and thin sections of skin are placed on the surface of a cutaneous ulcer as it represents a simple procedure which promotes healing and reduces pain [6]. In larger ulcers, skin grafting, and flaps are a treatment option [7].

Topical products in wound healing may be directed against the associated infections, including antimicrobials, such as iodine-based preparations and silver releasing agents. These products target the bacteria at different levels and may be used for multiple infectious agents. Glyceryl trinitrate represents a nitric oxide donor that is used as an ointment in the treatment of chronic anal fissures. As it causes vasodilatation, it may be used in cases of vasculitis as well. Zinc is used as a paste bandage in cases of infected leg ulcers, being an antioxidant agent. Phenytoin promotes wound healing by inhibiting enzyme collagenase and is mostly used for pressure ulcers. Retinoids cause angiogenesis, collagen synthesis and epithelization and topical tretinoin may be used in wound healing [4].

The use of specific devices in wound healing represents an ascending trend in wound healing and include various procedures such as negative pressure wound therapy, platelet-rich plasma infiltrations of the cutaneous ulcer, hyperbaric therapy, photodynamic therapy, radiant heat dressings, ultrasound therapy, laser therapy, hydrotherapy, electromagnetic therapy etc. [8].

Nonetheless, physiotherapy procedures may be required in cases of prolonged immobilization or after complex surgical interventions and impaired mobility and psychological treatments are used to alleviate stress to achieve a rapid and complete rehabilitation of the patient [9].

Considering the Training Requirements of Wound Healing for all Medical Specialties, in accordance with *European Standards of Postgraduate Medical Specialist Training,* on completion of this chapter, a trainee will be able to:

- Understand that treatment must be based on a diagnosis
- Understand that treatment must be evidence-based
- Understand that treatment must be patient-centered
- Assess the urgency of treatment
- Plan the treatment according to the aetiology and characteristics of the wound, taking into account other factors that have contributed to the wound and that are relevant in the care
- Evaluate products and methods used in the treatment, also based on the literature
- Carry out local treatment of acute and chronic wounds
- Generic groups of wound care products
- Negative-pressure wound therapy
- Choose the appropriate antibiotic to be used in the treatment of wound infection and prophylaxis, and justify their choice
- Manage pain
- Assess the treatment options realistically and determine the appropriate treatment limitations
- Identify the situations in which consultation of a specialist or other specialty is warranted.

This chapter illustrates the importance of adjuvant therapies in wound healing and describes the importance of systemic therapies, for example corticosteroids in managing wounds associated with inflammatory dermatoses such as pyoderma gangrenosum in the first case. The second case reemphasizes the importance of identifying the situations in which a multidisciplinary team is required, such as a vascular surgeon in cases of advanced peripheral arterial disease. Surgical treatment may be the best option in refractory cases, such as using the punch grafting technique, described in the next 2 clinical cases. And lastly, the necessity of using specific devices in wound healing was reiterated in the last three clinical cases presented in this chapter, which included the use of negative pressure wound therapy and autologous platelet rich plasma in treatment of cutaneous ulcers.

Case 12.1. The Role of Systemic Corticosteroids in the Management of Pyoderma Gangrenosum

Introduction

A 54-year-old female patient, with a history of ulcerative colitis, treated with mesalazine and azathioprine, presented to the clinic with giant, intensely painful ulcers (score 9 out of 10 on the Numeric Rating Scale), located on the right breast, evolving over one week, initially interpreted as a breast neoplasm. The ulcers had a purulent, necrotic base and violaceous margins (Fig. 12.1). The patient reported the onset of the condition as an erythematous papule surrounded by violaceous induration, initially located at the lower-lateral quadrant of the right breast, with rapidly progressive extension.

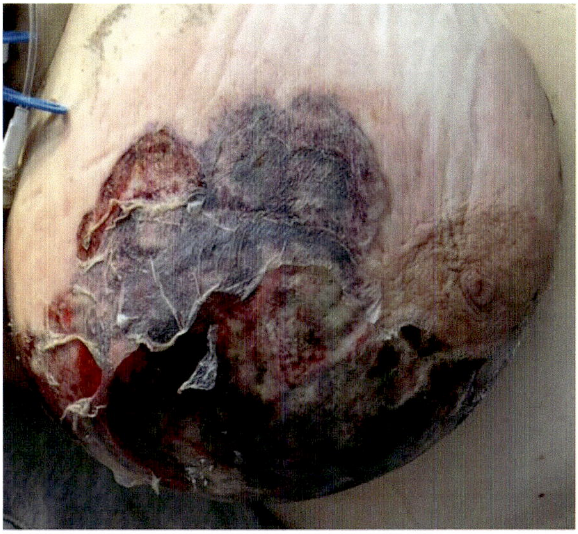

Fig. 12.1 Clinical aspect on the first visit

Differential Diagnosis

Considering the patient's history and clinical examination, bacterial infections (ecthyma gangrenosum, streptococcal gangrene), fungal infections (blastomycosis, coccidioidomycosis, paracoccidioidomycosis), parasitic infections (leishmaniasis), pyoderma gangrenosum, malignant conditions, vasculitis within autoimmune diseases, ulcerated necrobiosis lipoidica and necrotizing fasciitis were included in the differential diagnosis.

Treatment

Laboratory investigations were performed and revealed normochromic normocytic anemia and inflammatory syndrome. Based on clinical examination and paraclinical investigations, the diagnosis of pyoderma gangrenosum was established, supported by the onset of the disease (erythematous papule surrounded by a violaceous halo rapidly progressing to ulceration of the entire breast) and by the association with inflammatory bowel disease. During hospitalization, daily wound care was performed, including the application of topical antibiotics and hydroactive and bactericidal dressings, leading to the appearance of epithelialization buds. Systemic treatment included antibiotic therapy and corticosteroids (initially 1 mg/kg body weight equivalent to prednisone, with gradual dose reduction). The patient's progress was favorable, with lesion epithelialization occurring within 6 months from the onset, resulting in the formation of cribriform atrophic scars (Fig. 12.2).

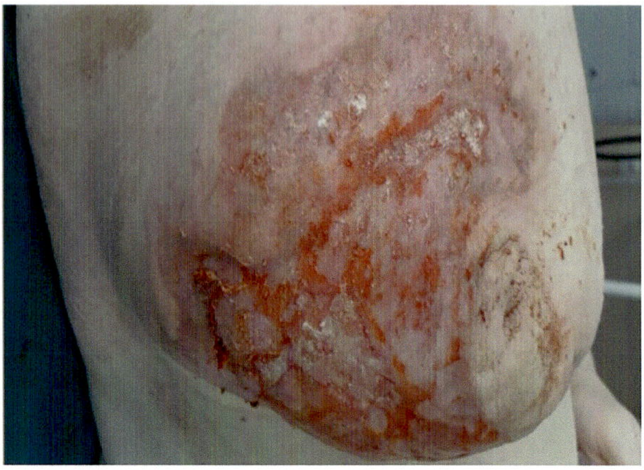

Fig. 12.2 Results after 4 months of systemic therapy

Discussions

Pyoderma Gangrenosum is a neutrophilic inflammatory dermatosis [10]. The most common presentation is an ulcerated skin lesion, intensely painful, with a violaceous-colored undermined edge and a purulent base [11]. Over 50–70% of patients develop PG in the context of an associated systemic disease such as inflammatory bowel disease, arthritis or hematologic diseases [12]. The treatment of PG aims to stop the extension of the inflammatory process and ulceration at the periphery, to prevent superinfection, to promote lesion epithelialization, and includes local wound treatment with antiseptics, antibiotics, and epithelizing agents, as well as systemic therapy with corticosteroids, immunosuppressants, and biological therapy [13]. Systemic corticosteroids play a major role in the healing process of an ulcer through several mechanisms: anti-inflammatory effects, immunosuppression and pain relief [14]. By reducing inflammation, it can help reduce oedema, redness, and pain associated with the ulcer and creates a more favorable environment for healing [15]. Corticosteroids suppress the immune system, which can be beneficial in conditions where the immune system is overactive or causing damage to tissues [16]. In the case of ulcers, especially those associated with immune-mediated diseases like pyoderma gangrenosum, corticosteroids can help reduce immunological damage to the surrounding tissues, allowing for better healing [17]. They also have analgesic properties that can help alleviate pain associated with ulcers, improving the patient's comfort during the healing process [18, 19]. In conclusion, it is important to properly select the treatment modalities for ulcers, taking into account the characteristics of the patient, the etiology of the ulcer and the possible complications [10].

Case 12.2. The Role of a Multidisciplinary Approach in Leg Ulcer Diagnostics and Management

Introduction

A 66-yeared-old male patient, smoker, with a background of stage III heart failure with left ventricular ejection fraction (LVEF) of 25%, atrial fibrillation and chronic obstructive pulmonary disease presented in the Dermatology Department with a history of three months of multiple ulcers on the lower left limb, at the malleolar level, extremely painful while exercising, at rest, or during the night (Fig. 12.3). Ulcers varied in size (between 1 to 5 cm in diameter), had a necrotic base and were covered by purulent secretions; on the posterior calf presented a well demarcated ulcer with full thickness skin loss extending down to fascia. Patient had pale and cold skin on the lower limbs, with no detectable pulse at the level of retro malleolar posterior tibial artery and slightly noticeable at the level of the popliteal artery. After the initial dermatological consultation, the patient was recommended to be evaluated by a vascular surgeon.

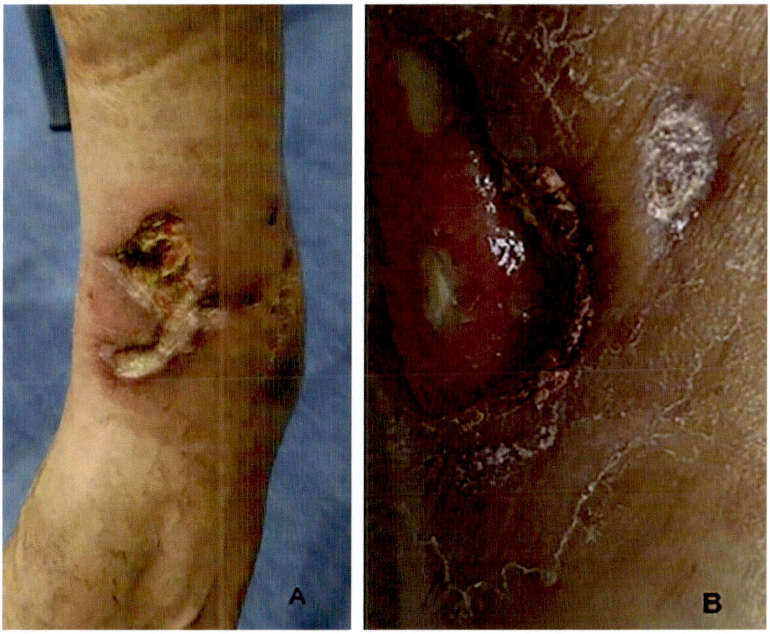

Fig. 12.3 Aspect of ulcers at the first dermatologic consultation (A)—anterior view of the left leg, (B)—posterior view of the left heel

Differential Diagnosis

Considering patient's history and the findings from the physical examination (intense pain, deep ulcerations, sharp edges and dry, cold, pale, shiny, hairless surrounding skin) there were excluded from the differential diagnosis other causes of chronic leg ulcers (chronic venous insufficiency, vasculitis, metabolic or neoplastic ulcerations) and the arterial disturbance was expressed as the etiological factor of this patient's leg ulcers.

Treatment

At first, dressings and treatment for the local infection were recommended. It was also decided to include a multidisciplinary approach with input from specialties of dermatology, vascular surgery, and cardiology. Doppler examination revealed barely perceptible arterial flow; possible occlusion on the distal left superficial femoral artery. The arteriography performed showed the presence of thrombotic occlusion of the left common iliac artery at the origin. Patient was referred to the Cardiovascular Surgery Service where he performed revascularization by extra-anatomic right-left common femoral bypass with Dacron prosthesis. On a 6 months follow-up, all the ulcerations were healed, with the presence of atrophic scars (Fig. 12.4).

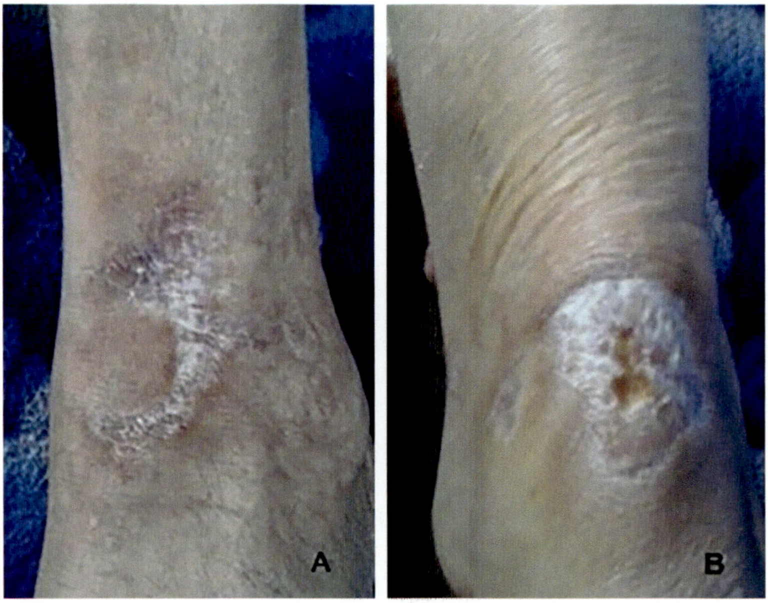

Fig. 12.4 Healed ulcers at the 6 months follow-up visit (A)—anterior view of the left foot, (B)—posterior view of the left heel

Discussions

Chronic wounds are becoming more prevalent as the population ages, given the underlying diseases and the slow process of wound repair as the body ages. With an estimated prevalence of 1.51 per 1000 population [20], leg ulcers generate considerable healthcare costs and substantial morbidity, sometimes with serious events such as limb amputations or even premature deaths. Due to the clinical presentation, chronic leg ulceration is a common condition found in Dermatology units, facing an extensive differential diagnosis. Considering that wound care is not a defined specialization, physicians often lack specialized training in the diagnosis and treatment of wounds therefore it is recommended to have different specialists such as dermatologists, endocrinologists, cardiologists, vascular surgeons, plastic surgeons, dietitian and geriatricians, involved to a different extent. The involvement of a multidisciplinary team in the management of chronic wounds has demonstrated an increase in the number of cases that achieve complete healing of ulcers, with a reduction in costs per case cured and a significant reduction in long-term complications (e.g. amputations) [21–23]. An appropriate knowledge of the lesion etiopathology is imperative as it provides the key to understand the diagnosis and approach its treatment reducing the risks associated with delayed diagnosis or inappropriate treatments. In the present case, the overall examinations performed by dermatologist, cardiologist and vascular surgery alongside imaging examinations allowed an accurate diagnosis to be made in a relatively short period of time. As indicated in the guidelines [24], revascularization through bypass surgery is the first line treatment which in this case was combined with conservative therapy (debridement, dressings, local infection control). Performing the appropriate treatment in a prompt manner allowed complete recovery of the patient without the need of any amputations. In conclusion, the successful management of patients with chronic wounds depends on a detailed assessment of each case and a close collaboration between specialists.

Case 12.3. The Role of Adjuvant Treatment with Dermal Micrografts in Martorell's Hypertensive Leg Ulcer

Introduction

A 67-year-old female patient, smoker, with a history of arterial hypertension, dyslipidemia, recanalized deep thrombosis of the left limb, under treatment with oral anticoagulants (acenocumarol) and venotonics (flavonoid fraction, purified and micronized), presented to the clinic with erythematous-violet plaque, with imprecisely defined edges, with trophic sclerotic changes, located on the left internal malleolus. That plaque presented on the surface millimeter-sized ulcers with a necrotic wound bed, evolving for about 5 months (Fig. 12.5). The lesion appeared after minor trauma and was associated with permanent severe pain (score 8 out of

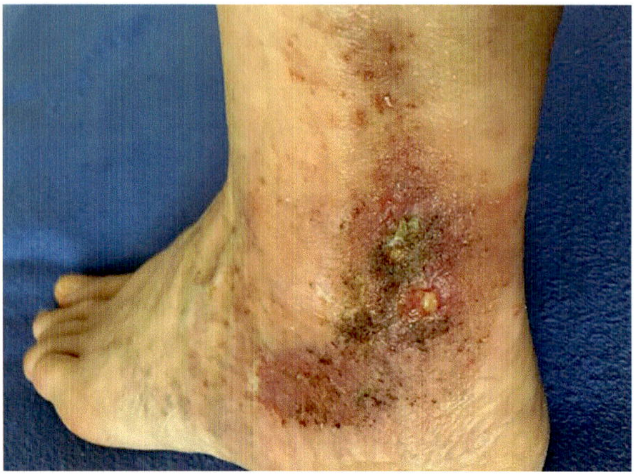

Fig. 12.5 Clinical aspect of the ulceration at the first visit

10 on the Numeric rating Scale). The patient had no history of intermittent claudication, and during the clinical examination, the perilesional skin was cold, but the peripheral arterial pulses of the posterior tibial and dorsal arteries of the leg were present. The patient underwent topical and systemic analgesic treatment without improvement of symptoms.

Differential Diagnosis

Considering the patient's history and the clinical examination, venous ulcer, arterial ulcer, Martorell's hypertensive ulcer, ulcer of mixed origin (arterial and venous), thromboangiitis obliterans, or livedoid vasculopathy were included in the differential diagnosis.

Treatment

The Doppler examination revealed normal arterial flow and recanalized deep venous thrombosis in the left lower limb. Associating the clinical and paraclinical data, we established the diagnosis of Martorell hypertensive ischemic ulcer with a venous component. Wound debridement was performed, followed by injection of suspension of dermal micrografts. After the detachment of the epidermis, an area of retroauricular skin the micrografts measuring 2 mm were collected, then 3.5 ml of saline solution was added. The sample was processed for 2 cycles of one minute each in a dedicated device (Rigenera™). The micro-graft suspension was collected with a syringe from the device and injected into the wound bed and wound edges. A local non-adherent dressing was applied, and the patient was reevaluated weekly for 6 weeks. The patient had a cardiological evaluation for hypertension treatment. Although the re-epithelialization of the ulcers was slow, during the 6 weeks, a significant decrease in pain was observed, with a score of 1 out of 10 on the NRS pain scale (Fig. 12.6).

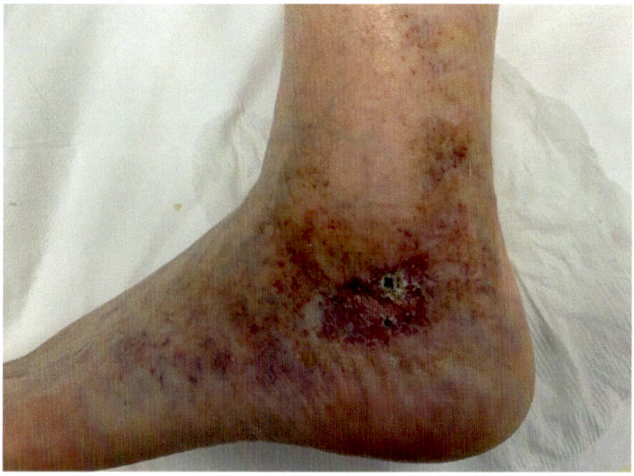

Fig. 12.6 Clinical aspect after 6 weeks

Discussions

Hypertensive ischemic leg ulcer (Martorell's or arteriosclerotic ulcer) has been described more frequently in women with cardiovascular comorbidities, being associated with intense pain and livedoid changes of the perilesional skin [25]. Early grafting of ulceration is considered the most effective treatment in reducing pain associated with ulceration [26]. The rapid evolution of ulcers occurs after trauma because the initial necrosis through arteriosclerosis caused by high blood pressure stimulates the inflammatory phase, causing necrosis, thus creating a vicious cycle. The skin graft has an angiogenic effect and decreases the local ischemic and pro-inflammatory environment, promoting healing and reducing pain [27]. In this case, the slow healing of the ulcer suggests the association of the venous component. The injection of the autologous dermal micrograft solution is a minimally invasive method, well tolerated by the patient, through which cells and growth factors necessary for healing are brought to the wound bed. This method promotes reducing wound size, decreasing pain, and therefore increasing the quality of life of patients [28]. Chronic ulcers are a financial burden on the health care system and a continuous development of treatment methods for these patients is necessary.

Case 12.4. The Role of Adjuvant Treatment with Dermal Micrografts in Neuropathic Leg Ulcer

Introduction

A 70-year-old male patient, smoker, with a history of ischemic coronary disease and type 2 diabetes mellitus, uncontrolled therapeutically (HbA1c 8%), diagnosed 20 years ago, presented for an ulceration with well-defined gray edges ("punched-out" appearance), with wound bed covered with granulation tissue, located on the amputation bed of the third left toe, on a pressure area (Fig. 12.7). The medical history revealed that the surgical amputation of the third toe was 3 weeks

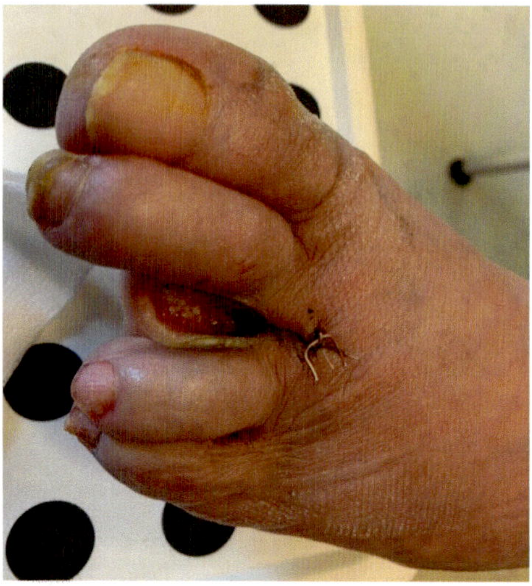

Fig. 12.7 Clinical aspect of the ulceration at the first visit

before presentation, as a result of gangrene developed from a neglected ulceration. During the clinical examination, the perilesional skin was xerotic and cold, with hypoesthesia, which determined frequent lower limb trauma.

Differential Diagnosis

Considering the clinical examination, the presumptive diagnosis was of neuropathic ulcer that appeared as a complication of the diabetic foot in the context of amputation. In the differential diagnosis, we included arterial ulcer, pressure ulcer, pyoderma gangrenosum, or amputation-related skin disease.

Treatment

Laboratory tests revealed elevated levels of glycemic values, the Doppler examination did not show arterial occlusion on the affected limb, and the X-ray had a normal appearance, excluding osteomyelitis. During the neurological examination, there was a loss of reflexes and a decrease in tactile and vibrational sensitivity in the lower limbs. The ulceration was classified as grade 1 on the Meggitt-Wagner classification with superficial ulcer (full-thickness) [29]. Ulcer debridement was performed. After detachment of epidermis, an area of ipsilateral retroauricular skin tissue, two punch biopsies of 2 mm were performed, sectioned, and inserted into a dedicated medical device (Rigenera®), containing saline solution. After the automatic processing of the sample, the micrograft solution was injected into the ulcer's edges and bed (4 mm deep) and covered with a sterile dressing. The dressing was changed weekly, and complete epithelization occurred after 4 weeks (Fig. 12.8).

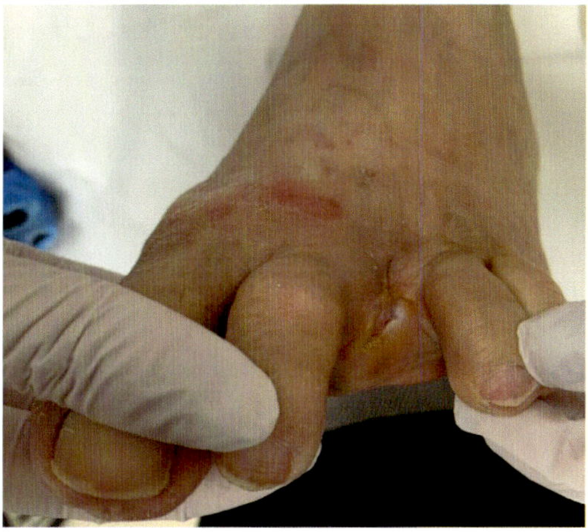

Fig. 12.8 Clinical aspect after 4 weeks

Discussions

Diabetic foot ulcers are some of the most common complications of therapeutically uncontrolled diabetes mellitus. The risk factors involved in the occurrence are diabetic polyneuropathy, peripheral vascular disease, macroangiopathy, microangiopathy, leg deformities, and external factors such as poor hygiene, the use of inappropriate shoes, or repeated trauma [30]. The treatment of diabetic foot ulcers represents approximately one-third of the total cost of diabetic care, is challenging, and requires a multidisciplinary team: dermatologist, diabetologist, general surgeon, cardiovascular surgeon, and podiatrist [31]. In the management of these patients, the control of glycemic values, as well as the assessment of peripheral vessels are important, because approximately 40% of diabetic patients associate peripheral arterial disease [32, 33]. Also, treating wound infections is vital, due to their risk for delayed healing and amputation. Skin grafting is a rapid method of healing skin ulcers compared to topical treatments. In the case of diabetic patients, a careful selection must be made because the method is burdened by the risks of delayed healing of both the graft site and the donor site, infections, and the impossibility of grafting if bones, tendons, or joints are exposed [34]. Micrograft treatment is a minimally invasive treatment that allows the mesenchymal stem cells with multi-lineage differentiation and immunomodulatory properties to stimulate ulcer healing by their ability to produce extracellular matrix and paracrine factors, promote angiogenesis, and even suppress inflammation [35].

Skin ulcers caused by diabetes increase morbidity and are burdened by local and distant complications. Thus, in this case, the autologous micrografts containing progenitor cells represented a fast and efficient method of promoting healing of the deep skin ulcer resulting from the amputation [36].

Case 12.5. A Giant Lower Leg Ulcer in a 61-Year-Old Male Treated with NPWT

Introduction

A 61-year-old male, from urban environment, with no significant medical personal or family history, presented for dermatological consultation with a giant ulceration (15 × 18 cm) on the anterior side of the left lower leg, covered by greenish yellow fibrino-purulent detritus and necrosis. Onset was 2 years prior, following a local trauma and the patient was previously treated by 3 procedures of skin grafting in a local Surgical Department, which resulted in secondary local infections and failure of treatment.

The physical examination revealed a giant ulcerated lesion, measuring 15 × 18 cm in diameter, covered by greenish yellow fibrino-purulent detritus and necrosis, on the anterior side of the left lower leg, in association with malodor and macerated surrounding skin (Fig. 12.9. Clinical aspect of the giant ulceration located on the anterior side of the left lower leg). Additionally, the patient presented bilateral varicose veins, atrophie blanche, ochre dermatitis in the contralateral lower leg, in association with local oedema.

Paraclinical investigations included bacteriological swabs, in association with cultures and antibiogram, which revealed the presence of *Pseudomonas spp*, sensible to systemic cephalosporins and arterial and venous Duplex ultrasonography, which identified great saphenous vein reflux, caused by saphenofemoral junction incompetence, without any abnormalities.

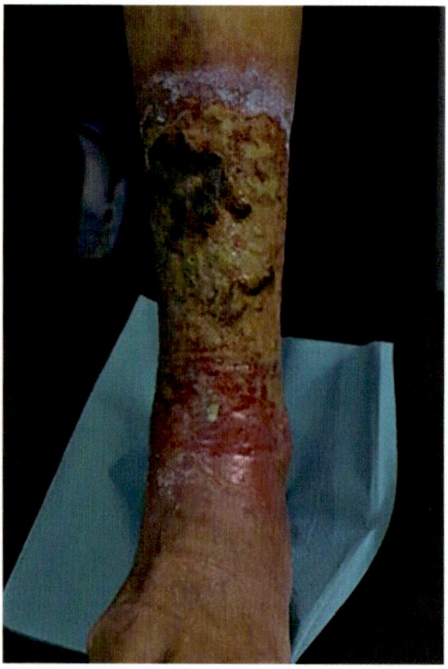

Fig. 12.9 Clinical aspect of the giant ulceration located on the anterior side of the left lower leg

Differential Diagnosis

Differential diagnosis of the cutaneous ulcer included peripheral arterial disease, diabetic ulcer, pyoderma gangrenosum and squamous cell carcinoma. Paraclinical investigations, including venous and arterial ultrasonography, in association with the clinical findings established the diagnosis of venous leg ulcer. Treatment was initiated and the favorable response postponed the decision of taking a punch biopsy.

Treatment

Treatment included systemic antibiotics as the ulcer associated significant purulent detritus and malodour and local cultures were positive for *Pseudomonas aeruginosa.* Management also included local surgical debridement with a curette, local dressings, such as mesh-type dressing, impregnated with neutral ointment and silver ions, with continuous release, in conjunction with hydroactive dressing and emollients in the periwound area. Following several weeks of local treatment, intermittent negative pressure wound therapy (NPWT) (70–125 mmHg) was initiated for 1 month, with a significant improvement of the ulcerated lesion with the appearance of granulation tissue. Local treatment was continued with gel impregnated dressing, promoting epithelization. After 4 additional months, the clinical aspect was significantly improved, with a decrease in size, odor and exudate of the ulcerated lesion, measuring 4×2 cm in diameter (Fig. 12.10. Clinical aspect of the ulcerated lesions after five months of therapy).

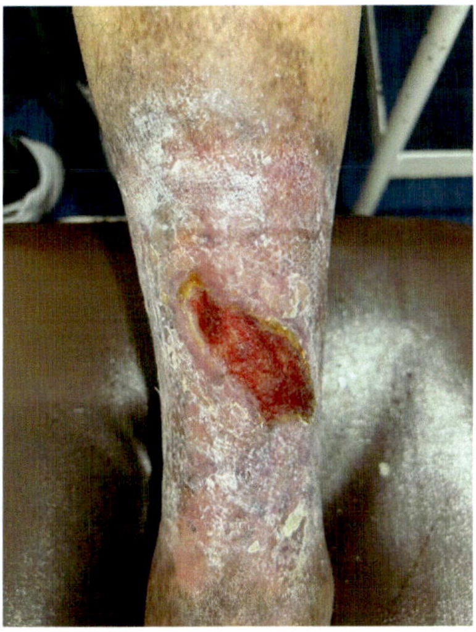

Fig. 12.10 Clinical aspect of the ulcerated lesions after five months of therapy

Discussion

Negative pressure wound therapy (NPWT) represents a versatile technique of managing wounds, first described in the nineteenth century. It implies the mechanism of applying sub-

atmospheric pressure to wounds in combination with a drainage system, which reduces the excessive inflammatory exudate and promotes the granulation of tissue. NPWT may be used continuously at pressures of 125 mmHg or intermittently at 125 mmHg for 4 min with 70 mmHg for 2 min. NPWT is indicated in cases of both acute and chronic wounds, including pressure ulcers, surgical wounds, burns, skin transplants, leg ulcer due to chronic venous insufficiency, diabetic ulcers and eschars. It is contraindicated in neoplastic processes, fistulas and necrosis [37].

Venous leg ulcers represent a clinical entity resulting from chronic venous insufficiency (CVI), following severe venous hypertension and tissue hypoxia. Clinically, the manifestations of CVI include oedema, hyperpigmentation, subcutaneous fibrosis and ulcer formation [38]. CVI represents the most common vascular disorder and the annual incidence ranges between 2–6% in females and 1.9% in males [39]. Risk factors of CVI are represented by obesity, smoking, alcohol consumption, increasing age, pregnancy, personal history of deep vein thrombosis, local trauma, family history of CVI and the female gender [40]. Regarding the etiopathogenesis of CVI, the most common pathway is the development of venous hypertension, which may be due to three main causes: obstruction to venous flow (in case of deep venous thrombosis), dysfunction of venous valves (which may be idiopathic or congenital) and failure of the venous pump system (in case of prolonged immobilization, obesity or through cardiac afflictions such as congestive heart failure or pulmonary hypertension) [40]. Clinical findings include local symptoms such as pain upon local palpation of affected tissue in the lower limbs, leg edema and discomfort described as a dull ache, throbbing or heaviness, or pressure sensation after prolonged standing [41]. Physical examination may reveal oedema, ochre dermatitis (local hyperpigmentation), lipodermatosclerosis, telangiectasia, reticular veins, varicose veins, atrophie blanche, acroangiodermatitis, septal acute panniculitis and venous leg ulcer [42]. Laboratory investigations may include duplex ultrasonography and ankle brachial index, bacteriological swab, culture and antibiogram, punch biopsy (for non-healing ulcers > 12 weeks), patch testing, plethysmography, phlebography [41]. Treatment of CVI includes endovenous treatment as the main option, as well as cleansing of the lesion, debridement, wound dressings (non-adherent dressing adapted to the evolution phase of the ulcers and the patients' needs), topical antimicrobials, in case of signs of infection, in single therapy or associated to systemic antibiotics, venotonics, aspirin, analgesics, moisturizing agents in the periwound area, compression therapy, negative wound pressure therapy, or other surgical techniques [43].

Case 12.6. The Role of Autologous Platelet-Rich Plasma as an Adjuvant Therapy for Non Healing Leg Ulcer in Chronic Venous Insufficiency

Introduction

A 56-year-old female patient with a history of chronic venous insufficiency and arterial hypertension, was referred to the Dermatology Department for an ulcerative lesion located on the left internal malleolus of the leg, evolving for 6 months. The clinical examination showed the presence of a poorly demarcated erythematous-violaceous plaque with poorly defined hyperpigmented margins, varicosities and two adjacent ulcers, measuring 1.0/0.7 cm and 1.5/1.2 cm with yellow discharge covering the wound bed (Fig. 12.11). The patient underwent several wound dressings and systemic treatment with venotonics (flavonoid fraction, purified and micronized) without any significant improvement of the lesions.

Differential Diagnosis

Through the patient's medical history and clinical examination, the differential diagnosis was considered between venous ulcer, arterial ulcer and livedoid vasculopathy. The established diagnosis was venous leg ulcer.

Treatment

A Doppler ultrasound was performed in order to confirm the aetiology of the ulcers and revealed the deep venous system of the limbs is patent and competent

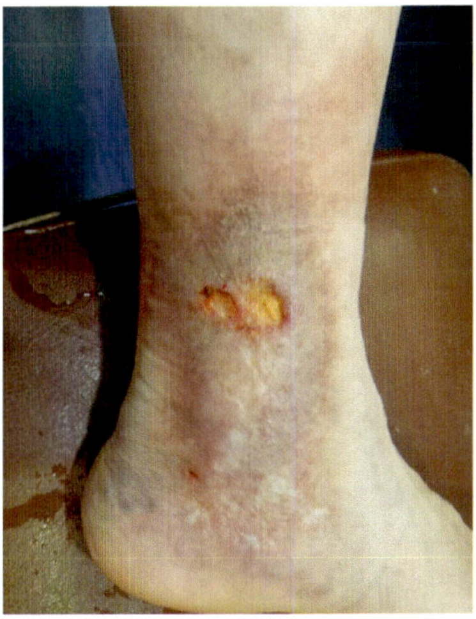

Fig. 12.11 Clinical aspect of the ulcers on the first visit

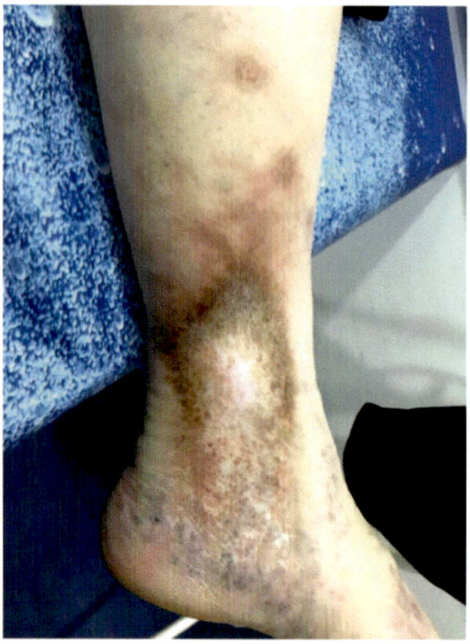

Fig. 12.12 Clinical aspect after 8 weeks

bilaterally, with the right and left great saphenous veins patent and competent, both small saphenous veins without reflux, three incompetent Cockett perforators, reflux in the right popliteal fossa perforator, and left femoropopliteal reflux with an incompetent Cockett perforator 1. After establishing the diagnosis of chronic venous insufficiency, the patient started the autologous platelet-rich plasma (PRP) treatment once a week, associated with debridement and dressing on the alternative days, for 6 consecutive weeks. A blood sample was taken from the patient and the separation of the platelets from red blood cells was performed by centrifugation. The supernatant plasma containing platelets was extracted from the tube and applied on the surface of the ulcers. The ulcers were covered with gauze for protection and the patient had a complete resolution of the leg ulcer after 8 weeks (Fig. 12.12).

Discussions

There are multiple treatment options for leg ulcers from dressings to skin substitutes or skin grafts. In our case, the small size of the ulcers and patient's compliance have allowed us to choose a minimally invasive treatment [44]. The use of platelet-rich plasma for the treatment of ulcers has been proved to promote wound healing with low complications rates. The mechanisms behind this technique include platelets degranulation and release of growth factors such as: platelet-derived growth factor (PDGF), insulin-like growth factor-1, epidermal growth factor, transforming growth factor-β, vascular endothelial growth factor, and fibroblast growth factors in order to promote collagen production and development of granulomatous tissue by stimulating fibroblasts and macrophages aggregation [45]. Unfortunately, there are neither enough data nor clear protocols available to support this effective, affordable and safe adjuvant therapy which can be useful in selected cases [46].

References

1. Team V, Chandler PG, Weller CD. Adjuvant therapies in venous leg ulcer management: a scoping review. Wound Repair Regen. 2019;27(5):562–90. https://doi.org/10.1111/wrr.12724.
2. Annamaraju P, Patel P, Baradhi KM. Pentoxifylline. StatPearls [Internet]. Treasure Island (FL): StatPearls Publishing; 2024. Available from: https://www.ncbi.nlm.nih.gov/books/NBK559096/.
3. Wee E, Kelly R. Pentoxifylline: an effective therapy for necrobiosis lipoidica. Australas J Dermatol. 2017;58(1):65–8. https://doi.org/10.1111/ajd.12420.
4. Enoch S, Grey JE, Harding KG. ABC of wound healing. Non-surgical and drug tratments. BMJ. 2006;332(7546):900–3. https://doi.org/10.1136/bmj.332.7546.900.
5. Beckman JA, Schneider PA, Conte MS. Advances in revascularization for peripheral artery disease: revascularization in PAD. Circ Res. 2021;128(12):1885–912. https://doi.org/10.1161/CIRCRESAHA.121.318261.
6. Conde-Montero E, de Farias KY, Pérez Jerónimo L, Vázquez AP, Marín LR, Guisado S, et al. Punch grafting for pain reduction in hard-to-heal ulcers. J Wound Care. 2020;29(3):194–7. https://doi.org/10.12968/jowc.2020.29.3.194.
7. Serra R, Rizzuto A, Rossi A, Perri P, Barbetta A, Abdalla K, et al. Skin grafting for the treatment of chronic leg ulcers—a systematic review in evidence-based medicine. Int Wound J. 2017;14(1):149–57. https://doi.org/10.1111/iwj.12575.
8. Fernández-Guarino M, Bacci S, Pérez González LA, Bermejo-Martínez M, Cecilia-Matilla A, Hernández-Bule ML. The role of physical therapies in wound healing and assisted scarring. Int J Mol Sci. 2023;24(8):7487. https://doi.org/10.3390/ijms24087487.
9. Robinson H, Norton S, Jarrett P, Broadbent E. The effects of psychological interventions on wound healing: A systematic review of randomized trials. Br J Health Psychol. 2017;22(4):805–35. https://doi.org/10.1111/bjhp.12257.
10. Ruocco E, Sangiuliano S, Gravina AG, et al. Pyoderma gangrenosum: an updated review. J Eur Acad Dermatol Venereol. 2009;23:1008.
11. Wong WW, Machado GR, Hill ME. Pyoderma gangrenosum: the great pretender and a challenging diagnosis. J Cutan Med Surg. 2011;15:322.
12. Powell FC, Hackett BC, Wallach D. Pyoderma gangrenosum. In: Goldsmith LA, Katz SI, Gilchrest BA, et al., editors. Fitzpatrick's dermatology in general medicine. 8th ed. New York: McGraw-Hill Companies, Inc.; 2012. p. 371.
13. Bennett ML, Jackson JM, Jorizzo JL, et al. Pyoderma gangrenosum. A comparison of typical and atypical forms with an emphasis on time to remission. Case review of 86 patients from 2 institutions. Medicine (Baltimore). 2000;79:37.
14. Bolognia J, Jorizzo JL, Schaffer JV. Dermatology, vol. 1. Philadelphia: Elsevier Saunders; 2012. p. 427.
15. Powell FC, Su WPD, Perry HO. Pyoderma gangrenosum: classification and management. J Am Acad Dermatol. 1996;34:395–409.
16. Adachi Y, Kindzelskii AL, Cookingham G, et al. Aberrant neutrophil trafficking and metabolic oscillations in severe pyoderma gangrenosum. J Invest Dermatol. 1998;111:259.
17. Farasat S, Aksentijevich I, Toro JR. Autoinflammatory diseases: clinical and genetic advances. Arch Dermatol. 2008;144:392.
18. Ahronowitz I, Harp J, Shinkai K. Etiology and management of pyoderma gangrenosum: a comprehensive review. Am J Clin Dermatol. 2012;13:191.

19. Maverakis E, Ma C, Shinkai K, et al. Diagnostic criteria of ulcerative pyoderma gangrenosum: a delphi consensus of international experts. JAMA Dermatol. 2018;154:461.
20. Martinengo L, Olsson M, Bajpai R, Soljak M, Upton Z, Schmidtchen A, et al. Prevalence of chronic wounds in the general population: systematic review and meta-analysis of observational studies. Ann Epidemiol. 2019;29:8–15.
21. Donnelly J, Shaw J. Developing a multidisciplinary complex wound care service. Br J Nurs. 2000;9(Suppl 3):S50–5.
22. Vu T, Harris A, Duncan G, Sussman G. Cost-effectiveness of multidisciplinary wound care in nursing homes: a pseudo-randomized pragmatic cluster trial. Fam Pract. 2007;24(4):372–9.
23. Gottrup F. A specialized wound-healing center concept: importance of a multidisciplinary department structure and surgical treatment facilities in the treatment of chronic wounds. Am J Surg. 2004;187(5 Suppl):S38–43.
24. Powers JG, Higham C, Broussard K, Phillips TJ. Wound healing and treating wounds: chronic wound care and management. J Am Acad Dermatol. 2016;74(4):607–25.
25. Mansour M, Afsaneh A. Martorell ulcer: chronic wound management and rehabilitation. Chronic Wound Care Manag Res. 2019;6:83–8. https://doi.org/10.2147/CWCMR.S172427.
26. Hafner J, Nobbe S, Partsch H, et al. Martorell hypertensive ischemic leg ulcer: a model of ischemic subcutaneous arteriolosclerosis. Arch Dermatol. 2010;146(9):961–8. https://doi.org/10.1001/archdermatol.2010.224.
27. Conde-Montero E, Pérez Jerónimo L, Peral Vázquez A, Recarte Marín L, Sanabria Villarpando PE, de la Cueva DP. Early and sequential punch grafting in the spectrum of arteriolopathy ulcers in the elderly. Wounds. 2020;32(8):E38–41.
28. De Francesco F, Graziano A, Trovato L, Ceccarelli G, Romano M, Marcarelli M, et al. A regenerative approach with dermal micrografts in the treatment of chronic ulcers. Stem Cell Rev Rep. 2017;13(1):139–48. https://doi.org/10.1007/s12015-016-9692-2.
29. Wang X, Yuan CX, Xu B, Yu Z. Diabetic foot ulcers: classification, risk factors and management. World J Diabetes. 2022;13(12):1049–65. https://doi.org/10.4239/wjd.v13.i12.1049.
30. Oliver TI, Mutluoglu M. Diabetic foot ulcer. [Updated 2023 Aug 8]. In: StatPearls [Internet]. Treasure Island (FL): StatPearls Publishing; 2024. Available from: https://www.ncbi.nlm.nih.gov/books/NBK537328/.
31. Everett E, Mathioudakis N. Update on management of diabetic foot ulcers. Ann N Y Acad Sci. 2018;1411(1):153–65. https://doi.org/10.1111/nyas.13569.PMID:29377202;PMCID:PMC5793889.
32. Tresierra-Ayala MA, García RA. Association between peripheral arterial disease and diabetic foot ulcers in patients with diabetes mellitus type 2. Med Univ. 2017;19:123–6. https://doi.org/10.1016/j.rmu.2017.07.002.
33. Prompers L, Schaper N, Apelqvist J, Edmonds M, Jude E, Mauricio D, et al. Prediction of outcome in individuals with diabetic foot ulcers: focus on the differences between individuals with and without peripheral arterial disease. The EURODIALE study. Diabetologia. 2008;51(5):747–55. https://doi.org/10.1007/s00125-008-0940-0.PMID:18297261; PMCID:PMC2292424.
34. Johnson TM, Ratner D, Nelson BR. Soft tissue reconstruction with skin grafting. J Am Acad Dermatol. 1992;27(2 Pt 1):151–65. https://doi.org/10.1016/0190-9622(92)70164-b. PMID: 1430351.
35. El Hage R, Knippschild U, Arnold T, Hinterseher I. Stem cell-based therapy: a promising treatment for diabetic foot ulcer. Biomedicines. 2022;10:1507. https://doi.org/10.3390/biomedicines10071507.
36. Trovato L, Failla G, Serantoni S, Palumbo FP. Regenerative surgery in the management of leg ulcers. J Cell Sci Ther. 2016;7:238.
37. Zaver V, Kankanalu P. Negative pressure wound therapy. [Updated 2023 Sep 4]. In: StatPearls [Internet]. Treasure Island (FL): StatPearls Publishing; 2024.
38. Santler B, Goerge T. Chronic venous insufficiency: a review of pathophysiology, diagnosis, and treatment. J Dtsch Dermatol Ges. 2017;15(5):538–56. https://doi.org/10.1111/ddg.13242. PMID: 28485865.

39. Al Shammeri O, AlHamdan N, Al-Hothaly B, Midhet F, Hussain M, Al-Mohaimeed A. Chronic venous insufficiency: prevalence and effect of compression stockings. Int J Health Sci (Qassim). 2014;8(3):231–6. https://doi.org/10.12816/0023975.
40. Bergan JJ, Schmid-Schönbein GW, Coleridge Smith PD, Nicolaides AN, Boisseau MR, Eklof B. Chronic venous disease. Minerva Cardioangiol. 2007;55(4):459–76 PMID: 17653022.
41. Labropoulos N. How does chronic venous disease progress from the first symptoms to the advanced stages? A review. Adv Ther. 2019;36(Suppl 1):13–9. https://doi.org/10.1007/s12325-019-0885-3.
42. Franks PJ, Barker J, Collier M, Gethin G, Haesler E, Jawien A, et al. Management of patients with venous leg ulcers: challenges and current best practice. J Wound Care. 2016;25(Suppl 6):S1–67. https://doi.org/10.12968/jowc.2016.25.Sup6.S1. PMID: 27292202.
43. Briggs M, Flemming K. Living with leg ulceration: a synthesis of qualitative research. J Adv Nurs. 2007;59:319–28.
44. Huber SC, de Moraes MB, Quintero M, de Paula LÍS, Cataldo JL, de Lima Montalvão SA, et al. A case series of platelet-rich plasma in chronic venous ulcers. Regen Ther. 2021;18:51–8. https://doi.org/10.1016/j.reth.2021.03.005.PMID:33869687;PMCID:PMC8027535.
45. Tsachiridi M, Galyfos G, Andreou A, Sianou A, Sigala F, Zografos G, et al. Autologous platelet-rich plasma for nonhealing ulcers: a comparative study. Vasc Specialist Int. 2019;35(1):22–7. https://doi.org/10.5758/vsi.2019.35.1.22.PMID:30993104;PMCID:PMC6453601.
46. Valencia IC, Falabella A, Kirsner RS, Eaglstein WH. Chronic venous insufficiency and venous leg ulceration. J Am Acad Dermatol. 2001;44(3):401–24.

Wounds and Ulcers Associated with Vascular Malformations—Embolization and Sclerotherapy

13

Arindam Bharadwaz

Abstract

Vascular anomalies are categorized into vascular malformations and vascular tumors. Skin defects and ulcerations occur in many vascular tumors (up to 25% in infantile hæmangiomas). Though rare in vascular malformations, superficial erosions (intertriginous dermatitis) are seen in lymphatic malformations and frank ulcerations can occur in arterio-venous malformation (AVM). These ulcerations are difficult to heal. Excision with skin grafting or Interventional Radiological (IR) approaches can be a treatment option. The efficiency of IR approach is illustrated in three patients with AVMs and in one case of venous malformation. In one case presentation, a large ulcer occurred on an amputated foot stump associated with a complex AVM. The treatment was by embolotherapy alone. In other two cases there were digital (finger) AVMs and in one case it was a venous malformation of the second toe. All lesions were associated with small punctate ulcers and were treated by sclerotherapy.

Keywords

Cutaneous ulcer • Wound healing • Vascular malformation • Sclerotherapy • Embolization

Introduction

It is difficult to estimate the exact incidence or prevalence of chronic wound /ulcers associated with vascular malformations. Epidemiological data for wounds associated with vascular malformations is scarce [1]. These ulcerations are difficult to

A. Bharadwaz (✉)
Radiology Department, Aarhus University Hospital, Aarhus, Denmark
e-mail: arinbhar@rm.dk

G.-S.Tiplica and K. Isoherranen (eds.), *Wound Healing*,
https://doi.org/10.1007/978-3-031-84579-6_13

heal. Excision with skin grafting is a surgical treatment option, but is very difficult and can result in amputation of the affected area. Interventional radiological (IR) approaches with embolo-sclerotherapy (embolization and/or sclerotherapy) are an effective limb- and tissue-preserving alternative therapy in these situations [2, 3]. Available literature suggests that AVM and complex vascular malformations such as Klippel Trenaunay Syndrome (KTS) or Park-Weber syndrome (PWS) are probably most commonly associated with chronic ulcers. But it can also occur with other types of vascular malformations, such as venous, capillary and lymphatic malformations [4].

AVM: Ulcers in AVM develop due to the increased venous pressure produced by the high flow from the artery to the vein in AVM. Other mechanisms include poor blood flow and tissue oxygenation in the affected area due to vascular steal phenomenon. Without adequate oxygen and nutrient supply, the tissues become vulnerable and may eventually ulcerate.

Syndromes and venous malformations: Abnormal dilatation, tortuosity and altered wall morphology led to blood pooling and venous stasis, and increased venous pressure in venous malformations, KTS and PWS. Venous insufficiency can also occur, leading to swelling, skin changes, and the development of venous ulcers. These may result in tissue breakdown and impaired healing mechanisms [5].

Capillary Malformations: Also known as port-wine stains, are abnormal clusters of capillaries near the surface of the skin. While they may not always lead to ulcers directly, they can contribute to chronic wounds if there is skin breakdown due to other reasons or if they are associated with other vascular abnormalities.

Lymphatic Malformations: These involve abnormal development of the lymphatic system, which can lead to lymphedema, oozing, bleeding and punctate ulcers, and impaired wound healing [6].

Treatment for ulcers and chronic wounds associated with vascular malformations often requires a multidisciplinary approach [7]. This may include:

- **Interventional Radiology:** Image guided sclerotherapy with or without embolization, aiming to obliterate the involved vascular space by injecting a sclerosant in the malformation. For most venous malformations this is an adequate treatment, but additional embolization is often required for AVMs. Interventional sclerotherapy is the standard mainstay of treatment of choice for vascular malformations. Surgery may be required to remove the residual tissue or sclero-embolotherapy-resistant malformations.
- **Compression Therapy:** Compression bandages, stockings or garments help improve blood flow and reduce swelling in venous ulcers.
- **Wound Care:** Proper wound care techniques, such as cleaning the wound, removing dead tissue, and applying dressings, are essential components of wound care and promote healing.

- **Laser Therapy:** Laser treatments can be used to target and reduce the size of certain vascular malformations, usually as an adjunct to other wound healing therapies.
- **Medication:** Medications may be prescribed to manage infections or inflammations associated with vascular malformations.

It should be noted that ulcers and wounds also occur in vascular malformations after sclerotherapy with or without embolization. Most ulcers occurring after treatment are self-limiting and heal without significant scar or deformity. However, sometimes they may require surgical procedures including skin grafting [8]. It's important for individuals with vascular malformations and associated ulcers or chronic wounds to receive ongoing medical care to prevent complications and promote healing [9]. A comprehensive treatment plan tailored to the specific needs of the patient can help improve outcomes and quality of life.

In this chapter we present some interesting cases of vascular malformations associated with ulcer-formations, a topic which is rarely discussed in the literature. Treatment approaches for these patients are not found in the guidelines or other available literature. The chapter includes short patient histories, differential diagnoses, treatment options, and how the cases were treated with positive outcomes. This, we hope, will help in your routine clinical practice regarding how to approach these specific groups of patients.

The medical trainee will learn

- How the patients with vascular malformations (AVM, venous malformations, KTS, PWS etc.) present with ulcers and wounds. Wounds of different aetiologies look different.
- Differential diagnoses and how to use the imaging modalities to arrive at the correct diagnosis.
- How to interpret the MR scanning (particularly the STIR sequence) showing flow-voids in AVMs and hyperintensities in venous malformation.
- Ultrasound (USG) reveals slow flow in venous malformation and high flow in AVM with arterialized outflow veins.
- How the treatment approaches are different and individualized in each case. A digital subtraction angiography (DSA) is always required for AVMs, but the injection route of embolizing/sclerosing material may be different in each case. Similarly, a phlebography for venous malformation is necessary, and may be performed by direct puncture and/or through a relevant vein.
- How to incorporate a routine, follow up regime for the patients in regular intervals to monitor the progress of wound healing, and take necessary steps to address any issues which may arise during the course of treatment and follow up.
- How to gain insight into the problem and know how interventional radiology has transformed the treatment and management of patients with vascular malformations in the last few decades.

Case 13.1. Embolization of Arteriovenous Malformation (AVM) with Amputation Stump Ulcer

Keywords: Arterio-venous malformation (AVM), ulcer, wound, sclerotherapy, embolization

Case history

A 60-year-old wheelchair-dependent woman was referred to the interventional radiology section with a non-healing ulcer of the amputation stump of the left foot. She is known with extensive vascular malformation in the left lower extremity, particularly AVM in the left foot, since childhood (diagnosed as Klippel Trenaunay variant in childhood). She had a forefoot amputation as a teenager. She has been using a prosthesis and a custom-made shoe for the left leg and foot. The amputation-stump ulcer was large, about 4–5 cm long and non-healing. Treatments at various wound-healing centres, surgical and medical units for a long time were without any clinical effect (Fig. 13.1a). She had been suffering from long-standing, severe and unbearable pain (9–10 on VAS/NRS). She had very limited physical activity and a profoundly restricted lifestyle. She was significantly mentally traumatized and psychologically affected because of the long clinical course without positive clinical outcome. Proximal amputation of the leg was considered as a treatment option.

Differential Diagnosis

MR scanning (STIR, T1WI, T2WI, dynamic angio sequence) showed a complex vascular lesion with multiple flow-voids from high-flow vessels particularly arterial feeders and engorged venous outflow, suggestive of an arterio-venous-malformation (AVM), though no definite central nidus was seen. Ultrasound with Doppler demonstrated multiple high flow areas and some arterialized draining veins. No solid areas were seen. The imaging findings were consistent with a type IV (tissue infiltrative) AVM (Fig. 13.2).

Treatment

Amputation was considered as a treatment option as the patient's ulcer did not respond to other forms of therapy. However, for a second opinion the patient was sent to the Interventional Radiology (IR) unit. After clinical evaluation, the patient was planned for endovascular therapy. Angiography was performed under general anæsthesia, which revealed a complex type IV AVM. The feeding arteries were approached with a coaxial microcatheter and microguidewire, and selectively embolized with a small quantity (about 0.1–0.2 ml) 700–900 μm

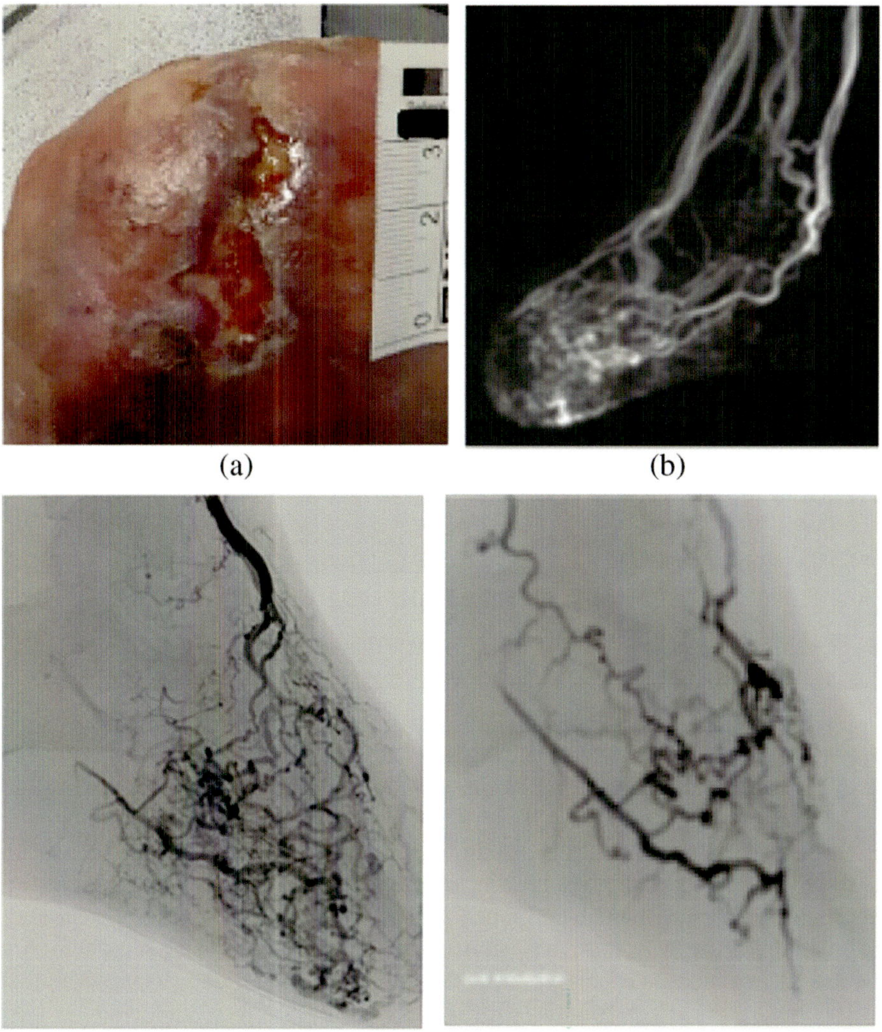

Fig. 13.1 Amputation stump ulcer at presentation (**a**). MR angiogram (**b**) and arteriography of the left foot (**c**) showing the extensive tissue-infiltrative AVM. Post-embolization devascularization of the AVM (**d**)

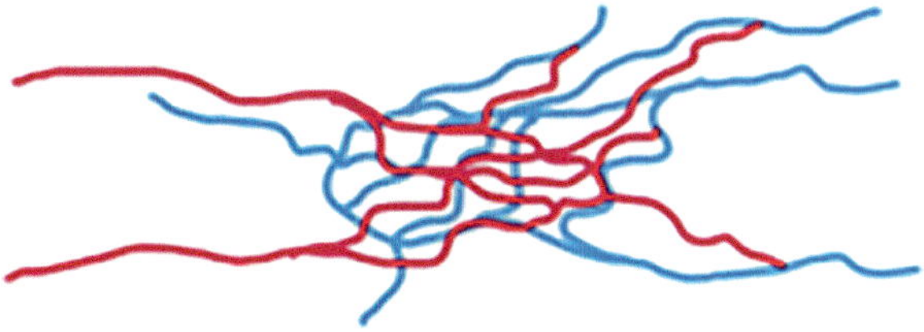

Fig. 13.2 Type IV (tissue-infiltrative) AVM

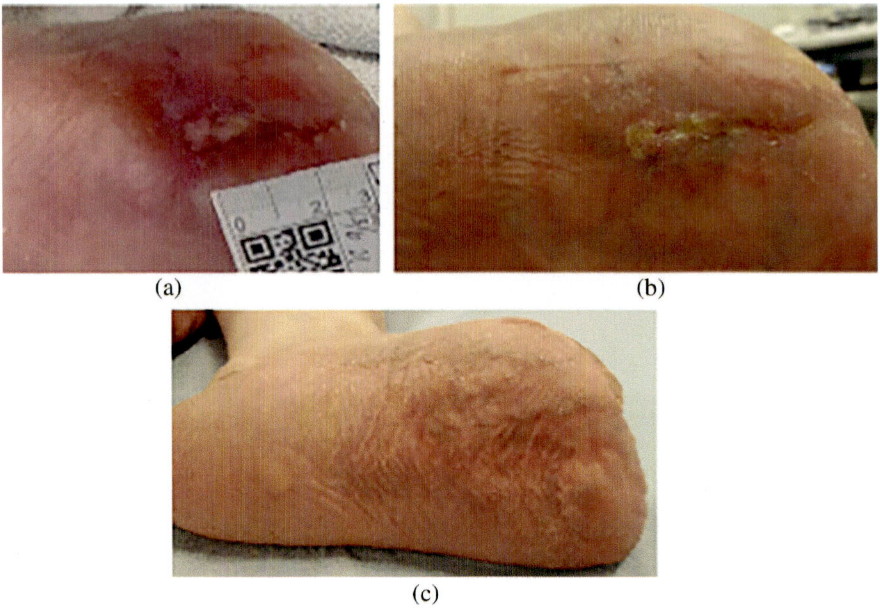

Fig. 13.3 Wound healing at 1 month (a), 2 months (b) and 3 months (c)

particles. Angiography revealed significant devascularization of the malformation (Fig. 13.1b–d).

At one month's follow up the wound started healing (about 2 cm compared to 5 cm before treatment), no pain (0 on VAS/NRS compared to 9 on before treatment on a scale from 0–10), and the patient started to walk with crutches. Follow up at 3 months showed complete healing of the stump-ulcer. She had no pain, and was walking normally, which continued till the recent last follow up 1½ year after the treatment. She was extremely satisfied with the outcome and scored 5 on a "patient-satisfaction on the effect of treatment" scale from 0 to 5, where 0 is least satisfied and 5 is extremely satisfied (Fig. 13.3a–c).

Discussions

AVMs are high flow vascular malformations, and can give rise to dermatological manifestations, such as eczematous reaction and angiodermatitis [10, 11]. Skin lesions including ulcerations and nodules related to underlying congenital AVM can occur, and is known as Stewart-Bluefarb syndrome or acroangiodermatitis and have been reported as pseudo-Kaposi's sarcoma [12, 13]. Skin ulceration associated with AVMs is difficult to manage [1]. It requires a multidisciplinary approach involving departments of Interventional Radiology (IR), dermatology, plastic surgery, vascular surgery, orthopedics, wound healing centre etc. Surgical removal and ligature of involved vessels have been reported, though it may require a multipronged therapy with surgery, medical antibiotic therapy, wound healing centres etc., takes a longer time to heal and leaves a relatively large skin defect and scar [14, 15]. IR therapy (embolization and/or sclerotherapy) can on the other hand be performed as an outpatient/day-care procedure, demand less healthcare resources and result in a better clinical outcome with complete healing of the wound, leaving no significant scar tissue. Klippel-Trenaunay syndrome usually has capillary, venous and lymphatic components, but AVM components can occur, particularly intracranially and in the lung [16, 17]. Peripheral AVM with leg ulcer associated with the syndrome has not been reported in the literature. Differentiation of KTS from Park-Weber syndrome (PWS) can be difficult as there is considerable phenotypic overlap between the two. PWS is a high-flow type of lesion associated with capillary malformation, AVM and limb overgrowth [18]. The IR approach with embolization in such a difficult situation can play an important clinical role and should be considered as a first line of treatment.

Abbreviations: VAS (Visual Analogue Scale)/ NRS (Numeric Rating Score) - from 0 – 10, 0 = no pain, 10 = worst possible pain

Learning points

1. Klippel Trenaunay syndrome associated with AVM of the extremities causing ulceration is rare and previously not reported in literature.
2. Wounds associated with AVMs are extremely difficult to treat by surgery, which entails risks of complications, including tissue loss and amputation.
3. IR treatment, including embolization, is a minimally invasive and highly effective procedure, can be performed as a day-care procedure, and can potentially avoid serious complications.
4. IR therapies should be done in a dedicated high-volume IR unit by experienced IR specialists routinely doing these procedures.

Case 13.2. Sclerotherapy for Venous Malformation of Right Second Toe with Intermittent Ulcer Formation

Keywords: Venous malformation (VM), ulcer, wound, sclerotherapy

Introduction

A 36-year-old young woman presented with a swollen right second toe, bluish discoloration and intermittent small ulcerations (Fig. 13.4a). The lesion was moderately painful (6–7 on VAS/NRS), and she had severe difficulty wearing shoes.

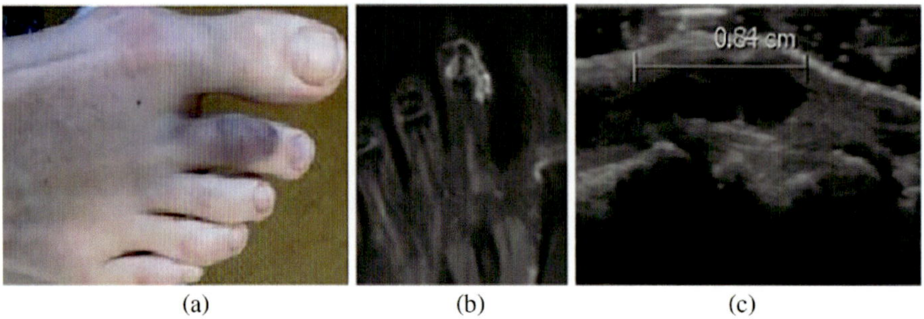

Fig. 13.4 Clinical (**a**) and imaging findings, MR (**b**) and USG (**c**) before treatment

There was very restricted dorsiflexion of the toe. The patient was moderately cosmetically affected (on a scale of mild - moderate - severe).

Differential Diagnosis

MR scanning with STIR sequence revealed a hyperintense lesion (Fig. 13.4b). No contrast-enhanced MR was available. Thus differential diagnoses of venous or lymphatic malformation were considered. USG showed slow-flow signals suggestive of a venous malformation (Fig. 13.4c). Absence of solid components ruled out a vascular tumor.

Treatment

Surgical treatment was possible, but associated with higher risks of significant tissue loss, nerve injury, a visible scar and probably amputation of the 2nd toe. Thus, the IR approach with endovascular sclerotherapy was considered as a first line therapy at a multidisciplinary team (MDT) meeting. The lesion was treated under local anesthesia with a small amount (0.5 ml) 3% Fibrovein (Sodium tetradecyl sulphate or STS/Sotradecol) as a foam prepared by mixing 2 ml STS with equal amount of atmospheric air and a small quantity of Lipiodol (about 1 ml) (Fig. 13.5a). Post-sclerotherapy ulcer formation occurred with neuralgia affecting the 2nd toe. The ulcer healed up in 4 weeks (Fig. 13.5b) and neural pain disappeared three months after the treatment. At 6 months follow up there was no trace of the malformation, no ulceration, no scar tissue, nor discoloration of the skin (Fig. 13.5c). There was full range of movement of the toe, including dorsiflexion, with complete absence of pain & neuralgia. She could comfortably put on any footwear/shoes without any difficulty and was extremely satisfied with the outcome (5 on scale from 0 to 5).

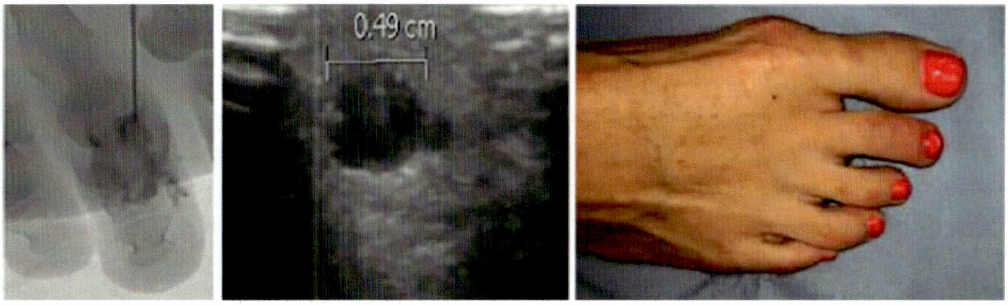

Fig. 13.5 Sclerotherapy (**a**), follow up USG at 4 weeks (**b**) and clinical outcome at 6 weeks (**c**)

Discussions

Venous malformations are the most common vascular malformations with an incidence of about 1–2 per 10,000 population and a prevalence of about 1% [19, 20]. However, the exact incidence of digital venous malformation is not known and probably a few cases with confusing nomenclature have been reported [21–23]. The exact incidence or prevalence of ulcers associated with digital venous malformation is unknown, and wound healing after sclerotherapy of venous malformations is not reported in the literature.

Learning points

1. Ulceration associated with digital venous malformations is extremely rare, and their treatment outcome is not reported in the literature.
2. Surgical treatment is possible but is associated with significant risks of complications including amputation, depending on the type of venous malformation.
3. IR (endovascular) sclerotherapy with direct puncture under local anæsthesia (for adults, and general anæsthesia for children) is a minimally invasive, effective treatment option resulting in long-term favorable clinical outcome.

Case 13.3. Direct Puncture Sclerotherapy for AVM of the Right Index Finger Tip

Keywords: Finger, digital Arterio-venous malformation (AVM), ulcer, wound, sclerotherapy

Introduction

A 51-year-old lady presented with a right index finger lesion, which according to the patient presumably started during her pregnancy. She was once surgically operated on about 30 years back. Current symptoms included increasing discomfort in the form of pain and burning sensation (VAS/NRS score between 4–7). The patient was unable to use the finger for her routine daily work. Pain relieved when she rested the finger on a cold surface. Small intermittent ulcers were being formed at the surface of the finger pulp. Her quality of life was severely affected (on a scale of mild - moderate - severe).

Diagnostic

CT and MR-angiography could be used for initial assessment, but spatial resolution at the fingertip would be sub-optimal. Pretreatment MR showed multiple flow-voids in the finger. Ultrasound with Doppler demonstrated the presence of A-V shunting, the nidus, turbulent high flow, and arterialisation of draining digital veins (Fig. 13.6a, b). However, detailed mapping overview of the lesion and reconstruction of the images were not possible by ultrasound. Pre-treatment digital subtraction angiography (DSA) was performed for detailed structural delineation and categorization of the AVM, and planning for therapy (Fig. 13.7).

Treatment

The patient was treated at two sessions of embolo-sclerotherapy through direct puncture of the nidus of the AVM with a thin butterfly needle (Fig. 13.8a–e). A few drops of 3% Sotradecol/STS foam (prepared by mixing 2 ml STS, 2 ml atmospheric air and about 0.5 ml Lipiodol) was injected under the guidance of simultaneous angiography through a coaxial microcatheter in the radial artery (Fig. 13.9a, b). The patient developed a post-treatment blackened area of pulp skin necrosis, which along with the pre-treatment ulcers healed up completely without any remaining scar tissue. Patient had significant improvement of pain and burning sensation (1–2 on VAS/NRS), and no wound formation. Patient was doing well 5 years after therapy.

Discussion

Most AVMs occur in the head and neck region. Isolated AVM/AVF of fingers are very rare. Actual prevalence is not known and only 24 cases of digital AVMs have been reported in the literature. Small AVMs may be asymptomatic, but large hemodynamically significant AVMs can lead to ulceration, bleeding, high output cardiac failure, embolic episodes, distal steal, and ischemia etc. [24–26]. AVMs by

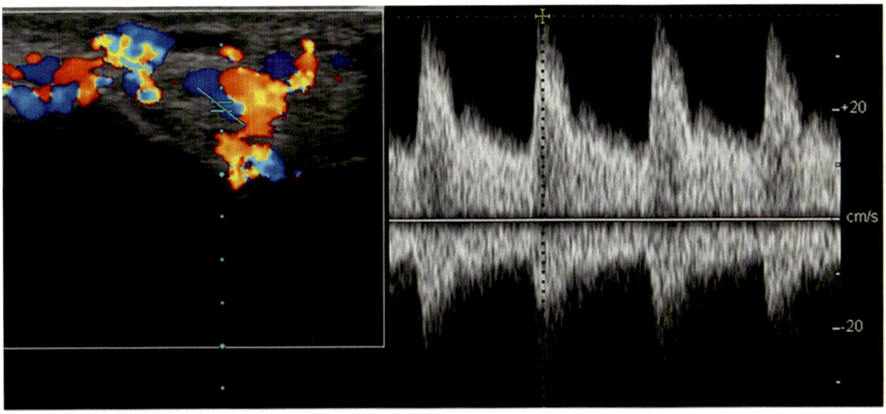

(a)

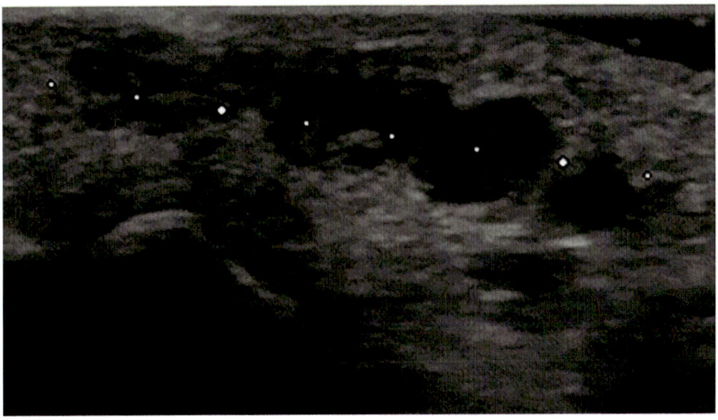

(b)

Fig. 13.6 USG with Doppler shows the finger-tip AVM (**a**) with dilated vascular spaces and turbulent high velocity flow (**b**)

definition are congenital. But digital AVMs are presumed to be acquired in nature. Both young and middle-aged patients with digital AVMs have been reported, where many of them do not reveal any history of trauma. There is no consensus on the modality of therapy and these lesions can be treated by reconstructive surgery, amputation or embolosclerotherapy [27, 28]. However, there are significant difficulties in treating these cases because of the necessity to preserve the finger and hand anatomy and hand/finger-function intact while treating the lesion adequately [29]. Besides, the technical challenges associated with endovascular therapy of digital AVMs are - inability to advance microcatheter into the nidus or close to the feeding arteries because of extremely narrow digital vessel calibre (smaller than the microcatheter itself) and tortuosity, cumbersome fixation of the finger during endovascular therapy, trouble choosing the suitable needle for direct puncture, significant risk of pulp tissue necrosis, and risk of non-target embolo-sclerotherapy

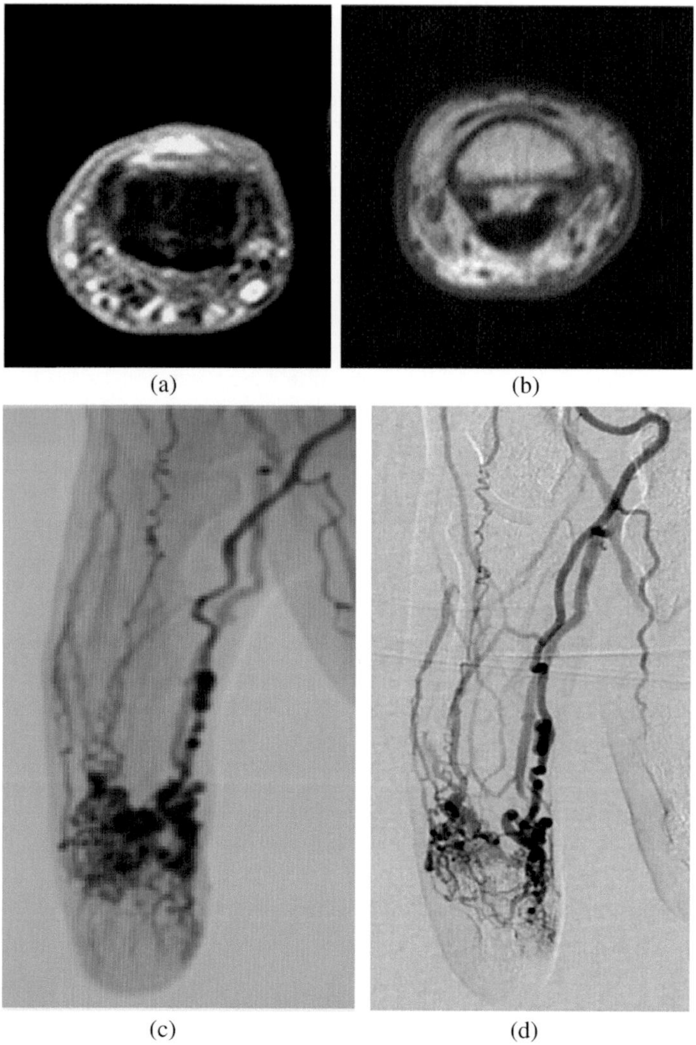

Fig. 13.7 MR scanning reveals flow-voids in the fingertip (**a**, **b**). Pre- and post-treatment angiography show AVM with nidus (**c**) and adequate devascularization after embo-losclero-therapy (**d**)

among others. Surgery may be an alternative to embolo-sclerotherapy, but it is associated with high risks of complications, takes long, time-consuming, laborious procedures, including microsurgery, venous, skin, nerve and muscle flap grafts, and possible repeat- or multistep-surgery. It leaves a large scar tissue with restricted functionality of the digit [15]. AVMs are one of the most difficult clinical conditions to treat and a complication rate of approximately 10% can be expected after sclero-embolo-therapy [30].

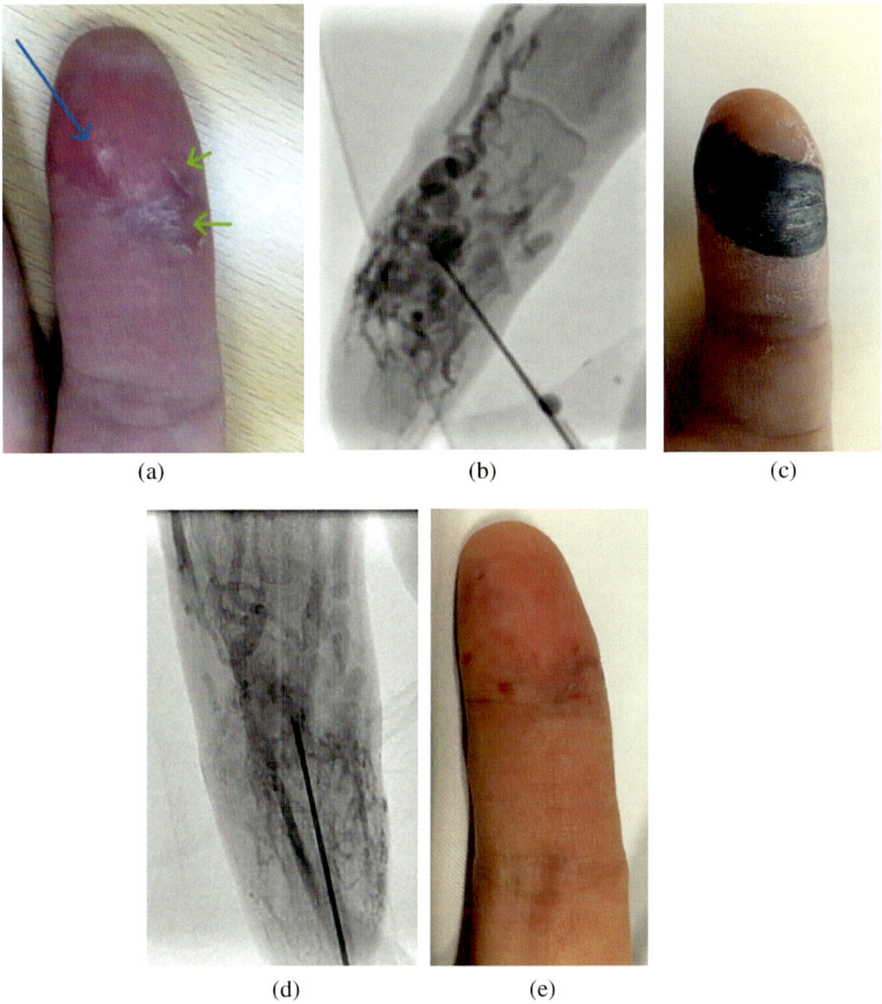

Fig. 13.8 Pre-treatment swelling (long blue arrow) and small ulcerated, excoriated area (short green arrows) in the fingertip (**a**), direct-puncture emboloscleotherapy (**b**), ischemic changes following first therapy (**c**), second session of direct-puncture emboloscleotherapy (**d**), and reduction of swelling and resolution of skin excoriation/ulcer formation (**e**)

Abbreviations: VAS (Visual Analogue Scale)/NRS (Numeric Rating Score) - from 0 – 10, 0 = no pain, 10 = worst possible pain.

Learning points

1. Digital AVMs are rare and only a handful of cases have been reported in the literature. Ulcers associated with digital AVM are extremely rare.

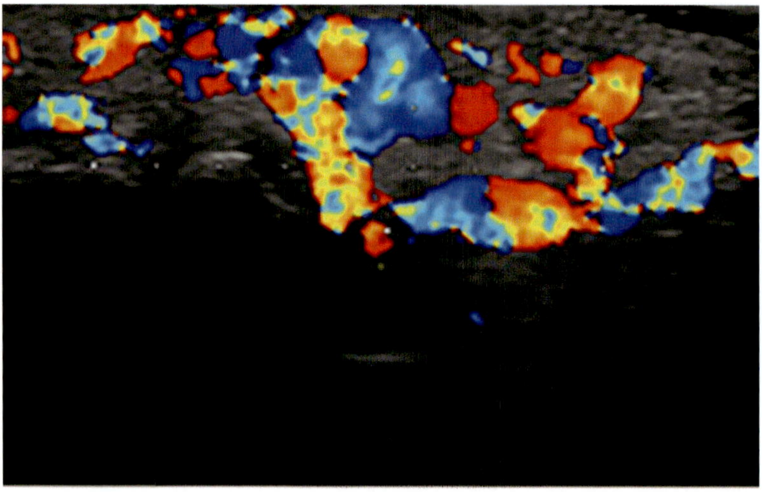

(a)

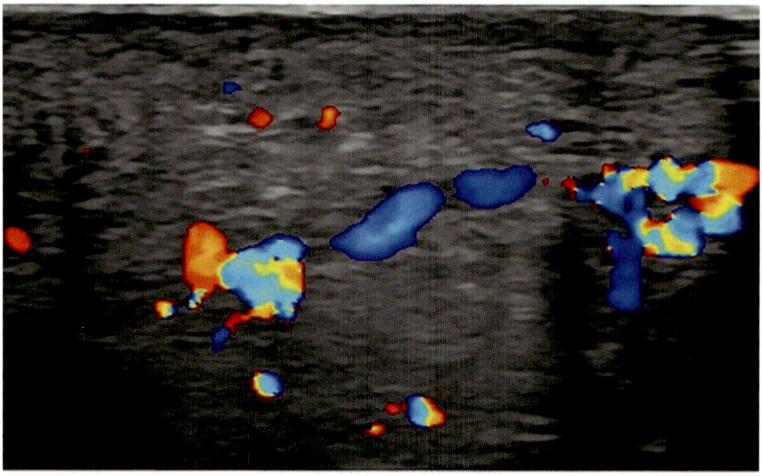

(b)

Fig. 13.9 Pre- (**a**) and pot-treatment (**b**) Doppler USG. Significant reduction of vascularity at the fingertip following treatment

2. They are very difficult to treat because of the complexity of the lesions and risks of significant complications.
3. Endovascular/IR treatment with direct puncture sclerotherapy is an effective treatment modality.

Case 13.4. Digital AVM with Right Little Fingertip Ulcerations Treated with Embolosclerotherapy

Introduction

A 62-year-old woman presented with a right little fingertip lesion for the last 15–20 years. She had several episodes of bleeding through tiny ulcers in the fingertip, including at least 3 episodes of violent pulsatile bleeding, which she had incredible difficulty in stopping. Previously treated twice with laser, without perceptible effect. She also had intermittent pain in the fingertip. The little finger had grown slightly bigger relative to the left side. She worked as a kindergarten teacher and she had to wash her hands several times a day and constantly bumps into various things that made it bleed from her fingertip, with the development of tiny ulcers.

Diagnostic

Ultrasound with Doppler demonstrated increased and turbulent flow, and arterialisation of draining digital veins, but could not delineate the detailed structure of the lesion. Pretreatment MR scanning was not done as MR was considered suboptimal for the lesion resolution. Patient's clinical history and USG was consistent with an AVM of the fingertip. A pretreatment digital subtraction angiography (DSA) was performed through the femoral route (Fig. 13.10a–f), where a selective catheter was placed in the brachial artery and a coaxial microcatheter was placed in the radial artery. Angiography helped in lesion mapping, categorization of the AVM and treatment planning.

Treatment

The lesion was accessed through direct puncture by a thin butterfly needle. Sclerotherapy was performed with foam produced by mixing 5 ml 3% Sotradecol (STS/Fibrovein) with 1 ml Lipiodol ultrafluid and 5 ml atmospheric air. Only a few drops of the foam were injected through a 2 ml syringe for embolosclerotherapy to avoid non-target ischemic complication of the finger.

Discussion

As discussed earlier, digital AVMs are presumed to be acquired in nature, which probably also apply to our case who was exposed to repeated trauma at her fingertips because of the nature of her daily work. However, what initiated or caused the lesion remained unknown. AVM of the fingers is a peculiar category pertaining to the superficial vascular anomaly group and was first described as digital

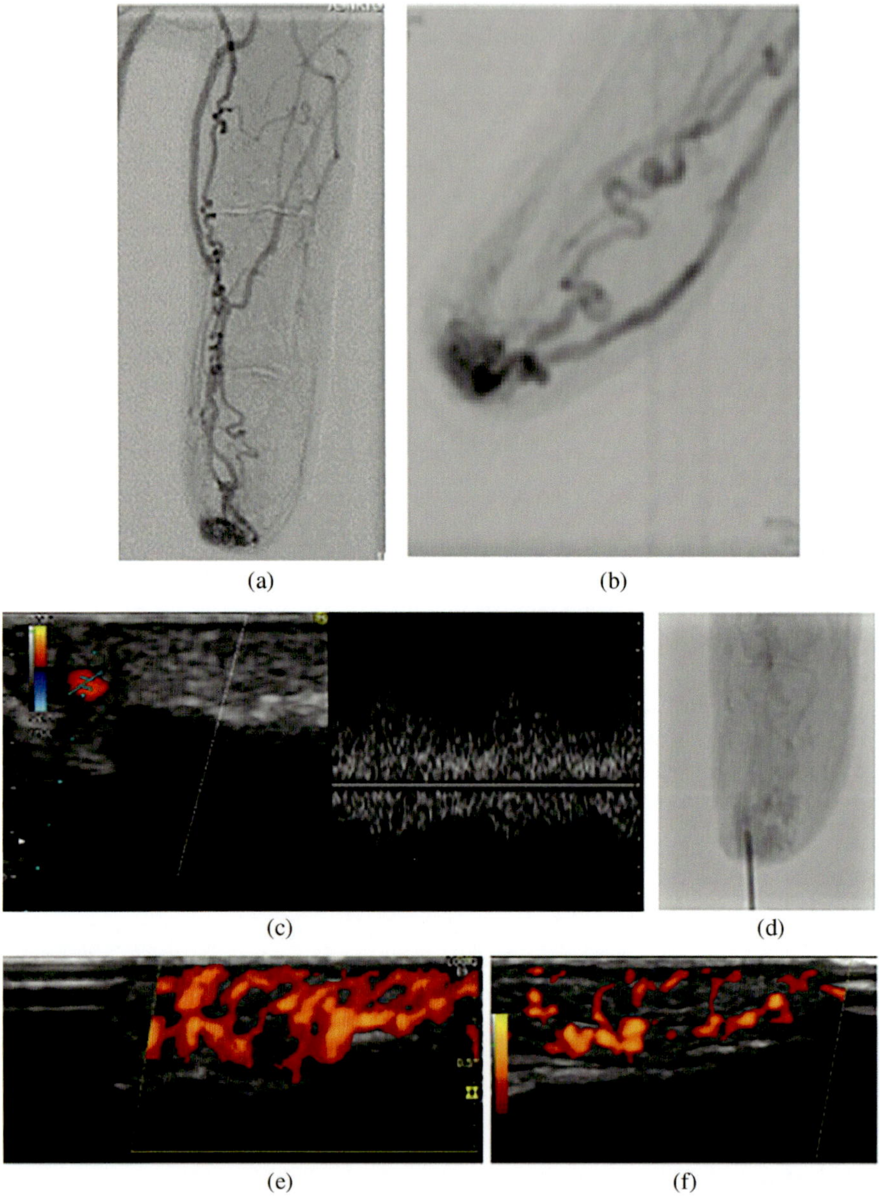

Fig. 13.10 Angiography shows the digital AVM with feeding artery and draining vein as well as the nidus (**a**), (**b**). Spectral Doppler USG reveals low-resistance arterial flow (**c**). Direct puncture embolo-sclerotherapy (**d**). Power-Doppler shows significant finger-pulp vascularity before treatment (**e**), reduced after sclerotherapy (**f**)

AVM in the late 90's [31]. It was earlier termed as cutaneous keratotic hemangioma [32, 33]. Histopathologically, epidermal hyperkeratosis, papillomatosis and prominently dilated subepidermal vascular elements are described. Thick- and thin-walled vessel-proliferations are found in the dermal and subcutaneous layers, without mitotic proliferation [4]. The patient had some symptoms at 3-months follow up after embolo-sclero-therapy, but at 1 year follow up she was almost asymptomatic. The patient is very satisfied with the therapy and has been doing well for the last 5 years after therapy.

References

1. Blaise J, Malloizel-Delaunay J, Nou M. Diagnosis of a chronic wound in the special case of a vascular malformation: a proposal of the wound and healing group of the French society of vascular medicine. JMV Journal de Médecine Vasculaire. 2024;49(2):103–11. https://doi.org/10.1016/j.jdmv.2024.03.003. https://www.sciencedirect.com/science/article.
2. Ueda T, Tanabe K, Morita M, Nakahara C, Katsuoka K. Leg ulcer due to multiple arteriovenous malformations in the lower extremity of an elderly patient. Int Wound J. 2016;13(2):226–30. https://doi.org/10.1111/iwj.12273. PMID: 24720817; PMCID: PMC7949821.
3. Jin Y, Yang X, Hua C, Lin X, Chen H, Ma G, et al. Ethanol embolotherapy for the management of refractory chronic skin ulcers caused by arteriovenous malformations. J Vasc Interv Radiol. 2018;29(1):107–13. https://doi.org/10.1016/j.jvir.2017.09.013. PMID: 29221921.
4. Akita S, Houbara S, Akatsuka M, Hirano A. Vascular anomalies and wounds. J Tissue Viability. 2013;22(3):103–11.
5. Oduber CEU, Van Der Horst CMAM, Hennekam RCM. Klippel-Trenaunay syndrome: diagnostic criteria and hypothesis on etiology. Ann Plast Surg. 2008;60(2):217–23.
6. Maari C, Frieden IJ. Klippel-Trénaunay syndrome: the importance of "geographic stains" in identifying lymphatic disease and risk of complications. J Am Acad Dermatol. 2004;51(3):391–8.
7. Garzon MC, Huang JT, Enjolras O, Frieden IJ. Vascular malformations. J Am Acad Dermatol. 2007;56(3):541–64.
8. Sreekar H, Dawre S, Petkar KS, Shetty RB, Lamba S, Naik S, et al. Diverse manifestations and management options in Klippel-Trenaunay syndrome: a single centre 10-year experience. J Plast Surg Hand Surg. 2013;47(4):303–7.
9. Gates PE, Drvaric DM, Kruger L. Wound healing in orthopaedic procedures for Klippel-Trenaunay syndrome. J Pediatr Orthop. 1996;16(6):723–6.
10. Bluefarb SM, Adams LA. Arteriovenous malformation with angiodermatitis. Stasis dermatitis simulating Kaposi's disease. Arch Dermatol. 1967;96(2):176–81.
11. Waterson KW Jr, Shapiro L, Dannenberg M. Developmental arteriovenous malformation with secondary angiodermatitis. Report of a case. Arch Dermatol. 1969;100(3):297–302.
12. Earhart RN, Aeling JA, Nuss DD, Mallette JR. Pseudo-Kaposi sarcoma. A patient with arteriovenous malformation and skin lesions simulating Kaposi sarcoma. Arch Dermatol. 1974;110(6):907–10.
13. Roach NK, Chow K, Lewis M. A non-healing ulcer with underlying radiologic findings: a case of Stewart-Blue Farb Syndrome. Austin J Clin Pathol. 2015;2(2):1030.
14. Işık M, Günerhan Y, Ege E. Chronic leg ulcer due to arteriovenous malformation: a case report. EJCM. 2018;6(2):76–9. https://doi.org/10.15511/ejcm.18.00276.
15. Shimizu F, Kato A, Uehara M, Oatari M. Successful reconstruction after radical resection of arteriovenous malformation of the finger and toe using microsurgery. JPRAS Open. 2015;6:34–40. https://doi.org/10.1016/j.jpra.2015.06.006.

16. Mall S, Sharma RK, Prajapat D, Gupta SK, Talwar D. Hemoptysis: Beyond routine chest computed tomography and bronchoscopy. Lung India. 2017;34(4):368–71. https://doi.org/10.4103/lungindia.lungindia_456_16. PMID: 28671169; PMCID: PMC5504895.
17. Ishikawa K, Yamamoto Y, Funayama E, Furukawa H, Sasaki S. Wound-healing problems associated with combined vascular malformations in Klippel-Trenaunay syndrome. Adv Wound Care. 2019;8(6):246–55. https://doi.org/10.1089/wound.2018.0835. PMID: 31832274; PMCID: PMC6906760.
18. Vikkula M, Boon LM, Mulliken JB. Molecular genetics of vascular malformations. Matrix Biol. 2001;20(5–6):327–35. https://doi.org/10.1016/S0945-053X(01)00150-0.
19. Eifert S, Villavicencio JL, Kao TC, et al. Prevalence of deep venous anomalies in congenital vascular malformations of venous predominance. J Vasc Surg. 2000;31(3):462–71. https://doi.org/10.1067/mva.2000.101464.
20. Yu J, Tran D, Newhard HM. Multicompartment intramuscular hemangioma of the foot: a case study. J Am Podiatr Med Assoc. 2014;104(2):203–7. https://doi.org/10.7547/0003-0538-104.2.203.
21. Mitsionis GI, Pakos EE, Kosta P, Batistatou A, Beris A. Intramuscular hemangioma of the foot: a case report and review of the literature. Foot Ankle Surg. 2010;16(2):e27–9. https://doi.org/10.1016/j.fas.2009.05.008.
22. Davies JL, Stone PA, McGarry JJ. Mixed cavernous and capillary intraosseous hemangioma of the foot. J Am Podiatr Med Assoc. 1997;87(10):478–82.
23. Yoon SY, Cho SH, Lee JD. Digital arteriovenous malformation. Acta Derm Venereol. 2006;86(1):82–3.
24. Sawani A, Huber K, Zibadi S, Payne WG. Diagnosis of arteriovenous malformation in the finger. Eplasty. 2017;17:ic10. PMID: 28507659; PMCID: PMC5408223.
25. Moye SJ, Billmire DA. Congenital arteriovenous malformation of the finger resulting in cardiac decompensation: A case report. J Hand Surg Am. 1992;17(5):887–91. https://doi.org/10.1016/0363-5023(92)90462-x. PMID: 1401800.
26. Kadono T, Kishi A, Onishi Y, Ohara K. Acquired digital arteriovenous malformation: a report of six cases. Br J Dermatol. 2000;142(2):362–5.
27. Darius KL, Hao-Yun Y, Luke HTT, Kiang-Hiong T, Chong TT. Case report of ethanol and cyanoacrylate embolisation of a recurrent uncontrollable torrentially bleeding arteriovenous malformation of the finger. EJVES Short Rep. 2018;39:40–3. https://doi.org/10.1016/j.ejvssr.2018.05.003. PMID: 29922724; PMCID: PMC6005803.
28. Park UJ, Do YS, Park KB, Park HS, Kim YW, Lee BB, et al. Treatment of arteriovenous malformations involving the hand. Ann Vasc Surg. 2012;26(5):643–8. https://doi.org/10.1016/j.avsg.2011.08.016. PMID: 22266239.
29. Shimizu F, Kato A, Uehara M, Oatari M. Successful reconstruction after radical resection of arteriovenous malformation of the finger and toe using microsurgery. JPRAS Open. 2015;5:34–40. https://doi.org/10.1016/j.jpra.2015.06.006.
30. Yakes WF, Rossi P, Odink H. Arteriovenous malformation management. Cardiovasc Intervent Radiol. 1996;19(2):65–71. https://doi.org/10.1007/BF02563895.
31. McCulley S, Fourie L, Hull SM. Spontaneous digital arteriovenous malformation in a 28-year-old pregnant female. Br J Dermatol. 1997;136(3):472–3.
32. Burge SM, Baran R, Dawber RPR, Verret JL. Periungual and subungual arteriovenous tumours. Br J Dermatol. 1986;115(3):361–6.
33. Yang CH, Ohara K. Acquired digital arteriovenous malformation: a report of three cases and study with epiluminescence microscopy. Br J Dermatol. 2002;147(5):1007–11.

Innovative Materials

14

Jan Plock, Bita Tafrishi, and Alina Samia Senn

Abstract

Chronic wounds present a significant burden on the healthcare systems worldwide, requiring innovative approaches for effective management. They pose a significant clinical challenge, often characterized by delayed healing, infection, and impaired tissue regeneration. This chapter highlights cases showcasing the successful utilization of novel technologies in the treatment of chronic wounds. The first case demonstrates the application of Spincare®, an electrospinning technology, in promoting wound healing following delayed healing after split-thickness skin grafting in a foot injury. The second case illustrates the efficacy of Novosorb/BTM®, a biodegradable temporizing matrix, in managing necrotizing fasciitis secondary to a skin injury in the lower leg. The following two cases show examples for chronic and complicated wound situations being treated with a decellularized fish skin from the Atlantic cod (Kerecis®), promoting wound healing in supporting cellular and vascular ingrowth. Through the integration of advanced technologies, significant improvements in wound healing and patient outcomes were achieved. These cases underscore the importance of adopting innovative approaches in chronic wound care to address the complexities associated with wound management and patient outcomes.

Keywords

Wound innovation • Biomaterials • Tissue engineering • Chronic wounds • Advanced dressings • Electrospinning • Biodegradable matrices • Healing technologies • Novel wound treatments • Tissue regeneration • Advanced wound care • Negative pressure wound therapy

J. Plock (✉) · B. Tafrishi · A. S. Senn
Department for Plastic Surgery and Hand Surgery, Cantonal Hospital Aarau, Aarau, Switzerland
e-mail: jan.plock@ksa.ch

G.-S.Tiplica and K. Isoherranen (eds.), *Wound Healing*,
https://doi.org/10.1007/978-3-031-84579-6_14

Introduction

Chronic wounds represent a growing significant healthcare challenge worldwide with implications for patient morbidity and healthcare costs [1]. They are characterized by prolonged healing times, frequent infections, and impaired tissue regeneration. These wounds are often complicated by comorbidities such as diabetes mellitus, peripheral vascular disease, and obesity [2]. Despite advances in wound care, managing chronic wounds remains complex, necessitating a multifaceted approach to address underlying pathophysiology and promote healing [3].

Multidisciplinary wound clinics that include infectious disease specialists, radiologists, dermatologists, surgeons, nutritionists etc. are more particularly suitable for treating complex chronic wounds. While the importance of multidisciplinary clinics is established, further research is needed to optimize the use of advanced technologies for individual patient care [4].

In recent years, there has been a growing interest in the development and application of novel technologies to address the complexities associated with chronic wound management. These include advanced wound dressings, bioactive materials, tissue engineering, and regenerative medicine [5].

One example of such innovative technology is the use of electrospinning technology as demonstrated by Spincare® in wound care. It enables the fabrication of customized nanofibers matrices that mimic the extracellular matrix, promoting tissue regeneration and creating an optimal environment for wound healing. It shows rapid and complete wound healing times ranging from 9 to 30 days with a low incidence of adverse events [6]. Its easy and quick dressing application (less than 10 min), excellent adherence, and potential early removal of secondary dressings suggest promising advantages for clinical practice.

Another innovative technology as seen in our case is the use of Novosorb®, a Biodegradable Temporising Matrix (BTM). It serves as a scaffold for cellular infiltration and neovascularization, facilitating wound healing. It has been used successfully to treat a variety of complex wound types, including those resulting from trauma, infection, and vascular disease [7].

In the last two cases of this chapter, Kerecis®, a fish skin technology, is presented. The natural properties and structure of the fish skin facilitates the healing of wounds and tissue damage. It is rich in omega-3-fatty acids and has a composition similar to human skin. With its advantage of no known bacterial or viral disease transmission risk to humans, it is an easy-to-handle acellular matrix with various clinical applications and thus has gained significant attention in the field of regenerative medicine [8].

In the following cases we present three novel wound management technologies to overcome the challenges of chronic wounds. By integrating evidence-based practices with innovative approaches, clinicians can enhance wound healing outcomes, reduce healthcare costs, and improve the quality of life for patients with chronic wounds.

Case 14.1

A 63-year-old patient sustained a skin injury with a log splitter on his dorsal lower leg. Despite daily disinfection, a small wound persisted on the lower leg, without any signs of infection.

The patient then traveled to Sri Lanka and engaged in sea swimming activities. Upon returning, the patient consulted the emergency room and reported symptoms suggestive of hyperglycemic diabetes mellitus with > 21 mmol/l, fever and increasing pain in the lower leg.

Upon initial clinical evaluation, we observed a 2×2 cm wound with perifocal redness and massive pain of the limb. Concurrently leukocytes were elevated (18G/L), C-reactive protein level massively increased (480 mg/l), both indicative of a systemic infection or sepsis.

Giving the clinical presentation of necrotizing fasciitis, we initiated immediate surgical treatment, sampling, and extensive debridement. Targeted antibiotics with Meropenem and Clindamycin were established. Microbiological analysis identified the presence of *Streptococcus pyogenes* and *Staphylococcus aureus.* We performed two more surgical debridements to remove necrotic tissue and establish a conducive environment for wound healing. For postoperative wound dressings Betadine®-soaked gauze was used.

During the fourth surgical revision wound conditions were considered clean (Fig. 14.1), and a temporizing dermal matrix (Novosorb/BTM®) and NPWT were applied (Fig. 14.2) [9]. A collaboration with endocrinology specialists facilitated the optimization of blood glucose control through tailored insulin dosages, addressing the underlying hyperglycemic state and promoting wound healing. Additionally nutritional counseling was provided, supplemented by Fresubin Protein Energy and Abound formulations, to address potential deficiencies and support tissue repair processes [4].

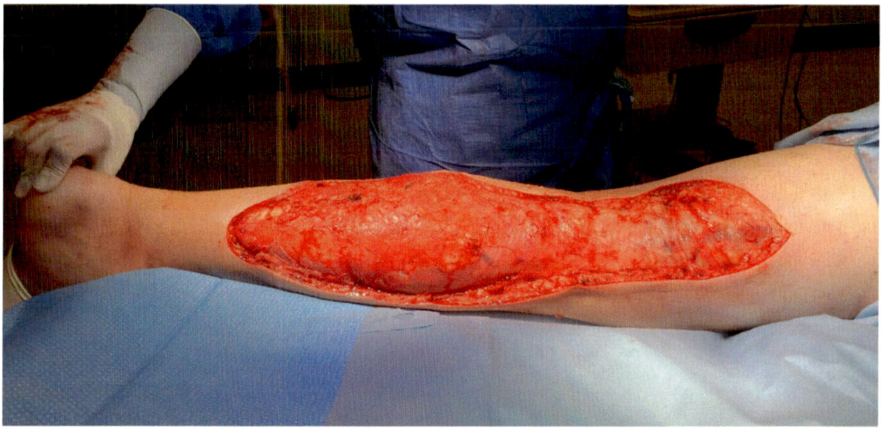

Fig. 14.1 Necrotizing fasciitis after radical surgical debridement on the left lower limb

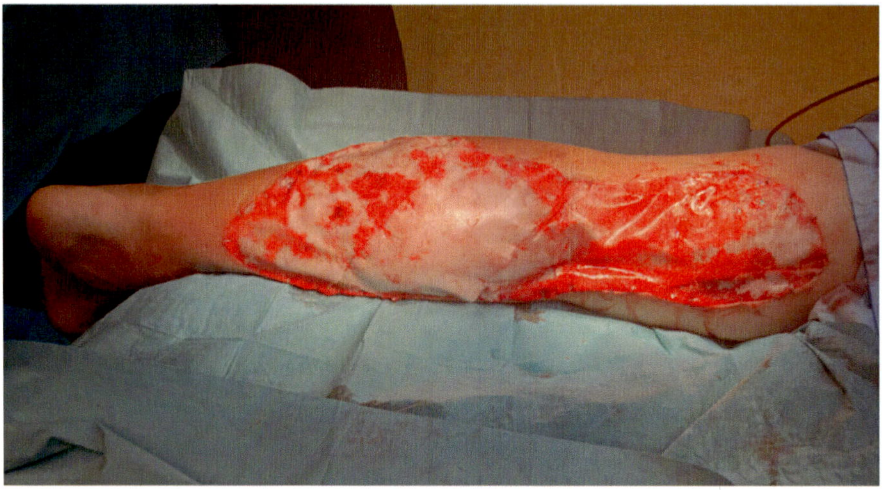

Fig. 14.2 Lamination with Novosorb® after the fourth surgical necrotic tissue removement

Four weeks after the operation a good vascularization with capillary refill was observed and we performed delamination of the dermal matrix followed by a split-skin grafting on the upper and lower left leg using grafts harvested from the right thigh and NPWT. Five days later the split-skin was found to be nicely adherent and healed [7]. The patient underwent outpatient wound therapy which involved immobilization in a bunny splint and dressing changes every 2 days. The wound was treated with Octenisept® disinfection, Bactigras®, absorbent cotton and an elastic bandage. Regular follow-up appointments enabled close monitoring of wound progress and adjustment of treatment strategies as warranted. Compression therapy was initiated. Currently, the scars have healed nicely, and the wound treatment is complete (Fig. 14.3).

Novosorb/BTM® (Biodegradable Temporizing Matrix) are synthetic dermal substitutes, based on polyurethane foam, used in wound care, providing a temporizing scaffold for cell ingrowth and tissue regeneration while gradually degrading over time [7, 10]. It is ultimately promoting wound healing by supporting granulation tissue formation and integration with the patient's own tissue as dermal substitute [11, 12].

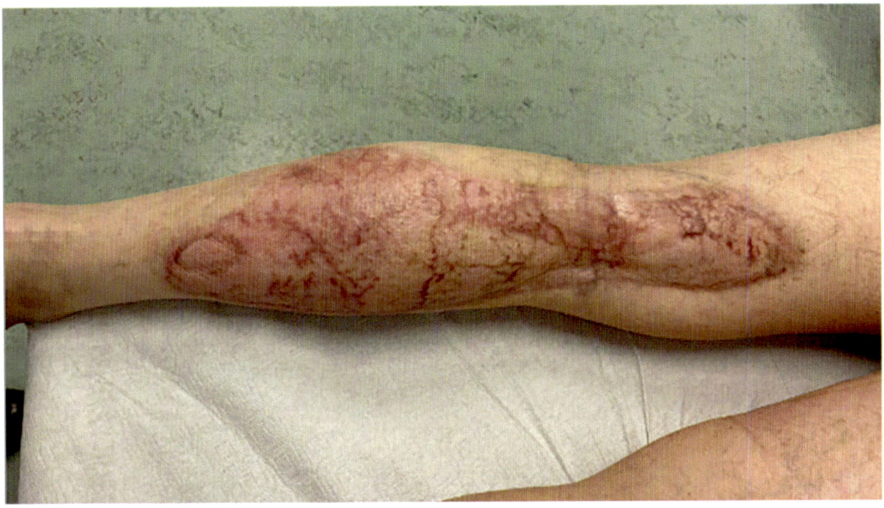

Fig. 14.3 6 months postoperative

Case 14.2

A 45-year-old patient initially sustained a full thickness skin wound while on vacation in Thailand. Conservative treatment failed under antibiotic treatment. Following surgical debridement after 9 days resulted in a 5 × 5 cm large wound with exposed extensor tendons on the dorsum of the foot.

A NPWT was applied to facilitate wound healing. The antibiotic therapy was changed to Cefepim 3 × 2 g i.v. according to microbiological results.

Microbiological analysis revealed the presence of *Myroides morgani* and the antibiotic therapy was continued. The attempt to cover the wound with a flap failed with partial flap necrosis and the wound was finally covered with split-thickness skin grafting.

Five days postoperatively, the NPWT device was removed, and the split skin appeared to be adherent. However, only partial healing could be observed (Fig. 14.4).

A dressing regime with Octenisept® disinfection, Prontosan® wound gel and Bactigras® was established. Eventually, due to increased moisture in the wound, Mepilex® dressings were used.

Despite regular dressing changes, wound healing stagnated, and the wound showed hypergranulation with only few epithelial islands. We debrided the fibrin deposits and covered the wound with Spincare® (Fig. 14.5). Nine days after

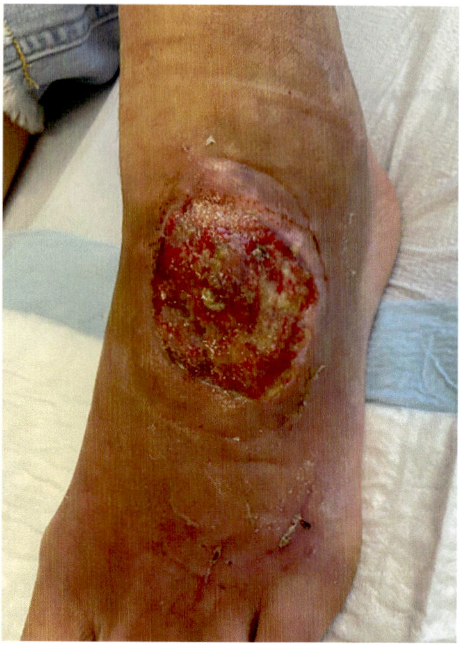

Fig. 14.4 Wound on the dorsal left foot after partial flap and split skin necrosis

the application increased epithelialization and reduced wound exudate were recognized Spincare® treatment was re-applied compression therapy of the left leg was initiated to improve venous return, reduce edema, and promote wound healing [6, 13, 14].

After 14 days full wound healing was achieved [15]. The daily wound care continued with Bepanthen® for scar care and to moisturize.

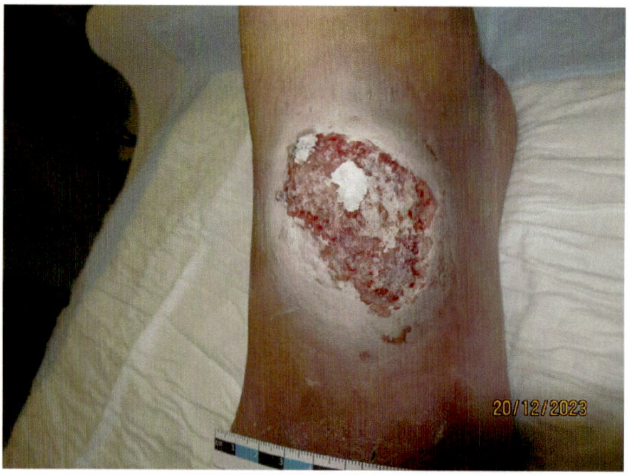

Fig. 14.5 Wound on the dorsal foot after the first application of Spincare®

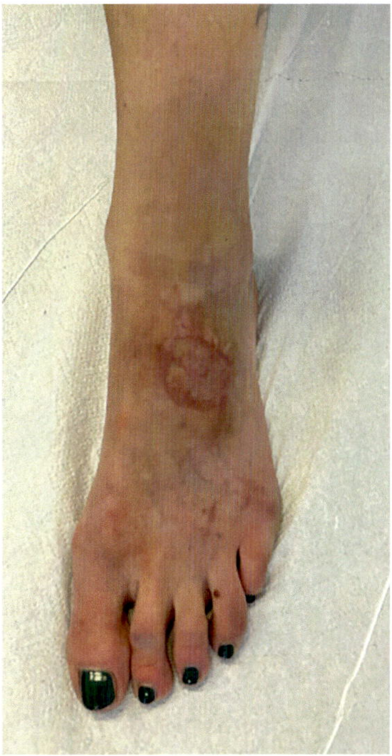

Fig. 14.6 Three months postoperative

The clinical check-up conducted three months postoperatively showed that the wounds had completely healed and displayed favorable cosmetic outcomes (Fig. 14.6).

Spincare® is an electrospinning technology that produces a semi-permeable membrane designed to provide a protective barrier over wounds resembling the extracellular matrix [15, 16]. It maintains a moist wound environment that promotes wound healing and also minimizes pain and trauma during dressing changes. The spider web-like matrix is spun with a gun device incorporating miniaturized electrospinning technology. The substrate is not further declared by the company [17].

Case 14.3

An 82-year-old patient presented with an infected wound on his right lateral malleolus after a minor trauma two weeks prior. The initial examination showed a full thickness skin defect (2 × 2 cm) with a surrounding infection of the superficial skin layers (erysipelas) (Fig. 14.7). Underlying bone (distal fibula) was still covered with soft tissue, and an x-ray showed no signs of osteomyelitis. An empirical antibiotic treatment with amoxicillin/clavulanic acid was administered. Diabetes and macroangiopathy were ruled out. Cardiac insufficiency and a chronic venous

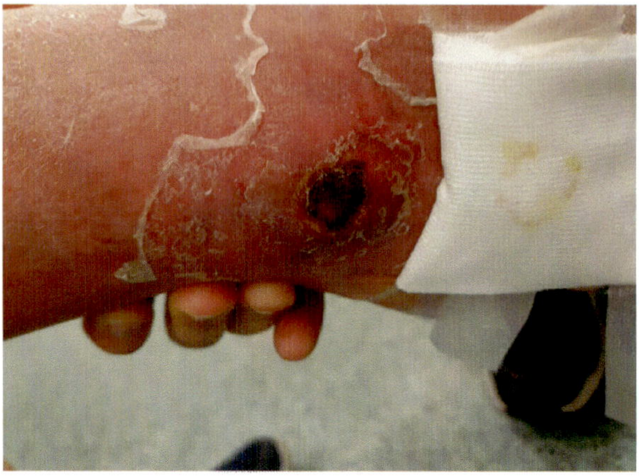

Fig. 14.7 Initial presentation of the wound with erysipelas and central full thickness defect at the right malleolus lateralis

insufficiency led to leg edema. A local compression therapy and modification of heart medication was performed.

Under antibiotic treatment the local infection was controlled (Fig. 14.8). As the patient was opposed to surgical treatment, conservative wound care was continued. Wound dressings were applied with hydrogel and a hydro fiber wound dressing (Aquacel®), and a silicone dressing (Biatain® Silicone) for coverage and absorbing exudate from the wound [18]. Fibrin layers were recurrently superficially debrided [19]. Over 11 weeks the wound was treated in the aforementioned regimen and the patient was seen in the outpatient wound clinic. In the end, the wound showed hypergranulation, but no signs of epithelialization [20]. The defect size decreased marginally (Figs. 14.9 and 14.10). Due to the stagnant findings, the decision was made to apply omega-III fish skin (Kerecis®) [21]. The fish skin was fixated with wound strips (Steri-Strip™). Coverage with silicone dressings (Biatain® Silicone) for protection was performed and exchanged when moist or detaching. The fish skin supported the cellular and vascular ingrowth. The wound epithelialized completely after 2 weeks of application (Fig. 14.11). For this chronic wound situation, the fish skin was a valid solution to reach epithelialization after weeks of management with conventional dressing materials in the outpatient wound clinic. It poses a great opportunity in tissue regeneration as an innovative, environmental neutral, time and resource saving material [8].

Kerecis® is decellularized fish skin from the Atlantic cod, rich in omega-3 fatty acids and has recently been shown to be efficient for enhanced wound healing in difficult wounds [22]. It can be used in chronic wounds, diabetic ulcers, pressure sores, burns, and large-scale wounds.

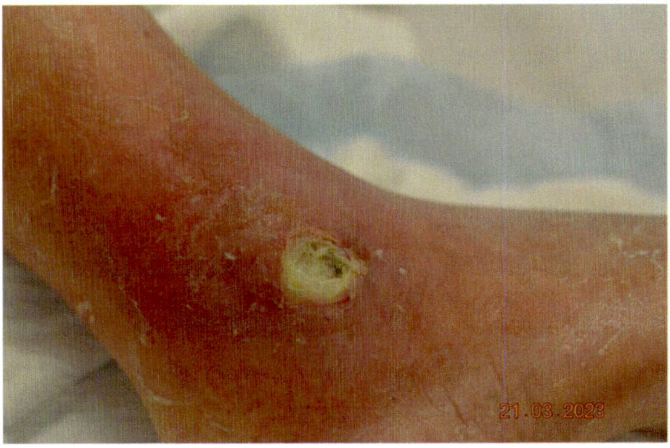

Fig. 14.8 Wound after infection regression with thick fibrin layer and intact wound surrounding

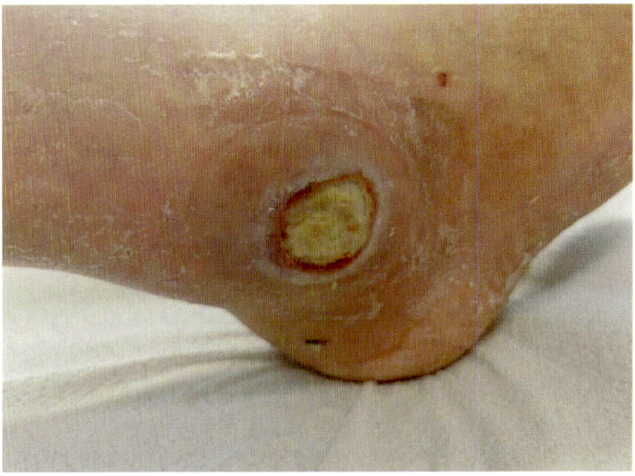

Fig. 14.9 Progression of the wound size under conventional wound treatment

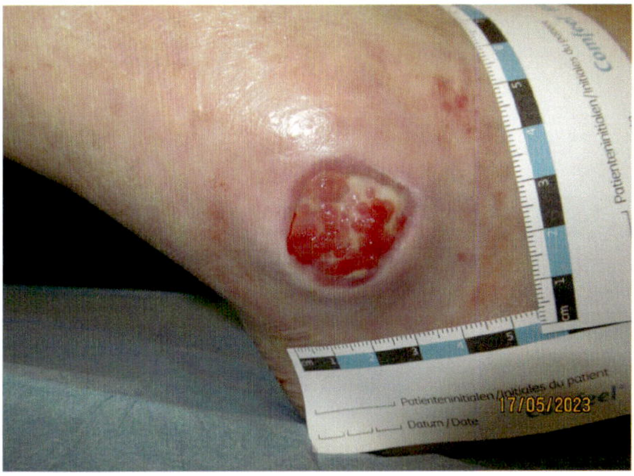

Fig. 14.10 Hypergranulating wound ground with stagnating epithelialization

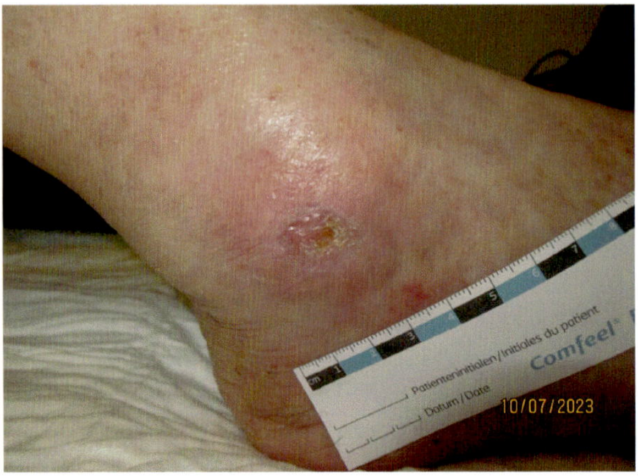

Fig. 14.11 Epithelialized wound 2 weeks after application of fish skin (Kerecis®)

Case 14.4

A 39-year-old patient underwent dermato-lipectomy after massive weight-loss. One week after the surgery, she presented with massive pain along the infected scar line and local pus secretion (Fig. 14.12).

To treat a suspected wound infection, limited surgical debridement of the wound and microbiological sampling was performed. To reach for a temporary wound closure a negative pressure wound therapy (NPWT) was applied. Empirical antibiotic (amoxicillin/clavulanic acid) therapy was started after the first debridement. After a second debridement, the wound showed progressive necrosis of the skin and the patient showed increasing inflammatory values without microbiological findings (Fig. 14.13). In review of all clinical symptoms and findings, pyoderma gangrenosum was suspected. Pyoderma gangrenosum is a dysregulation of neutrophil granulocytes and increased release of proinflammatory cytokines leading

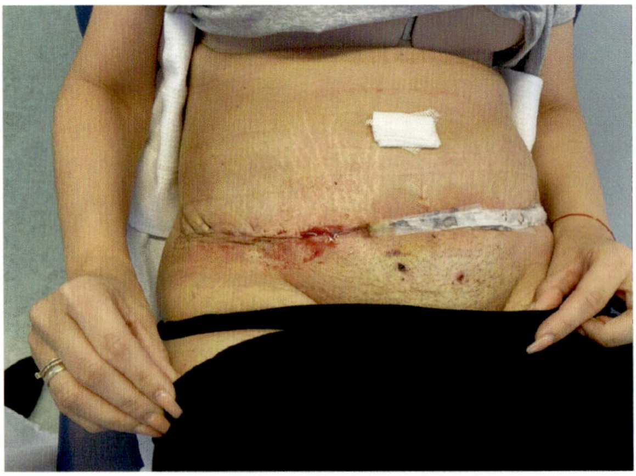

Fig. 14.12 Findings at initial presentation, highly suspicious for a wound infection

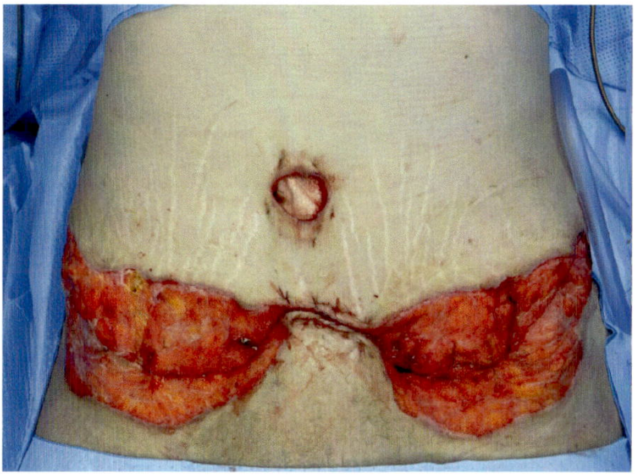

Fig. 14.13 Wound defect after multiple debridement's because of skin necrosis

to painful skin changes and development into deep necrosis [23]. The histology was affirmative exhibiting dermal necrosis and subcutaneous inflammation with infiltration of neutrophils and no detection of bacteria [24].

After initiation of high dose steroid therapy for immunosuppression, the wound showed early signs of healing [25]. As direct closure was not possible due to resulting defects until the level of the subcutaneous tissue and its size, a xenogeneic matrix (fish skin technology, Kerecis®) was applied to fill the remaining defect (Fig. 14.14). Further coverage with a negative wound pressure therapy (NPWT) was installed. Because fish skin shows no risk of viral disease transmission to humans, the fish skin can be applied as a temporary skin substitute with similar structure to human skin [8]. It functions as a barrier to protect the underlying tissue and improves wound healing in supporting cellular and vascular ingrowth. Wound healing is promoted by high levels of omega-3 fatty acids [26].

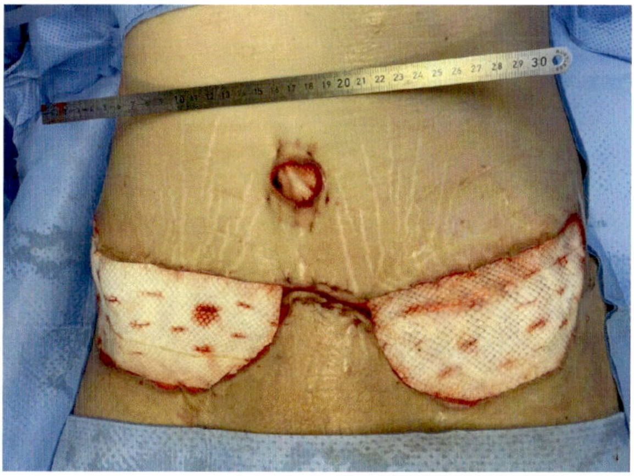

Fig. 14.14 Application of fish skin (Kerecis®)

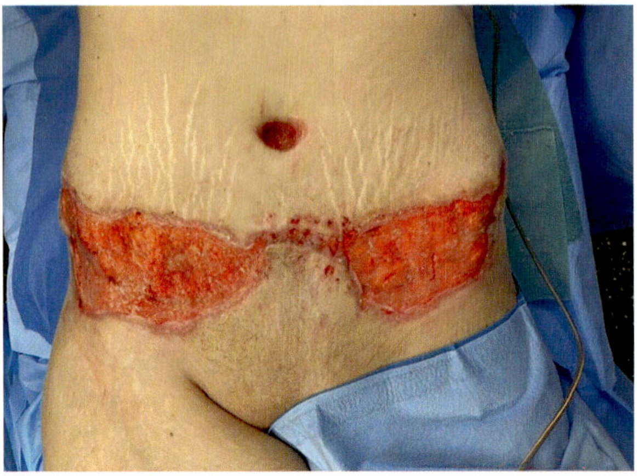

Fig. 14.15 Granulated wound before split-thickness skin graft transplantation

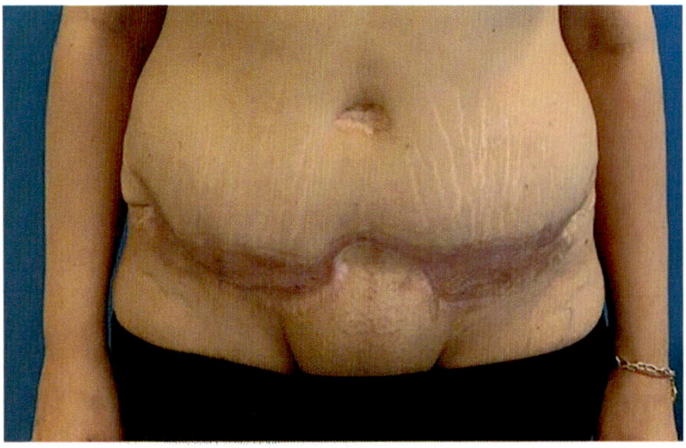

Fig. 14.16 Healed skin graft 6 weeks after transplantation

The NPWT was exchanged weekly until the remaining wound surface was conditioned. After 4 weeks, granulation had reached skin level (Fig. 14.15), and a split-thickness skin graft was performed. The rest of the healing processes showed no adverse events (Fig. 14.16).

Kerecis® is decellularized fish skin from the Atlantic cod, rich in natural omega-3 fatty acids. There is evidence for promotion of wound healing in difficult to treat wound situations and for balancing the wound bed in highly inflammatory environments [27].

References

1. Sen CK, Gordillo GM, Roy S, Kirsner R, Lambert L, Hunt TK, et al. Human skin wounds: a major and snowballing threat to public health and the economy. Wound Repair Regen. 2009;17(6):763–71. https://doi.org/10.1111/j.1524-475X.2009.00543.x.
2. Armstrong DG, Boulton AJM, Bus SA. Diabetic foot ulcers and their recurrence. N Engl J Med. 2017;376(24):2367–75. https://doi.org/10.1056/NEJMra1615439.

3. Falanga V, Isseroff RR, Soulika AM, et al. Chronic wounds. Nat Rev Dis Primers. 2022;8(1):50. https://doi.org/10.1038/s41572-022-00377-3.
4. Hayun Y, Yaacobi DS, Shachar T, Harats M, Grush AE, Olshinka A. Novel technologies in chronic wound care. Semin Plast Surg. 2022;36(2):75–82. https://doi.org/10.1055/s-0042-1749095.
5. Zhao R, Liang H, Clarke E, Jackson C, Xue M. Inflammation in chronic wounds. Int J Mol Sci. 2016;17(12):2085. https://doi.org/10.3390/ijms17122085.
6. Schulz A, Fuchs PC, Heitzmann W, Kanho CH, Schiefer JL. Our initial experience in the customized treatment of donor site and burn wounds with a new nanofibrous temporary epidermal layer. Ann Burns Fire Disasters. 2021;34(1):58–66.
7. Schlottmann F, Obed D, Bingöl AS, März V, Vogt PM, Krezdorn N. Treatment of complex wounds with NovoSorb® biodegradable temporising matrix (BTM)—a retrospective analysis of clinical outcomes. J Pers Med. 2022;12(12):2002. https://doi.org/10.3390/jpm12122002.
8. Baldursson BT, Kjartansson H, Konrádsdóttir F, Gudnason P, Sigurjonsson GF, Lund SH. Healing rate and autoimmune safety of full-thickness wounds treated with fish skin acellular dermal matrix versus porcine small-intestine submucosa: a noninferiority study. Int J Low Extrem Wounds. 2015;14(1):37–43. https://doi.org/10.1177/1534734615573661. Epub 2015 Mar 9 PMID: 25759413.
9. Zhang R, Zhang Y, Hou L, Yan C. Vacuum-assisted closure versus conventional dressing in necrotizing fasciitis: a systematic review and meta-analysis. J Orthop Surg Res. 2023;18(1):85. https://doi.org/10.1186/s13018-023-03561-7.
10. Cheng C, Kwiecien GJ, Rowe DJ, Gatherwright JR, Chepla KJ. Reconstruction of chronic wounds secondary to injectable drug use with a biodegradable temporizing matrix. Plast Reconstr Surg Glob Open. 2021;9(7):e3678. https://doi.org/10.1097/GOX.0000000000003678.
11. Kidd T, Kolaityte V, Bajaj K, Wallace D, Izadi D, Bechar J. The use of NovoSorb biodegradable temporising matrix in wound management: a literature review and case series. J Wound Care. 2023;32(8):470–8. https://doi.org/10.12968/jowc.2023.32.8.470.
12. Li H, Lim P, Stanley E, et al. Experience with NovoSorb® biodegradable temporising matrix in reconstruction of complex wounds. ANZ J Surg. 2021;91(9):1744–50. https://doi.org/10.1111/ans.16936.
13. Romano I, Summa M, Heredia-Guerrero JA, et al. Fumarate-loaded electrospun nanofibers with anti-inflammatory activity for fast recovery of mild skin burns. Biomed Mater. 2016;11(4):041001. https://doi.org/10.1088/1748-6041/11/4/041001.
14. Woo KM, Chen VJ, Ma PX. Nano-fibrous scaffolding architecture selectively enhances protein adsorption contributing to cell attachment. J Biomed Mater Res A. 2003;67(2):531–7. https://doi.org/10.1002/jbm.a.10098.
15. Haik J, Ullmann Y, Gur E, et al. Spincare® system demonstrates safety and efficacy in treating partial thickness burns. J Burn Care Res. 2024. https://doi.org/10.1093/jbcr/irae024.
16. Vasella M, Cirebea J, Gousopoulos E, et al. Outcome of facial burn injuries treated by a nanofibrous temporary epidermal layer. J Clin Med. 2023;12(16):5273. https://doi.org/10.3390/jcm12165273.
17. Chappidi S, Buddolla V, Ankireddy SR, Lakshmi BA, Kim YJ. Recent trends in diabetic wound healing with nanofibrous scaffolds. Eur J Pharmacol. 2023;945:175617. https://doi.org/10.1016/j.ejphar.2023.175617. Epub 2023 Feb 24. PMID: 36841285.
18. Nuutila K, Eriksson E. Moist wound healing with commonly available dressings. Adv Wound Care. 2021;10(12):685–698. https://doi.org/10.1089/wound.2020.1232. Epub 2021 Feb 11. PMID: 32870777; PMCID: PMC8568799.
19. Powers JG, Higham C, Broussard K, Phillips TJ. Wound healing and treating wounds: chronic wound care and management. J Am Acad Dermatol. 2016;74(4):607–25 (quiz 625–6). https://doi.org/10.1016/j.jaad.2015.08.070. PMID: 26979353.
20. Mitchell A, Llumigusin D. The assessment and management of hypergranulation. Br J Nurs. 2021;30(5):S6–10. https://doi.org/10.12968/bjon.2021.30.5.S6. PMID: 33733836.

GPSR Compliance

The European Union's (EU) General Product Safety Regulation (GPSR) is a set of rules that requires consumer products to be safe and our obligations to ensure this.

If you have any concerns about our products, you can contact us on ProductSafety@springernature.com

In case Publisher is established outside the EU, the EU authorized representative is:

Springer Nature Customer Service Center GmbH
Europaplatz 3
69115 Heidelberg, Germany

Batch number: 10756376

Printed by Printforce, the Netherlands